The precautionary principle is proving of unusual significance as new forms of biotechnology and chemical synthesis offer tantalizing contradictions as to any proof of associated harm for all manner of exposed populations now and in the long-term. This is even more politically salient as fresh trade agreements are being sought between nations with many differing interpretations of precaution. Levente Szentkirályi offers a brilliant, case study rich analysis of a new moral position of a reasoned duty of care on all creators of possible risks, both established and still untried. Would that his prescriptions be followed.

***Tim O'Riordan**, Professor Emeritus of Environmental Sciences, University of East Anglia, Norwich, UK, and editor of two books on the precautionary principle across the world*

In *The Ethics of Precaution*, Dr. Szentkirályi offers perhaps the most complete and compelling moral philosophical defense available for use of the precautionary principle in environmental, health, and safety regulation. But the book does much more than this: It also engages with law, history, economics, environmental science, and a range of other relevant bodies of expertise to advance its argument. The result is a powerful philosophical case for the precautionary principle and an exemplary work of interdisciplinary scholarship.

***Douglas Kysar**, Joseph M. Field '55 Professor of Law, Yale University, USA, and author of* Regulating from Nowhere: Environmental Law and the Search for Objectivity

The Ethics of Precaution

Thousands of substances are manufactured in the United States to which the public is routinely exposed and for which toxicity data are limited or absent. Some insist that uncertainty about the severity of potential harm justifies implementing precautionary regulations, while others claim that uncertainty justifies the absence of regulations until sufficient evidence confirms a strong probability of severe harm.

In this book, Levente Szentkirályi overcomes this impasse in his defense of precautionary environmental risk regulation by shifting the focus from how to manage uncertainty to what it is we owe each other morally. He argues that actions that create uncertain threats wrongfully gamble with the welfare of those who are exposed and neglect the reciprocity that our equal moral standing demands. If we take the moral equality and rights of others seriously, we have a duty to exercise due care to strive to prevent putting them in possible harm's way.

The Ethics of Precaution will be of great interest to researchers, educators, advanced students, and practitioners working in the fields of environmental political theory, ethics of risk, and environmental policy.

Levente Szentkirályi is a teaching faculty member at the University of Colorado at Boulder, where he teaches discipline-specific academic writing and problems of social justice. Broadly trained in political science and philosophy, his interdisciplinary research interests bridge normative political theory with environmental policy and broadly consist of environmental justice, moral responsibility, and the ethics of risk. Dr. Szentkirályi's appreciation for scholarship that intersects different disciplines has deeply influenced his student-centered pedagogy and has shaped substantive research interests in teaching and learning in political science.

The Ethics of Precaution

Uncertain Environmental Health Threats and Duties of Due Care

Levente Szentkirályi

Routledge
Taylor & Francis Group
NEW YORK AND LONDON

First published 2020
by Routledge
52 Vanderbilt Avenue, New York, NY 10017

and by Routledge
2 Park Square, Milton Park, Abingdon, Oxon, OX14 4RN

Routledge is an imprint of the Taylor & Francis Group, an informa business

Library of Congress Cataloging-in-Publication Data
A catalog record for this book has been requested

ISBN: 978-0-367-19374-4 (hbk)
ISBN: 978-0-429-24431-5 (ebk)

Typeset in Times New Roman
by Apex CoVantage, LLC

Contents

List of Tables and Figures ix
Preface x

1 Paradigm Shift in Risk and the Necessity of Precaution 1

1.1 Motivation Behind the Precautionary Principle 3
1.2 Paradigm Shift in Environmental Risk Management 5
1.3 Plan of the Book 8

2 Precautionary Risk Regulation as a Matter of Right 19

2.1 Complexities of Environmental Harms 20
2.2 Contemporary Formulations and Common Objections 28
2.3 Efforts to Answer Common Objections 36
2.3.1 Precaution as Minimizing Harm 37
2.3.2 Precaution as Deliberative Policy Making 42
2.4 Alternative Rights-Based Formulation 46

3 Uncertain Environmental Threats as Objective Wrongs 69

3.1 On the Association Between Obligation and Culpability 70
3.2 From Moral Equality to Duties of Due Care 72
3.2.1 A Kantian Commitment to Equality 73
3.2.2 Argument for Due Care in Brief 75
3.3 Uncertain Threats and Autonomous Standing 77
3.4 From Reasons to Duties 81

4 Uncertain but Culpable 92

4.1 Moral Responsibility and Causal Responsibility 93
4.2 Ethics of Risk and Unreasonable Risk Impositions 97

4.3 Moral Luck and the Epistemic Limitation Excuse 102
4.4 Initial Objections 111

5 Obligations of Due Care Under Uncertainty 127

5.1 When Risk can be Deduced 129
5.2 When Risk can be Scientifically Verified 130
5.3 When Risk Remains Unverifiable 134
5.4 Context-Dependent Mitigating Factors 137
5.5 Rejoinders to Standard Objections to Precaution 143

6 Feasibility of a Precautionary Standard of Due Care 161

6.1 Tetraethyl Lead: A Brief History 162
6.2 "Intentional Externalizing" and the Orchestrated Failure to Protect Public Health 164
6.3 Motivating the Need for a Standard of Due Care 170
6.4 Exercising Due Care 175

7 Demanding Higher Standards of Corporate Responsibility 186

7.1 Taking Responsibility for Uncertain Threats of Environmental Harm: An Overview 187
7.2 Recent Developments 191
7.3 Implications and Prospects for Future Research 192

Index 196

Table and Figures

Table

2.1 Forms of Uncertainty 21

Figures

5.1 Discharging the Industrial Standard of Due Care 132
5.2 California Proposition 65 Warning Content 139
5.3 Breyers' Growth Hormone–Free Label for Tamper Band (2015) 139
5.4 Breyers' Growth Hormone–Free Product Labels (2016) 140
5.5 Examples of Existing Consumer Protection Labels 141
5.6 Proposed Uncertain Threat Warnings 141
6.1 Correlation Between Lead Phase-Out and Reduced Environmental Exposure 169
6.2 Reduced Environmental Exposure in Children During Leaded Gasoline Phase-Out 170
6.3 Facts About Ethyl Gasoline Advertisement 174

Preface

This book is written in memory of my late father, classical pianist and composer, professor, photographer, and Hungarian freedom fighter, Dr. András Szentkirályi. Days before my father died from complications of a heart attack, as he lay in critical condition on a gurney waiting to be helicoptered to an area hospital, in what would prove to be the last lucid exchange I would have with him, my father took my hand and reminded me to pay our utility bill on time with the check he had left on his desk in his study. Even in that tense moment, I recall being puzzled how he could be concerned with such trivial matters as avoiding a late fee when his life was in the balance. Admittedly, my family always struggled financially, so even modest unexpected expenses created difficulties for us. Further, having endured many hardships—not the least of which included surviving the Second World War in Budapest, having his life shaken by the 1956 Hungarian revolution, and losing his first son to leukemia—my father took very little for granted. In retrospect, however, this exchange with my father had neither to do with our finances nor a reluctance to accept the gravity of his situation, but rather testified to his perseverance and his deep sense of responsibility for his family.

Unexpectedly drawn into Hungary's armed resistance against Soviet oppression (in which his older sister, a young nurse, was shot and killed while aiding victims of a street battle), after surviving one of the violent street battles of the uprising, my father was seized by Soviet forces and Hungarian secret police, detained for several days, interrogated, and beaten. What ultimately saved him from certain execution was his youth: for in a time of moral bankruptcy, the Soviets oddly refrained from killing revolutionaries who were not yet legally adults. Understanding, however, that upon his 18th birthday he would be re-apprehended for his known support of the resistance, my father was compelled to abandon his family and he escaped to Austria—soon after which he settled in Rome, only to enlist with the U.S. Army in 1959 to immigrate to the United States with hope in a better future. Overcoming both language and financial barriers to continuing his education and musical training, he earned degrees from premier music conservatories and research institutions in the country. My father's doctoral studies and pursuit of a college teaching career required a great many sacrifices of him and our family, which made his wrongful termination as an assistant professor by the Music Department at Bowling Green State University, as well as his subsequent failure to return to academia, that much harder to bear. Forced to table his talent and passion for composing and teaching classical music, after years of accepting whatever work he could secure to support his family, my father finally settled into photography—turning what had once been a hobby into his new profession—and he struggled the rest of his life as a small business owner. Yet he never bemoaned his circumstances, or became resentful, or projected his disappointments and frustrations onto others. He simply did what was necessary to persevere. And despite the unreasonable concessions life imposed on him, my father fostered an optimistic and cheerful disposition, finding purpose in his family and joy in life's simple pleasures—an enduring testament to his integrity and strong character.

He should have survived the heart attack. He should have met his delightful grandchildren. He should have seen his kids grow into devoted parents and counseled them through their own hardships. He should have enjoyed greater professional success and achieved the life of quiet contentment he had sought in his later years. He should have grown old with my mother and continued to fill their home with music and laughter. For he was deserving.

When we lose a loved one whose life is unfairly cut short, no justification can allay our heartache, and no such a loss can ever be made right. Yet, we may find some solace in honoring our loved ones in what ways we can, in striving to keep their history and memory alive for ourselves and for our progeny, and in learning from their mistakes and striving to live a life they would be proud of. It is in this vein that what began as a haphazard ambition of mine to earn an advanced degree soon evolved into a way for me to help carry on my late father's legacy and to share with him, in spirit at least, the sacrifices and rewards of completing my doctoral studies and settling into a career as a university teaching faculty member. I believe my father would have taken pride in these accomplishments and that he would have been humbled to know that my work in the ethics of precaution and my research in problems of social justice are deeply rooted in our unique family history and his experience as a revolutionary—which have cemented my broader interests to better understand the moral obligations we have to protect others from harm and injustice and which ground this book project on safeguarding our communities against potential environmental health risks.

My father's memory has motivated me these last years to overcome the challenges of balancing a full-time teaching career with finishing this manuscript and also caring for my young son as a part-time stay-at-home dad. Yet, just as deontology is at once backward-looking (as we judge the character of our actions) and forward-looking (as moral duties intend to shape our future actions), so too is my motivation for writing this book—which, in this case, is bookended by my five-year-old son, András Szentkirályi.

As parents, we diligently work to protect the welfare of our children and to make informed and prudent decisions to afford them a healthy and promising future. However, prevailing uncertainty about the threats of environmental harm that this book explores undermines our ability and responsibility to do so. Scholars and commentators have focused extensively on the battery of interrelated, complex, and exigent problems of global climate change that our younger generations have inherited—the nuances of which we have come to better understand in the three decades following the first Intergovernmental Panel on Climate Change (IPCC) report. And this attention is not undeserved. For instance, we face the increased prevalence of climate change–related extreme weather events, such as hurricanes, floods, prolonged droughts, heatwaves, and forest fires, which not only leave human lives in their wake but also threaten our infrastructure and food systems. With global warming, we have observed the spread of emerging infectious diseases, whose mobility and resistance to traditional antibiotics make all countries vulnerable to epidemics. The world's oceans are not only freshening because of the melting polar icecaps, which alters their chemistry and the direction of ocean currents, but our oceans also act as carbon sinks, absorbing much of the carbon that is emitted into the atmosphere—all of which have profound effects on these aquatic environments and regional climates. And with the melting of the polar icecaps comes sea level rise, which not only threatens coastal lands and island communities, but also results in the salinization of our limited inland freshwater sources. Similarly jeopardizing our access to safe, potable water are large algal blooms and the untenable strain on water treatment facilities that floods create—which, in turn, also jeopardize our food security. Accordingly, some have argued that global warming constitutes the greatest public health crisis in environmental history.

However, it is not just the foreseeable crises of climate change that threaten the futures of our youth. Equally concerning are the overlooked or understated possibilities of environmental harm that our children are exposed to on a daily basis—many of which have become commonplace because our lack of knowledge of their actual risks to human health casts doubt on the legitimacy of regulatory measures and undercuts momentum for social reform. Added sugars in processed foods and in kids' drinks, estrogen-mimickers in plastic water bottles, innumerable pesticide residues on raw and in processed foods, genetically-engineered foods, genetically engineered foods, synthetic growth hormones and antibiotics in conventional dairy products, aerosol vapors in e-cigarettes, formaldehyde in shampoos, total dissolved solids in public drinking water, outgassing volatile organic compounds in countless consumer goods in our homes and schools, and so on and so forth. Many such ordinary threats of environmental harm remain unresolved and poorly regulated. As some scholars and policy analysts have bemoaned, within the dominant framework of environmental risk management in the United States, until a preponderance of scientific evidence corroborates actual risks of harm, environmental health issues are not ripe for resolution. We do not need to invoke high-profile cases of environmental harm, like the recent water crisis in Flint, Michigan, that exposed a community of children to high levels of lead in drinking water (whose effects we know quite well) to affirm how tolerant of environmental risk and harm policy-makers and regulators have become, even when we know that children are uniquely vulnerable to harm upon exposure to effluents. Given the complexity of many environmental harms—whose effects are commonly deferred, following years of low-level, cumulative exposure to and bioaccumulation of diverse pollutants—delaying regulation until a preponderance of evidence is achieved fails to adequately prevent against injury.

Consequently, this book is also dedicated to my son, his generation, and the youngsters who may follow, all of whom have the right not to be harmed, which depends on the exercise of our collective right to know the dangers we face so that we may better insulate ourselves and our children from potential, undeserved, and avoidable injury—rights that impose correlative duties on emitters (be they individuals, corporations, or governments) to implement reasonable precautionary measures to safeguard against possible harm, and to strive to eliminate uncertainty about the actual risks to public health that their emissions beget. Championing these rights and substantiating these duties by defining a reasonable and practical standard of due care may help to shape meaningful policy reform—reform that we owe to our youth as their guardians and advocates.

Like raising a child, any scholarly research is inherently a collective effort, and I would be remiss if I did not acknowledge several people who were instrumental in the completion of this manuscript. I am indebted to Ben Hale, David Mapel, and Sam Fitch, my former dissertation advisors, for their collective wisdom, their patience with my progress on improving this project, and their constructive comments on earlier chapter drafts. Astute, forthright and yet forgiving, and selfless with their time, these three individuals epitomize for me the sort of advisor, mentor, and colleague I aspire to be. I am also grateful to William Boyd, Krister Andersson, Steve Vanderheiden, Kerry Whiteside, Carolyn Raffensperger, Tim O'Riordan, Joel Tickner, Ted Schettler, and the anonymous reviewers for Routledge and *Ethics, Policy, and Environment* for their constructive feedback on earlier versions of different excerpts of this manuscript. They posed difficult challenges to the arguments I develop here, some of which I have not yet found adequate solutions to, but which I trust will galvanize future research projects. My sincere thanks are also owed to Paul Bowman, Matthew Heller, Craig White, and Moonhawk Kim, who generously gave of their time and offered helpful perspectives on various aspects of this work in progress, as well as to my dear friend and graphic designer, Adam Schlosser, who worked with me to create the uncertainty consumer protection label—one of the practical policy proposals the book explores. Finally, I owe great deal to my beloved wife, Dr. María Fernanda Enríquez Szentkirályi, who is certainly pleased that this project is now behind me. Her patience through the countless evenings and weekends I spent researching and writing gave me the time and focus necessary to finish this project, whereas her support and friendship helped to keep me grounded—reminding me of my greater purpose in this life as father and husband.

1 Paradigm Shift in Risk and the Necessity of Precaution

The discovery in 1939 that DDT (dichlorodiphenyltrichloroethane) had potent insecticidal properties was trumpeted as a laudable scientific innovation, due in no small measure to its capacities to protect public health from various diseases, such as malaria and typhus,[1] and to safeguard the agricultural industry against the myriad pests that threaten crop yields.[2] Prior to the late 1950s, little was known about the adverse health effects of DDT exposure. However, the reality of the pesticide's impact on public health and the natural environment were soon realized[3]—culminating in the Environmental Protection Agency's (EPA's) ban of the suspected carcinogen in 1972, prompting substantive revisions to the Federal Insecticide, Fungicide, and Rodenticide Act (FIFRA) to improve protections against the use of and exposure to DDT[4] and motivating the Supreme Court to declare that "substantial evidence" of the hazards to public health warranted the substance's prohibition.[5] Such examples stand as testimony to the potentially harmful consequences of our ignorance, they illustrate missed opportunities to preventatively regulate the release of substances that have the potential to cause harm, and they press us to consider what the benefit of hindsight should teach us about environmental risk management.

In circumstances when uncertainty is eliminated and replaced by the knowledge that exposure is likely to entail adverse human health effects, we may question whether the resulting harms could have or should have been avoided. For instance, before the data on DDT existed, before regulators could determine the harmful consequences of exposure and the probability that it would cause injury—that is, before we knew the actual risks that DDT posed, when the threat to public health was unknown—would regulators have been justified in exercising precaution and restricting the use of the substance? More strongly, considering the large-scale production and widespread use of DDT, which reached roughly 80 million pounds annually in the United States by the late 1950s (an amount equivalent to the weight of the volume of water of nearly 15 Olympic-sized swimming pools),[6] did legislators and environmental regulators have a *pro tanto* responsibility to regulate the pesticide to proactively try to mitigate the uncorroborated potential for harm to the public? And what of corporations involved in the manufacture and sale of the chemical substance, or individuals who purchased related products and applied the pesticide: did they have a duty to prevent exposing others to the uncertain threats of environmental harm that their actions entailed? If so, on what grounds?

Some insist that uncertainty about the severity of potential harm or the probability the harm will occur justifies implementing precautionary regulations. Conversely, others claim that uncertainty justifies the absence of regulations until sufficient evidence verifies a strong probability of severe harm. By engaging arguments in both environmental policy and normative ethics, which claim that in the absence of a preponderance of evidence verifying a probable risk of severe harm to public health, preventatively regulating the emission of such substances is unjustified, this interdisciplinary book project overcomes this impasse in its defense of exercising precaution by shifting the focus from how to manage uncertainty to what it is we owe each other morally. Specifically, this book argues that actions that create what we might call "uncertain threats of environmental harm"—possibilities of harm that remain uncorroborated because both the consequences of exposure and the probability that exposure will result in physical injury are unknown—wrongfully gamble with the welfare of those who may be exposed and neglect the reciprocity that our equal moral standing demands. Consequently, if we take the moral equality and rights of others seriously, then despite our lack of knowledge of the actual health effects of exposure, emitters are obliged to take reasonable precautionary measures to prevent exposing others to potentially harmful emissions.

These conclusions challenge diverse policy arguments that reject the merits and plausibility of precautionary risk regulation, as well as traditional normative theories of moral responsibility, and conventional arguments from moral luck and the ethics of risk, which all deny (explicitly or by implication) that we have any such obligations when this combination of outcome and probability uncertainty obtains. It should be clarified at the outset, however, that this book's defense of precautionary measures to safeguard the public against potential, albeit uncorroborated, environmental health threats is qualified: it should *not* be understood as entailing a fundamental policy shift to a strictly precautionary system of risk management (which would involve blanket prohibitions of all risky behavior that involves the emission of effluents whose health effects are unknown), and it should *not* be understood as implying that all risky behavior whose outcomes and probability of causing harm remain unknown are morally objectionable (which would also involve paralyzing prohibitions on the range of actions we would be free to perform). Either of these implications would be wildly implausible and should be rejected out of hand.

More modestly, this book's defense of our obligation to exercise precaution focuses on a particular subset of environmental risks: namely, those that do not permit us to ascertain the outcome of exposure and the statistical likelihood that exposure will cause material harm. That is, the subset of effluents for which we lack complete toxicity profiles: empirical findings from a standard series of toxicological studies that determine how different forms ("pathways"), doses (intensities), durations, and timings of exposure can adversely affect human health. Moreover, it is only when emitters neglect to take reasonable strides to mitigate the potential for harm to others when outcome and probability uncertainty obtain that their actions are morally impermissible. This is to say that so long as due care is exercised, which will take different forms in different contexts, it is permissible for emitters to continue to release substances into the environment that pose empirically unverified threats to public health.

1.1 Motivation Behind the Precautionary Principle

These qualifications diverge from the original justification for the precautionary principle and its adoption in the United States as a policy tool to manage environmental risk. As some scholars have argued,[7] the precautionary principle emerged as part of a broader reaction to heightened awareness of the pervasiveness of pollution-related public health threats, especially those that were suspected to cause cancer. As late as 1958, for instance, only four known carcinogens had been documented, and yet within two decades, nearly 40 had been cataloged, as well as hundreds of substances known to cause cancer in animals.[8] This improved understanding of the myriad dangers we face outdoors, in the workplace, and in our homes was facilitated by advances in the toxicological sciences, which enhanced our ability to discern trace levels of a given substance and to test the long-term effects of this low-level exposure. According to some estimates, for instance, "the sensitivity of detection methods for monitoring chemicals in food increased by 'between two and five orders of magnitude,' an improvement that allowed the detection of carcinogens at the parts per trillion level."[9] Supplanting earlier, less-nuanced ("clinical") methods of diagnosing demonstrable health effects of acute exposure (via "insensitive toxicity indicators")[10] were more sophisticated methods capable not only of detecting variation in adverse health effects at different intensities (doses) of exposure but also of ascertaining variation resulting from different pathways of exposure (inhalation, ingestion, absorption through the skin), durations of exposure, timings of exposure (e.g., prenatal, infancy, adolescence, or in conjunction with an intervening causal factor), and physiological dispositions or vulnerabilities to being harmed upon exposure.[11] These superior testing capabilities also began to reveal a complex and disquieting tapestry of causal relationships that commonly define environmental harms: trace levels of effluents persisting and accumulating in our bodies creating deferred health problems (as with mercury and lead),[12] exposure to multiple effluents creating amplified cumulative effects (as with the diverse air pollutants),[13] and some effluents only causing injury when interacting with other exogenous substances (as with smoking and asbestos-related lung cancers).[14]

With this enhanced understanding came heightened public concern, due in no small measure to several high-profile cases of environmental harm and to vocal critics of existing environmental policies. For instance, as leaded gasoline went into mass production in the 1920s and workers in lead additive research and processing plants fell victim to severe lead poisoning, public health scientists like Alice Hamilton and Yandell Henderson—who warned that lead emissions from vehicle exhaust would be detrimental to public health—indicted the oil and automotive industries for neglecting to pursue safer alternative fuel additives and for proactively stalling the implementation of mandatory emission standards.[15] Similarly, at the height of DDT production and application in the early 1960s, environmentalists like Rachel Carson—whose popularized research proved to be pivotal in highlighting the extensive harm that synthetic pesticides were causing—underscored the inadequacies of extant environmental protections.[16] As such, for a brief period, exercising precaution became the guiding intuition of socially responsible environmental policy: to adequately protect an alarmed public from the battery of possibly harmful effluents with which it interacted on a daily basis. The public's fear over being enveloped by environmental risk and its general distrust of industry combined with our improved awareness of the potential for harm—yet our concurrent lack of understanding of many of the actual dangers to public health, given the limits of dose-response testing capabilities and the tenuousness of subsequent inferences about tolerance and threshold values and "reasonable" risk—all served as catalysts to the early adoption of a humble, precautionary approach to U.S. environmental risk management.

Consider, for instance, one of the paradigmatic examples of precautionary risk regulation: the 1958 Federal Food, Drug, and Cosmetics Act (and what has come to be referred to as the Delaney Clause). This legislation aimed to protect the nation's food supply by enacting a blanket ban of any food additive (§409 (c)(3)(A)), color additive (§721 (b)(5)(B)), or animal drug (§512 (d)(1)(I)) that was "found to induce cancer in man or animals," regardless of the magnitude of exposure or "how small that risk of cancer might be."[17] This "zero-tolerance," or zero-risk, standard meant that industry shouldered the burden of demonstrating empirically that its additives were safe to public health before it was permitted to manufacture the substances. The intuition here was that exposure to a substance known to cause harm in one context is likely to cause similar harm in other contexts: that it would be unreasonable not to act preventatively to safeguard the public against foreseeable harm. Motivated by an analogous intuition that with substances known to cause harm at acute levels of exposure, it is both reasonable to infer that exposure at lower doses will likely beget adverse health effects and also unreasonable therefore to expect regulators to refrain from protecting the public from foreseeable harm, the ruling in *Ethyl Corporation* v. *EPA* (1976)[18] is a hallmark defense of precautionary, health-based standards.

As public health scientists and regulators started to better understand the causes of the epidemic of "pediatric lead poisoning" in the United States (attributable chiefly to lead paint in older homes and tetraethyl lead exhaust in the ambient air),[19] the question before the D.C. Circuit Court of Appeals in 1976 was whether exposure to leaded gasoline posed a "significant" risk of harm to public health. Yet the court ruled that an "endangerment finding"—which requires corroborating a "significant risk of harm"—need not be empirically precise and that a credible threat of harm can warrant precautionary regulatory decisions to prevent the perceived threat.[20] This is to say that *Ethyl Corp. v. EPA* established a precedent that even in the absence of actual injury or a preponderance of evidence of an imminent risk of harm to public health, regulation can be justified: that prevailing uncertainty did not justify inaction.

1.2 Paradigm Shift in Environmental Risk Management

These developments paralleled

> early pesticide cancellations [like DDT], the precautionary thrust of the Clean Air and Clean Water Acts, [other] rulings of the D.C. Circuit and other appellate courts in many of the early environmental cases [including *Reserve Mining Company v. EPA* (1975)[21]], and OSHA's quest for a generic cancer policy.[22]

Yet such efforts to institute precautionary standards were and continue to be met with strong resistance, in large part because of the perceived inflexibility and impracticality of these standards, as well as a firm commitment to the ideas that risk can be quantified,[23] that regulatory decisions must be able to withstand the scrutiny of cost–benefit analysis (CBA), that the human body can tolerate some baseline threshold of exposure to pollutants without suffering health problems,[24] and that the nonscientific assessments of risk—or what some disparagingly refer to as "intuitive toxicology"—that substantiate precautionary risk regulations are subjective, irrational, inflated, and thus are highly unreliable.[25] The Delaney Clause, for example, with its unqualified intolerance of even minute exposure to known carcinogens (what we might call trivial or *de minimis* risks), was criticized not only by industry but also by advocates of formal risk assessment and CBA in our legislatures, regulatory agencies, and courts for ignoring statistical realities of actual dangers to public health and tolerating economically implausible standards. The U.S. Court of Appeals leveled a ringing indictment against the Delaney Clause in *Public Citizen* v. *Young* (1987),[26] directed perhaps at precautionary measures more broadly, declaring that regulations that do not limit their purview to credible risks and exempt trivial risks are "absurd or futile," since inherent to all human behavior is some risk of harm to others, and since the costs of blanket prohibitions of risk are economically unfeasible. Moreover, the court insisted that such regulatory decisions are also "directly contrary to the primary legislative goal" of promoting "human safety," since the enforcement of the Delaney Clause would permit imposing higher risks of actual harm on the public through exposure to known toxic substances so long as these substances were noncarcinogenic.[27]

The inability of proponents of precaution to adequately respond to these charges of inefficiency, implausibility, counter-productiveness, and irrationality (which persist in contemporary critiques of the precautionary principle), coupled with the apparent paralysis of industry and commerce that a commitment to precaution would entail—given the considerable number of substances that improved detection capabilities had revealed could be harmful and would therefore be subject to severe restriction or prohibition—cemented a paradigm shift in environmental risk management, and the adoption of formal or quantitative risk assessment (QRA) and CBA. This meant that when faced with uncorroborated public health threats, before any legislative or regulatory decision could be justified, a credible and unreasonable risk to human health had to be verified, and it had to be demonstrated that other available alternatives were less cost-effective (that comparable health safety standards could not be achieved through cheaper means, or that the costs are proportionate to the benefits). Moreover, the regulatory agencies were charged with meeting these burdens of proof. It is important to note that these precedents trace back to the 1925 conference of oil and automotive industries, concerned industrial hygienists, and the Surgeon General of the Public Health Service, who had gathered to discuss whether the manufacture of tetraethyl lead (TEL) in gasoline and its emission into the ambient air warranted regulation. Given TEL's ability to extend the life of internal combustion engines and to make engines more fuel efficient, industry executives exploited growing fears of oil shortages and underscored the economic benefits that would be forfeited if use of the additive was restricted. And in an effort to thwart mandatory emission standards, industry executives proposed to self-regulate leaded gasoline: to proactively cease all production of TEL if it could be verified empirically that exposure posed a danger to public health—which effectively absolved industry of the need to demonstrate the relative safety of TEL and instead shifted the burden of proof to the public.[28]

This shift toward requiring quantitatively verifiable risks and cost-effective risk regulations, which broadly define the United States' current approach toward environmental risk management, was cemented in precedent-setting cases like *Industrial Union Dept., AFL-CIO v. American Petroleum Institute* (1980)[29] and *Corrosion Proof Fittings v. EPA* (1991).[30] The former case, which involved occupational exposure to benzene (a known carcinogen), both redefined the notion of what is "safe" and insisted that efforts must be made to quantify the risk of harm given the "best available evidence" and to weigh economic considerations in setting enforcement standards. Specifically, the court clarified that "safe" work environments should not be understood as free of all risk, but rather as involving "acceptable" levels of risk, and it required the Occupational Safety and Health Administration (OSHA) to meet its burden of proof and demonstrate empirically that workers were exposed to "unsafe" or significant risks of harm.[31] The court also established that the regulatory agency (here, the Secretary of Labor) must weigh the costs and benefits of any proposed permanent standard before its institution and enforcement are justified—achieving both economic and technological feasibility. In *Corrosion Proof Fittings*, which concerned the EPA's authority under the Toxic

Substances Control Act (Section 6) to ban all products containing asbestos (another known carcinogen), the court rejected the agency's justification for the ban—concluding that the EPA had failed to show quantitatively that no alternative regulation would be superior to the status quo or the total ban the EPA endorsed. In other words, the court insisted that the EPA had failed to demonstrate that the proposed ban was, in fact, the least burdensome alternative: "In its zeal to ban any and all asbestos products, [the EPA] basically ignored the cost side of the TSCA equation."[32]

Similarly, the Food Quality Protection Act (1996) amended the "food additives" provision of the Delaney Clause, discarding the previous strict and burdensome zero-risk, health-based standard for pesticide residues on raw foods (processed foods had been exempt), and issued a relaxed standard of "reasonable certainty" of no harm—that is, "reasonable certainty that no harm will result from aggregate exposure to the pesticide chemical residue."[33] This new standard was also extended to raw foods "on which a much wider range of pesticides typically are used than the 80–100 chemicals used on processed foods."[34] The act does preserve some precautionary elements, including a tenfold increase in protection standards to account for uncertainty and for variation in exposure by the public, as well as an emphasis on ensuring the safety of more vulnerable populations (such as infants and children) and its special attention to consumption patterns and the cumulative effects of consumption. Nevertheless, these three examples speak to evolving perceptions of risk as probabilistic, trust in the reliability of scientific methods to assess environmental risk, and commitment to utilitarian cost–benefit balancing.

As suggested at the outset, these considerations continue to be the crux of contemporary debates over precautionary risk regulation. Critics maintain that in the absence of a preponderance of evidence to verify that exposure to a given effluent entails an actual risk to public health—with the *public* bearing the burden of proof—we should refrain from restricting its use and emission: uncertainty precludes regulation. (Conventional normative arguments in moral responsibility, moral luck, and the ethics of risk make analogous claims against imposing restrictions until the evidence is in.) Proponents argue antithetically that in the absence of a preponderance of evidence to confirm that exposure to a given substance is safe to public health—with *industry* bearing the burden of proof—we should preventatively safeguard the public against potential harm: uncertainty necessitates regulation. The problem, however, is that both groups wrongly assume that their respective policy approaches alone can constitute an effective system of environmental risk management, and their diametrically opposed and staunchly held views would suggest that the choice between the precautionary principle and formal risk assessment is mutually exclusive. Moreover, both proponents and opponents of precaution (in both the policy and normative ethics circles) ground their arguments in the mistaken narrow conception of uncertainty as *probability* uncertainty, where what is unknown is only the probability that exposure will materialize in harm. In its defense of a precautionary risk regulation, this book denies all three assumptions and argues that a viable system of managing environmental risk requires both approaches. These paradigms of risk or regulatory regimes are complementary, not incongruous, for the danger to public health that many environmental threats pose cannot be quantified (demonstrating the limited applicability of QRA), and formal risk assessments *can* successfully account for many environmental risks when we know that exposure will be harmful and what remains uncertain is the probability that exposure will cause injury (demonstrating the limited applicability of precaution). This implies both that it is imprudent to dismiss the merits of a precautionary approach and that any feasible defense of the precautionary principle must constrain the purview of precaution—and this book argues that it is primarily when we do not know the outcome of exposure or the probability for harm that preventative measures are justified.

There are two other significant ways this book departs from conventional policy-oriented arguments about precaution. First, central to the normative defense of exercising precaution developed in the subsequent chapters is the rejection of the inclination of proponents of QRA to treat environmental risk in scientific and statistical abstraction.[35] At stake are neither "statistical casualties"[36] nor quantifiable costs of risks and harms in the aggregate, but rather the welfare of real people who bear the actual consequences of risk impositions and environmental harms. Our deliberations and regulatory decisions about whether or not to restrict emissions that may cause harm to public health should not ignore our accountability to particular individuals and vulnerable groups. Second, this book's defense of precaution rejects conventional justificatory appeals to epistemic uncertainty that proponents of precaution commonly make. Since prevailing uncertainty about the potential for harm is the very same reasoning that critics of precaution use to substantiate the absence of regulation, appealing to uncertainty is a nonstarter, which means that most arguments for precaution are untenable. By proposing a novel normative foundation for risk regulation that is independent of what we can or cannot know, this book not only strives to vindicate the plausibility of precautionary standards, but it also challenges us to reevaluate our preconceptions about environmental risk and to reframe the fundamental objectives of managing threats of environmental harm.

1.3 Plan of the Book

Chapter 2 begins by detailing several relevant forms of uncertainty (including outcome, probability, causal, and scientific uncertainty) in order to underscore the complexity of environmental harms and to illustrate how scholars of environmental policy and normative ethics have largely misconstrued what uncertainty consists of—treating it narrowly, as stated earlier, as probability uncertainty: where what is unknown is the likelihood that harm may come to pass. The notion of "genuine" uncertainty is introduced to complicate these existing conceptions and treatments of uncertainty and to preface the chapter's central charge—that defenses of precautionary risk regulation, as well as opposing arguments supporting formal risk assessment, are incomplete and flawed. As noted earlier, it is misguided for critics to dismiss the merits of precaution and to assume that QRA can address all potential environmental health threats, and it is misguided for proponents to overestimate the purview of a precautionary approach to managing environmental risk. While the exercise of precaution is a viable and necessary response to many threats of environmental harm, it is primarily when we face both outcome and probability (or genuine) uncertainty that preventative safeguards are justified.

Chapter 2 also explains that because the central justification defenders of precaution appeal to—namely, our prevailing epistemic limitations—is turned on its head by critics to justify the opposite conclusion (and vice versa), there is only one plausible alternative to vindicate the precautionary principle: to ground precaution in something *other than* our epistemic limitations. After demonstrating that existing arguments in support of precautionary risk regulation do not successfully refute common objections, Chapter 2 sketches an alternative, normative justification for requiring precautionary safeguards under conditions of uncertainty. Namely, that individuals have a right, as a matter of moral equality, not to have others gamble with their welfare by putting them in potential harm's way.

The deontological argument in support of this claim is constructed in Chapters 3 and 4. Briefly, Chapter 3 argues that the equal moral standing of others demands that we respect them as ends in themselves, as autonomous moral agents. Yet to expose others to uncertain environmental threats without first trying to mitigate the potential for harm is to gamble with their welfare, and therefore to disrespect their moral standing. In this way, to avoid wrongdoing, we are obliged to take reasonable measures to strive to prevent exposing others to potential harm. After exploring the Kantian foundation for this argument, this chapter also delineates two qualifications that are necessary to justify the book's proposed *pro tanto* duty to exercise due care. The first qualification is that not all uncertain threats are the same: outcome and probability uncertainty vary across contexts and can be more or less pronounced, which determines when an obligation of due care exists and how strong the duty is. To clarify this notion, a distinction is drawn between having reasons to exercise due care and having those reasons translate into a duty of due care. The second qualification is that a feasible standard of due care must be sensitive to context, which implies that what precaution may require will vary across contexts and actors. Despite the relevance of context, however, Chapter 3 underscores that our duty of due care is universal (in the Kantian sense) and does not permit exceptions.

This argument for due care also requires showing that existing accounts of moral responsibility, the ethics of risk, and moral luck, and their respective treatments of uncertainty, do not adequately explain how uncertain threats of environmental harm are morally permissible. To this end, Chapter 4 explains how conventional theories of moral luck mistakenly treat uncertainty narrowly as probability uncertainty and argue that it is only when a strong probability of severe harm exists that an imposition of risk is unreasonable and merits interdiction. Consequently, since uncertainty undermines our ability to discern consequences and probabilities, theories of moral responsibility should have us believe that all uncertain threats are morally permissible. In contrast, arguments from moral luck claim that we cannot be culpable for the uncertain threats we author or any subsequent injuries they beget, since our ignorance under conditions of uncertainty is unavoidable and, therefore, excusable. Paralleling theories of moral responsibility, arguments in the ethics of risk entail that uncertain threats are trivial, highly improbable, and/or would result in negligible harm. The implication of this starting assumption is these unquantifiable and uncorroborated threats amount to reasonable risks, which is to say that exposing others to uncertain threats is morally permissible.

After explaining how these conventional accounts are based on problematic assumptions that undercut the plausibility of their arguments that uncertain threats are morally innocuous (permissible or excusable), Chapter 5 centers on the second qualification in Chapter 3 noted earlier and explores how degrees of uncertainty, the extent to which we can eliminate uncertainty, and the alternatives available to us all shape what due care consists of and how the obligation can be discharged. Moreover, the chapter introduces a number of morally relevant context-dependent factors that can either amplify or diminish one's duty to exercise precaution. Some of these factors include the availability of feasible substitutes, the involvement of vulnerable populations (like infants, children, industrial workers, the poor, or minority communities), the volume of production and emission of the substance that poses the uncertain threat, and an emitter's history of delinquency with existing environmental regulations or of social irresponsibility with regard to the uncertain threat. For instance, if an uncertain environmental threat that an emitter authors puts a vulnerable population in the way of possible harm, or if the emitter engages in socially irresponsible practices like withholding information, or manufacturing doubt, or misleading the public about the actual risks to human health that exposure to his emissions would entail, the standard of due care to which we should hold the emitter would be higher than in the absence of these criteria. Conversely, if an emitter had a history of complying with existing environmental standards or utilized an available alternative (substance or course of action) to mitigate the potential for injury from exposure to an uncorroborated threat of harm, her obligation to exercise due care would be diminished.

Returning to the battery of policy-oriented and normative objections from Chapter 2 against the plausibility of the precautionary principle—including claims that precautionary regulatory decisions tolerate severe restrictions on mere speculative and subjective risks; that precautionary policies are vacuous, incoherent, self-defeating, and paralyze all policy making; and that precautionary standards fail to balance the benefits with the costs of regulation—Chapter 5 closes by arguing that the proposed rights-based account of precaution can withstand these diverse charges. With regard, for instance, to the objection that the precautionary regulations are too burdensome and unduly hamper industry, not only does the proposed normative argument for exercising precaution stipulate that a precautionary approach should only aim to augment, *not* supplant, a risk assessment–based regulatory regime, but it also stipulates that preventative measures to safeguard against uncorroborated environmental threats are only justified with a particular subset of environmental risk (when both outcome and probability uncertainty prevail). Moreover, in emphasizing the significance of moral equality and reciprocity, this reformulation and normative defense of the precautionary principle makes plain that we must reconcile the right of those who wish to exercise their autonomy and perform actions that entail the discharge of potentially harmful substances with the right of those who are exposed to the potentially harmful consequences of these actions to *not* have others gamble with their welfare and put them in potential harm's way. And in this vein, it is also emphasized that any viable defense of an obligation of due care under uncertainty must prescribe reasonable and context-dependent precautionary standards, such that if the uncertain threat ultimately proves to cause no actual harm, we would not retrospectively find the measure unwarranted.

These considerations reappear in Chapter 6, which examines a high-profile case of an uncertain threat of environmental harm: the protracted public health hazard that the manufacture and emission of TEL and leaded gasoline involved for more than five decades. This case testifies to the negative consequences of failing to exercise precaution—consequences we should want to avoid and which thus emphasize the necessity of precautionary standard of due care. TEL was commonly used as a gasoline additive to prevent engine knocking and improve automotive efficiency. In the early 1920s, as the additive began to be mass-produced, little was known about the health effects of exposure to lead in the ambient air. With its mass production and subsequent increased workplace exposure, various high-profile instances of acute lead poisoning surfaced, which affirmed for many the danger to the broader public.[37] Yet opportunistic corporations like General Motors, DuPont, and Standard Oil Company of New Jersey, which had strong vested interests in the continued and expanded production of TEL and leaded gasoline, capitalized on the prevailing uncertainty to block initiatives to implement mandatory emission standards for more than 50 years.[38]

These companies enjoyed proprietary rights to the scientific data that could corroborate the health effects of exposure to leaded gasoline exhaust, which was purposefully withheld from regulators, consumers, and the general public. Moreover, these corporations commonly misrepresented the dangers of exposure, funded industry-led studies to cast doubt on the empirical findings of public health scientists who confirmed that exposure to TEL had adverse health effects, and ignored safer alternative additives that could have served the same purpose—though, perhaps, with a less profitable return—without endangering the public. Consequently, this example illustrates the intuition behind precautionary risk regulation, the harm to public health and welfare that can result from the absence of exercising due care, and how reasonable precautionary measures could have promoted greater corporate social responsibility and prevented this public health threat.

These considerations also underscore that any proposed precautionary standard must be amenable to changes in context. For example, the manufacture of the gasoline additive and exposure to lead from vehicle exhaust involved two vulnerable populations: namely, industrial workers (who experience intense exposure) and infants and children (who are physiologically predisposed to being harmed). Also, feasible alternative additives were available to the oil and automotive industries whose effects were known. However, the market for alternative blended fuels (using alternative anti-knocking additives) was not perceived to be as lucrative. Further, while the oil and automotive industries engaged in public disclosure initiatives, which seem, *prima facie*, to align with the proposed precautionary standard that Chapter 5 develops in detail, these initiatives deliberately aimed to mislead the public about the dangers of exposure to TEL and to introduce uncertainties about the possibility for harm—since these corporations knew that the absence of a preponderance of evidence confirming the actual health effects would preclude any mandatory emission standard. While such considerations might warrant amplifying industry's obligations of due care in this case, with other examples of uncertain environmental threats, some of these factors may well not obtain.

Consider briefly, for instance, the example of bisphenol A (BPA), an endocrine disruptor or estrogen mimicker used in countless consumer goods. As late as 2008, exposure to BPA was not a public health concern. And while the prolonged and cumulative health effects of low-dose exposure—especially among vulnerable populations like infants and children—are still uncorroborated and contentious, and while the Food and Drug Administration postponed issuing any formal ban of BPA in consumer products, several manufacturers pulled certain products containing BPA as early as 2009 and altered their manufacturing processes to offer BPA-free versions of many of their consumer goods. For example, companies like Philips AVENT, Gerber, and Playtex preventatively removed a host of plastic baby bottle and baby food packaging products (for the sake of retaining their respective market shares) and in effect worked to mitigate the potential threat to consumers and the general public. These efforts prompted a general trend of phasing out BPA in consumer goods by corporations like General Mills and Nalgene despite the lack of federal or state regulations requiring them to do so.

In this way, let us suppose for the sake of argument that the industry-initiated phase-out of BPA and the willingness to absorb these costs, as well as corporations' decisions to use alternative substances in the manufacture of their consumer goods—despite the fact that these initiatives and their apparent effect on public health have come under scrutiny—may approximate the sort of responsible corporate behavior that a precautionary standard of due care intends to promote. Moreover, industry's proactive implementation of a comprehensive "BPA-free" labeling scheme serves to disclose information to the public about the possibility for harm, which similarly seems to satisfy the standard of due care delineated in Chapter 5. So while the case of BPA *did* involve particularly vulnerable populations (pregnant women, infants, and children), since industry utilized substitutes whose effects were known (given a new and lucrative market for "BPA-free" products), and if we assume for the sake of argument that their public disclosure initiatives were not underhanded, these considerations might warrant diminishing industry's duties of due care. Accordingly, applying the same precautionary standard of due care in both instances would not be appropriate and would either yield too stringent of policies and undue burdens on corporations, in the BPA example, or too lax of policies and undue burdens on the public, in the TEL example. (Admittedly, these cursory remarks on the example of BPA overlook the public scrutiny that has since followed regarding the rash implementation of poorly studied substitutes to BPA and the profit-driven motives of these corporations that obscure their commitment to transparency and public health—considerations that cast doubt on whether this case can serve as a paradigmatic example of industry exercising due care. Nevertheless, the case of BPA still motivates the idea that a defensible duty of due care must be context dependent.)

Finally, following the discussion in Chapter 6 of the case of TEL, which emphasizes the feasibility and necessity of the proposed rights-based standard of due care, the book closes with a brief discussion of the implications of this normative defense of precaution on broader social injustices, including food justice and environmental discrimination, global environmental inequities, and climate ethics.

Notes

1. Environmental Protection Agency (EPA), "DDT, a Review of Scientific and Economic Aspects of the Decision to Ban Its Use as a Pesticide," *Prepared for the Committee on Appropriations of the U.S. House of Representatives*, EPA-540/1-75-022, July 1975: www2.epa.gov/aboutepa/ddt-regulatory-history-brief-survey-1975.
2. This is true among some policy analysts even today, with knowledge of the harmful effects of DDT exposure (see, e.g., Aaron Wildavsky, *But Is It True? A Citizen's Guide to Environmental Health and Safety Issues* (Cambridge: Harvard University Press, 1995) and Indur Goklany, *The Precautionary Principle: A Critical Appraisal of Environmental Risk Assessment* (Washington, DC: Cato Institute, 2001)).
3. See, e.g., Rachel Carson, *Silent Spring* (Boston: Houghton Mifflin, 1962).
4. EPA, "DDT, a Review of Scientific and Economic Aspects of the Decision to Ban Its Use as a Pesticide."
5. *Environmental Defense Fund Inc. v. EPA*, 489 F. 2d 1247, United States Court of Appeals, District of Columbia Circuit, Decided 13 December, 1973.
6. EPA, "DDT, a Review of Scientific and Economic Aspects of the Decision to Ban Its Use as a Pesticide." With a capacity of 660,000 gallons of water, since 1 gallon of water weighs approximately 8.3 pounds, the volume of water in one Olympic-sized swimming pool weighs approximately 5.5 million pounds.
7. See, e.g., Joel Tickner, ed., *Precaution, Environmental Science, and Preventive Public Policy* (Washington, DC: Island Press, 2003); Douglas Kysar, *Regulating from Nowhere: Environmental Law and the Search for Objectivity* (New Haven: Yale University Press, 2010); William Boyd, "Genealogies of Risk: Searching for

Safety, 1930s–1970s," *Ecological Law Quarterly* 39 (2012): 895–988; and David Vogel, *The Politics of Precaution: Regulating Health, Safety, and Environmental Risks in Europe and the United States* (Princeton: Princeton University Press, 2012). See also Poul Harremoës et al., eds., *Late Lessons from Early Warnings: The Precautionary Principle 1896–2000*, Environmental Issue Report, No. 22 (Copenhagen: European Environment Agency, 2001).

8. Boyd, "Genealogies of Risk," 944; William Boyd, "Environmental Law, Big Data, and the Torrent of Singularities," *UCLA Law Review Discourse* 64 (2016): 549, fn. 10; see also Richard Wilson, "Risks Caused by Low-Levels of Pollution," *Yale Journal of Biology and Medicine* 51 (1978): 37, 48.
9. Food and Drug Administration, "Chemical Compounds in Food Producing Animals: Criteria and Procedures for Evaluating Assays for Carcinogenic Residues," *Federal Register* 44 (1979): 17070, 17075; Boyd, "Genealogies of Risk," 944.
10. Sven Hernberg, "Lead Poisoning in a Historical Perspective," *American Journal of Industrial Medicine* 38 (2000): 247–8.
11. Finn Bro-Rasmussen, "Risk, Uncertainties, and Precautions in Chemical Legislation," in *Precaution: Environmental Science and Preventative Public Policy*, Joel Tickner, ed. (Washington, DC: Island Press, 2003): 94; Kristin Shrader-Frechette, *Taking Action, Saving Lives: Our Duties to Protect Environmental and Public Health* (Oxford: Oxford University Press, 2007): 99–100; Judith Layzer, "Love Canal: Hazardous Waste and the Politics of Fear," in *The Environmental Case: Translating Values into Policy*, 3rd ed. (Washington, DC: CQ Press, 2012): 69–70; Boyd, "Genealogies of Risk," 914.
12. John Drexler et al., "Issue Paper on the Bioavailability and Bioaccumulation of Metals," EPA, Risk Assessment Forum (2003); Yingcun Xia and Howell Tong, "Cumulative Effects of Air Pollution on Public Health," *Statistics in Medicine* 25 (2006): 3548–59; EPA, "Framework for Metals Risk Assessment," EPA-120/R-07/001, March 2007: https://epa.gov/sites/production/files/2013-09/documents/metals-risk-assessment-final.pdf; Toronto Public Health, *Health Assessment for the Cumulative Air Quality Modelling Study: Wards 5 and 6* (Toronto: TPH 2014); EPA, "Basic Information about Lead in Drinking Water," https://epa.gov/ground-water-and-drinking-water/basic-information-about-lead-drinking-water, last updated December 12, 2016.
13. David Carpenter et al., "Understanding the Human Health Effects of Chemical Mixtures," *Environmental Health Perspectives* 110 (2002): 25–42; Ken Sexton and Stephen Linder, "Cumulative Risk Assessment for Combined Health Effects from Chemical and Nonchemical Stressors," *American Journal of Public Health* 101 (2011): S81–8.
14. Agency for Toxic Substances and Disease Registry, "Toxicological Profile for Asbestos" (Atlanta: U.S. Department of Health and Human Services, 2001): 6; Marilyn Browne et al., "Cancer Incidence and Asbestos in Drinking Water, Town of Woodstock, New York, 1980–1998," *Environmental Research* 98 (2005): 229; John Gamble, "Risk of Gastrointestinal Cancers from Inhalation and Ingestion of Asbestos," *Regulatory Toxicology and Pharmacology* 52 (2008): S148–9.
15. Alice Hamilton et al., "Tetra Ethyl Lead," *Journal of the American Medical Association* 84 (1925): 1481–6; U.S. Public Health Service, "Proceedings of a Conference to Determine Whether or Not there Is a Public Health Question in the Manufacture, Distribution, or Use of Tetraethyl Lead Gasoline," in *Public Health Bulletin No. 158* (Washington, DC: Government Publishing Office, 1925): 62; David Rosner and Gerald Markowitz, "A 'Gift of God'?: The Public Health Controversy Over Leaded Gasoline During the 1920s," *American Journal of Public Health* 75 (1985): 344, 349; Hernberg, "Lead Poisoning in a Historical Perspective," 246.
16. Carson, *Silent Spring*.

17. Food, Drug, and Cosmetics Act, 21 U.S.C. §342 (1958), Goklany, *The Precautionary Principle*, 4; see also Donna Vogt, *The Delaney Clause Effects on Pesticide Policy* (Washington, DC: Congressional Research Service, 1995); and Robert Percival et al., *Environmental Regulation: Law, Science, and Policy*, 6th ed. (New York: Aspen Publishers, 2009): 244, 283–8.
18. *Ethyl Corp v. EPA*, 541 F. 2d 1 (D.C. Circuit 1976).
19. Hernberg, "Lead Poisoning in a Historical Perspective," 249.
20. See also *Massachusetts v. EPA* 549 U.S. 497 (2007), where the same issue was at stake.
21. *Reserve Mining Company v. EPA*, 514 F. 2d 492 (8th Circuit 1975).
22. Boyd, "Genealogies of Risk," 985. A generic cancer policy would identify the lowest permissible level of exposure to the set of known carcinogens—an approach that would sidestep the time-consuming and costly process of establishing a baseline threshold of exposure chemical by chemical.
23. The distinction and significance between "measurable risk" and "unmeasurable uncertainty" (or that which we do not know) were made as early as the 1920s: see Frank Knight, *Risk, Uncertainty, and Profit* (Boston: Houghton Mifflin Co., 1921): 19–20, 233. See also John Maynard Keynes, "The General Theory of Employment," *Quarterly Journal of Economics* 51 (1937): 209, 214; Sunstein, *Risk and Reason: Safety, Law, and the Environment* (Cambridge: Cambridge University Press, 2002), chapters 3, 5, 7; Cass Sunstein, *Laws of Fear: Beyond the Precautionary Principle* (Cambridge: Cambridge University Press, 2005): chapters 5–6.
24. And that if no tolerance threshold (or safe level of exposure) can be established, as with the cumulative effects of exposure to lead or radiation, then it is acceptable to determine and implement "permissible" levels of exposure.
25. Sunstein, *Risk and Reason*, 35; Sunstein, *Laws of Fear*, 83.
26. *Public Citizen v. Young*, 831 F. 2d 1108 (D.C. Circuit 1987).
27. *Public Citizen v. Young*, majority opinion, §21; Percival et al., *Environmental Regulation*, 284–5.
28. Jerome Nriagu, "Clair Patterson and Robert Kehoe's Paradigm of 'Show Me the Data' on Environmental Lead Poisoning," *Environmental Research* 78 (1998): 73–4; Public Health Service, "Proceedings of a Conference to Determine Whether or Not there is a Public Health Question in the Manufacture, Distribution, or Use of Tetraethyl Lead Gasoline;" U.S. Public Health Service, "The Use of Tetraethyl Lead Gasoline and Its Relation to Public Health," *Public Health Bulletin No. 163* (Washington, DC: Government Publishing Office, 1926).
29. *Industrial Union Dept., AFL-CIO v. American Petroleum Institute*, 448 U.S. 607 (1980).
30. *Corrosion Proof Fittings v. EPA*, 947 F.2d 1201 (5th Cir. 1991).
31. Percival et al., *Environmental Regulation*, 201–2.
32. Ibid., 258.
33. Ibid., 288.
34. Ibid.
35. Shrader-Frechette, *Taking Action, Saving Lives*, 3–7, 76–8, 113–7, 150–2; Boyd, "Genealogies of Risk," 923, 927.
36. Shrader-Frechette, *Taking Action, Saving Lives*, 79.
37. Percival et al., *Environmental Regulation*, 184, 192.
38. Alan Loeb, "Birth of the Kettering Doctrine: Fordism, Sloanism and Tetraethyl Lead," *Business and Economic History* 24 (1995); Bill Kovarik, "Charles F. Kettering and the 1921 Discovery of Tetraethyl Lead in the Context of Technological Alternatives" (working paper), *Presented to the Society of Automotive Engineers Fuels and Lubricants Conference*, Baltimore, MD, 1994 (revised in 1999); Jamie

Lincoln Kitman, "The Secret History of Lead," *The Nation*, March 2, 2002: www.thenation.com/article/secret-history-lead; Gerald Markowitz and David Rosner, *Deceit and Denial: The Deadly Politics of Industrial Pollution* (Berkeley: University of California Press, 2002).

References

Agency for Toxic Substances and Disease Registry. "Toxicological Profile for Asbestos." Atlanta: Department of Health and Human Services, 2001.

Boyd, William. "Genealogies of Risk: Searching for Safety, 1930s–1970s." *Ecological Law Quarterly* 39 (2012): 895–988.

———. "Environmental Law, Big Data, and the Torrent of Singularities." *UCLA Law Review Discourse* 64 (2016): 546–70.

Bro-Rasmussen, Finn. "Risk, Uncertainties, and Precautions in Chemical Legislation." In *Precaution: Environmental Science and Preventative Public Policy*, edited by Joel Tickner, 87–102. Washington: Island Press, 2003.

Browne, Marilyn, et al., "Cancer Incidence and Asbestos in Drinking Water, Town of Woodstock, New York, 1980–1998." *Environmental Research* 98 (2005): 224–32.

Carpenter, David, et al. "Understanding the Human Health Effects of Chemical Mixtures." *Environmental Health Perspectives* 110 (2002): 25–42.

Carson, Rachel. *Silent Spring*. Boston: Houghton Mifflin, 1962.

Corrosion Proof Fittings v. Environmental Protection Agency, 947 F.2d 1201 (5th Circuit 1991).

Drexler, John, et al. "Issue Paper on the Bioavailability and Bioaccumulation of Metals." U.S. Environmental Protection Agency, Risk Assessment Forum, 2003.

Environmental Defense Fund Inc. v. EPA, 489 F. 2d 1247 (D.C. Circuit 1973).

Environmental Protection Agency. "DDT, a Review of Scientific and Economic Aspects of the Decision to Ban Its Use as a Pesticide." Prepared for the *Committee on Appropriations of the U.S. House of Representatives*. EPA-540/1-75-022, July 1975. www2.epa.gov/aboutepa/ddt-regulatory-history-brief-survey-1975.

———. "Basic Information about Lead in Drinking Water." Last updated December 12, 2016. https://epa.gov/ground-water-and-drinking-water/basic-information-about-lead-drinking-water.

Ethyl Corp. v. EPA, 541 F. 2d 1 (D.C. Circuit 1976).

Food and Drug Administration. "Chemical Compounds in Food Producing Animals: Criteria and Procedures for Evaluating Assays for Carcinogenic Residues." *Federal Register* 44 (1979).

Gamble, John. "Risk of Gastrointestinal Cancers from Inhalation and Ingestion of Asbestos." *Regulatory Toxicology and Pharmacology* 52 (2008): S124–53.

Goklany, Indur. *The Precautionary Principle: A Critical Appraisal of Environmental Risk Assessment*. Washington: Cato Institute, 2001.

Government Publishing Office. Food, Drug, and Cosmetics Act. 21 U.S.C. §342 (1958).

Hamilton, Alice, et al. "Tetra Ethyl Lead." *Journal of the American Medical Association* 84 (1925): 1481–6.

Harremoës, Poul, et al., eds. *Late Lessons from Early Warnings: The Precautionary Principle 1896–2000*, Environmental Issue Report, No. 22. Copenhagen: European Environment Agency, 2001.

Hernberg, Sven. "Lead Poisoning in a Historical Perspective." *American Journal of Industrial Medicine* 38 (2000): 244–54.

Industrial Union Dept., AFL-CIO v. American Petroleum Institute, 448 U.S. 607 (1980).

Keynes, John Maynard. "The General Theory of Employment." *Quarterly Journal of Economics* 51 (1937): 209–23.

Kitman, Jamie Lincoln. "The Secret History of Lead." *The Nation*, March 2, 2002. http://thenation.com/article/secret-history-lead.

Knight, Frank. *Risk, Uncertainty, and Profit*. Boston: Houghton Mifflin Co., 1921.

Kovarik, Bill. "Charles F. Kettering and the 1921 Discovery of Tetraethyl Lead in the Context of Technological Alternatives." Presented to the *Society of Automotive Engineers Fuels and Lubricants Conference*, Baltimore, Maryland, 1994.

Kysar, Douglas. *Regulating from Nowhere: Environmental Law and the Search for Objectivity*. New Haven: Yale University Press, 2010.

Layzer, Judith. *The Environmental Case: Translating Values Into Policy*, 3rd edition. Washington: CQ Press, 2012.

Loeb, Alan. "Birth of the Kettering Doctrine: Fordism, Sloanism and the Discovery of Tetraethyl Lead." *Business and Economic History* 24 (1995): 72–87.

Markoitz, Gerald and David Rosner. "Corporate Responsibility for Toxins." *Annals of the Academy of Political and Social Science* 584 (2002): 159–74.

Massachusetts v. EPA, 549 U.S. 497 (2007).

Nriagu, Jerome. "The Rise and Fall of Leaded Gasoline." *Science of the Total Environment* 92 (1990): 13–28.

Percival, Robert, et al. *Environmental Regulation: Law, Science, and Policy*, 6th edition. New York: Aspen Publishers, 2009.

Public Citizen Health Research Group v. Young, 831 F.2d 1108 (D.C. Circuit 1987).

Public Health Service. "Proceedings of a Conference to Determine Whether or Not There Is a Public Health Question in the Manufacture, Distribution, or Use of Tetraethyl Lead Gasoline." *Public Health Bulletin No. 158*. Washington: Government Publishing Office, 1925.

———. "The Use of Tetraethyl Lead Gasoline and Its Relation to Public Health." *Public Health Bulletin No. 163*. Washington: Government Publishing Office, 1926.

Reserve Mining Company v. EPA, 514 F. 2d 492 (8th Circuit 1975).

Rosner, David and Gerald Markowitz. "A 'Gift of God'?: The Public Health Controversy over Leaded Gasoline during the 1920s." *American Journal of Public Health* 75 (1985): 344–52.

Sexton, Ken and Stephen Linder. "Cumulative Risk Assessment for Combined Health Effects from Chemical and Nonchemical Stressors." *American Journal of Public Health* 101 (2011): S81–8.

Shrader-Frechette, Kristin. *Taking Action, Saving Lives: Our Duties to Protect Environmental and Public Health*. Oxford: Oxford University Press, 2007.

Sunstein, Cass. *Risk and Reason: Safety, Law, and the Environment*. Cambridge: Cambridge University Press, 2002.

———. *Laws of Fear: Beyond the Precautionary Principle*. Cambridge: Cambridge University Press, 2005.

Tickner, Joel, ed. *Precaution, Environmental Science, and Preventive Public Policy*. Washington: Island Press, 2003.

Toronto Public Health. *Health Assessment for the Cumulative Air Quality Modelling Study: Wards 5 and 6*. Toronto: TPH, 2014.

Vogel, David. *The Politics of Precaution: Regulating Health, Safety, and Environmental Risks in Europe and the United States*. Princeton: Princeton University Press, 2012.

Vogt, Donna. *The Delaney Clause Effects on Pesticide Policy*. Washington: Congressional Research Service, 1995.

Wildavsky, Aaron. *But Is It True? A Citizen's Guide to Environmental Health and Safety Issues*. Cambridge: Harvard University Press, 1995.

Wilson, Richard. "Risks Caused by Low-Levels of Pollution." *Yale Journal of Biology and Medicine* 51 (1978): 37–51.

Xia, Yingcun and Howell Tong. "Cumulative Effects of Air Pollution on Public Health." *Statistics in Medicine* 25 (2006): 3548–59.

2 Precautionary Risk Regulation as a Matter of Right[1]

Decisions whether or not to regulate environmental threats of harm whose impacts are unknown have commonly turned on the scientific uncertainty that obscures the health effects of exposure. They have been grounded, in other words, in our inabilities to confirm the severity of the adverse consequences of exposure, or the probability that this projected harm will occur, or the causes of manifest harms. Both advocates *and* opponents of regulating environmental threats under conditions of uncertainty have conventionally appealed to these epistemic limitations, to the lack of scientific evidence, to justify their antithetical policy positions. Those who believe that environmental risk regulation should err on the side of caution insist that prevailing uncertainty requires that we implement precautionary regulations to safeguard the public against the possibility of harm.[2] Conversely, those who believe that scientific corroboration of a strong probability of severe harm to the public is a necessary condition of any legitimate risk regulation[3] insist that prevailing uncertainty—when the evidence "remains unavailable, uncertain, or controversial"[4]—requires that we *refrain* from restricting activities whose effects remain indeterminate.[5] This places contemporary debates about how to respond to uncertain threats of environmental harm, about whether to regulate activities that entail possible albeit uncorroborated risks of harm to public health, at an untenable impasse.

This impasse permits but two alternatives. One is to accept that this stalled debate entails that *no* uncertain threat of environmental harm merits being regulated. After all, how can we be persuaded by a call for preventative regulation that can be turned on its head to yield a contradictory conclusion? The other is to ground an argument for exercising precaution in something *other than* uncertainty and what we can or cannot know. If we take seriously the concern that the welfare of others may be jeopardized by our failure to regulate environmental threats under conditions of uncertainty, and if we acknowledge that environmental history is rife with examples of how the emission of substances once thought to be benign proved to be deleterious, then the first alternative must be rejected. The absence of compelling reason in support of some conclusion does not itself constitute justification for its rejection. As Shrader-Frechette notes, "from flawed or incomplete evidence—ignorance—no conclusion follows," for "failure to have evidence does not prove anything, one way or the other."[6] Accordingly, this chapter begins to develop an alternative justification for precautionary risk regulation, which is further developed and defended in subsequent chapters: a justification that shifts the discussion from the implications of our epistemic limitations to what individuals who may be exposed to uncertain threats of environmental harm are owed as a matter of their equal moral standing to emitters.

Section 2.1 explains that in the debate over the merits of precautionary risk regulation, uncertainty has conventionally been misconceived as having only to do with the probability of harm to public health. In detailing several different forms of uncertainty, Section 2.1 also stipulates that precautionary measures are justified only under broader conditions (or higher "degrees"[7]) of uncertainty. That is, the precautionary approach to risk regulation applies only to a subset of environmental health risks. Section 2.2 introduces existing formulations of the precautionary principle and explores several perennial policy-oriented and normative objections to these formulations, which deny the viability of a precautionary approach to regulating environmental risk. Section 2.3 demonstrates that key efforts to refute these objections are problematic, lending credence to a substantive reformulation of the principle that this book aims to defend. The common objections highlighted in Section 2.2 can be avoided and precautionary risk regulation can be defended by recasting the precautionary principle *not* as a way of managing the uncertainty of risks of harm and *not* as a policy approach grounded in scientific knowledge about risk, but rather as a normative principle that preserves moral equality and as a policy tool founded on the right against being exposed to potentially harmful and preventable environmental threats. While the arguments for these claims are developed later in Chapter 5.4, briefly introduces this rights-based interpretation of the precautionary principle, gesturing toward the normative defense of our moral obligation to exercise due care (precaution) under conditions of uncertainty that is developed in Chapters 3 and 4.

2.1 Complexities of Environmental Harms

It is necessary to begin by clarifying what uncertainty means, for current scholarship in environmental policy and normative ethics often presupposes a narrow conception of uncertainty and thus can problematically assume we have greater knowledge of the potential for harm than we really do. As an aside, the reader should note that the aim of this section is neither to detail a comprehensive taxonomy of uncertainty, as scholars like Hansson have attempted,[8] nor to explore the many complex facets of the distinction between risk and scientific uncertainty (or between probability and predictability), as scholars like Steel have done.[9] Rather, with a two-fold aim, this section explores select forms of uncertainty that consistently reappear in environmental policy literature on the precautionary principle and philosophical literature on risk and responsibility but that are often treated quite loosely by scholars—if not left implicit in their writing. The first objective is to underscore that uncertainty is a complicated concept that is often oversimplified (as Hansson and Steel aptly demonstrate), which has both generated misunderstanding of the unique moral problems that uncertainty entails and prompted questionable conclusions about how we should respond to these moral problems. The second objective is to narrow the purview of the precautionary principle, for it is alleged later that a precautionary approach to environmental risk management is only appropriate when certain forms of uncertainty are achieved. Table 2.1 denotes four distinct forms of uncertainty, which the following discussion explains in turn.

Environmental harms are often deferred, far-reaching, and cumulative and are caused by long-term, low-level exposure to pollutants.[10] Consider, for instance, our exposure to various pesticides, whose toxic residues are commonly found on raw foods and in processed foods, in municipal drinking water, in a host of garden and lawn care products, and in diverse public spaces (parks, pools, lakes, hospitals, schools, day care centers, etc.). Given the pervasive use of pesticides, the potential for harm is widespread, with exposure generally occurring at low levels over long periods of time and often entailing a mixture of pesticides that create a cumulative risk.[11] While the effects of direct, shorter-term, higher-dose exposure are often known (i.e., the toxicity of a given pesticide can usually be corroborated), the likelihood of exposure and the probability that exposure will cause harm remain uncorroborated. It is this

Table 2.1 Forms of Uncertainty

Type	*Description*	*Examples*
Outcome	Severity and/or permanency of immediate or long-term effects of exposure is unknown.	BPA, GMOs, rBGH, e-cigarettes (present) Saccharin artificial sweetener (1980s) DES synthetic estrogen (1970s) DDT pesticide (1950s) Tetraethyl lead fuel additive (1920s)
Probability	Likelihood that exposure will be harmful is unknown.	Diverse physiological dispositions. Low-level exposure and deferred effects.
Causal	Outcome of exposure is known to be harmful, yet complex causal chains of events obscure whether manifest harms are associated with exposure.	Various pathways of exposure. Indirect and cumulative health effects. Low-level exposure and deferred effects. Early warning signs.
Scientific	Capacity to test and verify health effects is constrained, and/or scientific community is divided on findings of existing tests.	Discipline-specific measures and protocols. Extrapolation from epidemiological studies. Corruption of science. Reliance on industry safety assessments.

particular conception of uncertainty—what Table 2.1 refers to as "probability uncertainty," which is the form of uncertainty that conventional definitions of "risk" adopt—that informs existing interpretations of and criticisms against the precautionary principle, as well as the impasse noted earlier.

The Environmental Protection Agency (EPA), for instance, treats the "risk" of any given pesticide as a combination of the substance's toxicity and "the likelihood of people coming into contact with it."[12] Toxicity is determined by "dose-response assessments," which consist of exposing lab animals in controlled environments to different doses of a potentially harmful substance, determining the minimum dose at which harm is observed, and then extrapolating from these data the likely effects of comparable exposure to human health.[13] And when a substance is determined to be "nontoxic," that is to cause no harm, the EPA maintains that no level of exposure constitutes a risk to human health. Conversely, when a substance is found to be detrimental to human health, then the risk is defined by the likelihood of exposure.[14] The most commonly cited version of the precautionary principle (as propounded by the UN Environment Programme) also endorses a conception of uncertainty as probability uncertainty. The Rio Declaration states that "where there are threats of serious or irreversible damage, the lack of full scientific certainty shall not be used as a reason for postponing cost-effective measures to prevent environmental degradation."[15] This language of "serious or irreversible damage" implies that the effects of exposure are known or can reasonably be estimated, and consequently that what remains unknown, what justifies the exercise of precaution, is uncertainty about the probability that these harmful outcomes will come to pass.

Yet probability uncertainty is *but one* of several relevant forms of uncertainty, and to understand how the proposed rights-based interpretation of the precautionary principle departs from conventional justifications of precautionary risk regulation, it is necessary to explore what else uncertainty means. Proponents of precaution commonly ground preventative regulations in the *prima facie* possibility for nontrivial (or substantive) and irreparable harm to public health and the subsequent responsibility to safeguard against these *foreseeable* harms. However, in the rights-based account, it is chiefly when both probability *and* outcome uncertainty are obtained that precautionary measures are justified.

Despite the narrow conception of uncertainty as probability uncertainty that many scholars of environmental policy and risk theory adopt, in many cases, "outcome uncertainty" also is achieved, such that we also lack knowledge of (are unable to foresee) the severity and/or permanency (irreversibility) of immediate or long-term consequences of exposure.[16] For instance, prior to the 1920s, the health effects of (low-level) exposure to tetraethyl lead (a popular fuel additive) in the ambient air from vehicle exhaust were poorly studied and largely unknown (see Chapter 6).[17] Analogously, until the 1950s, the toxicological effects of dichlorodiphenyltrichloroethane (DDT) were poorly understood and were severely overshadowed by the synthetic insecticide's apparent benefits.[18] The same is true of diethylstilbestrol (DES), a synthetic estrogen commonly prescribed to pregnant women before the early 1970s "to prevent miscarriages and avoid other pregnancy problems"—for the injuries to those who were exposed to DES while in utero (taking the form of various cancers) took decades to manifest.[19]

Among the diverse examples of substances whose public health effects are presently unverified and, thus, whose continued use remains controversial include bisphenol A (BPA) and recombinant bovine growth hormone (rBGH), which is alternatively known as recombinant bovine somatotropin (rBST). BPA is an industrial chemical used in countless consumer goods—from sales receipts, to plastic containers, to canned foods—and acts like an endocrine disruptor or estrogen mimicker. As late as 2008, exposure to BPA was not a public health concern. While the prolonged and cumulative consequences of low-dose exposure—especially among vulnerable populations like fetuses and infants—still remain unverified and contested,[20] and while the U.S. Food and Drug Administration (FDA) postponed issuing any formal ban of BPA in consumer products,[21] several manufacturers pulled certain BPA-containing products as early as 2009 and altered their manufacturing processes to offer BPA-free versions of many of their consumer goods.[22] Growth hormones, on the other hand, are commonly used as catalysts for lactating dairy cattle to produce greater volumes of milk, and traces of rBGH residues have been found in all possible dairy products produced with milk from rBGH-treated cattle. What is more, because cattle given rBGH are more prone to develop infections of their udders, they are also given higher levels of antibiotics than non–rBGH-treated cattle, the ingestion of which may pose further long-term health risks to consumers.[23] The FDA has denied the potential adverse health effects of consuming rBGH-treated dairy and maintains that there is no salient difference between milk from treated and untreated cows.[24] At one time the FDA even insisted that dairy producers choosing to label their products as made from milk of untreated cows should include a disclaimer that "No significant difference has been shown between milk derived from rBST-treated and non-rBST-treated cows," so as to avoid confusing or misleading consumers.[25] Nevertheless, the findings of current studies remain contested. For instance, in its 2010 rejection of the constitutionality of state bans of hormone-free labeling initiatives, an Ohio federal court explicitly denied the FDA's long-standing claim that no substantive difference exists—underscoring, in part, what researchers had already revealed: that milk from rBGH-treated cows contains higher levels of a particular "insulin-like growth factor" hormone (IGF-1) as compared to milk from untreated cattle.[26] And although the FDA has argued that exposure to this hormone has benign health effects (poses "no appreciable risk"),[27] this conclusion ignores limits on our capacity to test for these effects.

Consider, for example, the admission by Cornell University's Program for Breast Cancer and Environmental Risk Factors (BCERF) that we are unable to discriminate between hormones found naturally in cattle from the synthetic growth hormones injected into the animals and that this limitation undermines the ability of scientists to accurately establish the proportion of the total hormones detected in dairy products that should be attributed to rBGH treatments.[28] Consider, moreover, that according to the American Cancer Society (ACS), which cautiously admits to an uncorroborated, albeit possible, connection between heightened levels of IGF-1 and health problems like cancer, recent studies have "failed to confirm" but have *not* been able to demonstrate the falsity of earlier scientific findings that purported that higher IGF-1 levels increase the probability of developing various cancers.[29] The ACS also explains that the harmful effects of rBGH to cattle *have* been scientifically corroborated, which may lend credence to the potential harm to humans, and that the health effects of the possible transmission of antibiotics from rBGH-treated cows to humans through consumption of rBGH-treated dairy products remains "unclear." Further still, the ACS claims that because there has been no empirical study that examines the variation of IGF-1 levels in people who consume rBGH-treated versus untreated dairy products, it is neither clear that consuming dairy with trace residues of rBGH increases one's level of the IGF-1 hormone nor that increased IGF-1 blood levels cause harmful health effects.[30] Consequently, in contrast to the FDA's definitive claims, the ACS concludes that "[t]he evidence for potential harm to humans is inconclusive" and that further scientific research is necessary to verify actual health effects of exposure.[31]

These concerns allude to a third salient form of uncertainty, which has to do with our ability to verify the consequences of exposure to a potentially harmful environmental threat: what is referred to in Table 2.1 as "scientific uncertainty." This uncertainty can be understood as resulting either from constraints on the scientific community's capacity to test and corroborate actual health effects of exposure or from disagreement within the scientific community about the meaning and implications of the best available evidence derived from available methods of analysis. With regard to the former source of scientific uncertainty, as some scholars have noted, toxicity studies suffer from "inadequacies in . . . observational methods"[32]—relying heavily on epidemiologic tests on animals (generally rodents, rabbits, and monkeys), from which the likely effects to human health are then extrapolated or inferred. Uncertainty in these findings persists, at least in part, because exposure occurs and health effects are observed in sterile, controlled environments, which do not resemble the more complex and less predictable environments in which humans are exposed to environmental threats. Similarly, these experiments test the effects of short-term, high-dose exposure as opposed to examining the long-term, low-dose exposure that characterizes most environmental threats to which humans are exposed. Further, not only does the physiology of humans differ substantively from lab animals, these experiments commonly involve "adolescent to middle-age-animals" that are less vulnerable to exposure than their "neonatal" counterparts.[33] Yet even if we table these concerns and accept that we can approximate the actual human health effects of exposure to potentially harmful substances with animal testing, toxicity studies still have difficulty accounting for the causal complexities of environmental threats: diverse intervening causal factors; cumulative exposures; different pathways, timings, and lengths of exposure; varying physiological dispositions or vulnerabilities to exposure; and so on—considerations that can alter the kind, magnitude, consistency, and observability of demonstrable harm. This is to say that like "tipping points," thresholds beyond which ecosystems are unable to absorb the effects of anthropogenic environmental change and invariably decline, which scholars have argued "often 'cannot be forecast by existing science,'"[34] current toxicology is similarly hampered by "causal uncertainty"—a fourth form of uncertainty that is explored below.

With regard to the latter source of scientific uncertainty, fractures within the scientific community commonly follow from the politicization of science or the incongruous standards and methods of analysis across the relevant scientific disciplines. The vulnerability of science to being co-opted by private interests, and political influence is no new phenomenon. Scholars like Pielke or Oreskes and Conway, for instance, have argued that science is all too often married to the values and political agendas that shape public policy making[35]—with proponents of precautionary risk regulation like Shrader-Frechette pointing specifically to the corruption of toxicology.[36] Indicting "privatized science"[37] for purposefully producing, if only irresponsibly tolerating, commonly flawed and incomplete and hence misleading empirical studies, Shrader-Frechette denies both the alleged objectivity of toxicity studies and the claim that scientists and policy-makers are less prone to misconceive and distort actual risks.[38] Underscoring the normative and policy problems with a "technocratic" approach toward environmental risk management, which leaves the scientific community to decide what risks are credible, unreasonable, and warrant regulation, Shrader-Frechette and Whiteside both lament that regulators commonly defer to the safety assessment findings of private industry-led toxicity studies.[39] While this is largely because regulatory agencies often lack the resources to conduct independent tests, this clear conflict of interest means that risk regulation standards are directly shaped by the very actors they are intended to regulate. Yet even when science is not co-opted in this way, different scientific disciplines employ "different measures and different experimental protocols," which makes the comparison and compilation of data from different relevant fields (such as geology, hydrology, chemistry, etc.) quite difficult.[40] Toxicology is a complex science, requiring, some would say, collaborative or interdisciplinary efforts, and because scientific consensus can be "elusive," so, too, can our understanding of the health effects of exposure to environmental threats.[41]

As the foregoing suggests, these different forms of uncertainty are not mutually exclusive. Scientific uncertainty, for example—as the upshot of our inability to accurately test and corroborate health effects of exposure—entails or produces outcome and/or probability uncertainty, since these difficulties with empirical tests obscure the conclusions we can draw about the likely consequences of exposure, or the likelihood of being exposed to the environmental threat. Concomitantly, scientific uncertainty—as the upshot of disagreement within the scientific community about the meaning and implications of existing safety assessment data—can be the product of outcome uncertainty and/or probability uncertainty, since difficulties with discerning the likely consequences of exposure or the probability of exposure will obscure the warrant for the conclusions we draw from existing empirical tests and data. Moreover, the degree to which the scientific community may be divided over the risk assessment data can also be influenced by "causal uncertainty." Under conditions of causal uncertainty, the outcomes of exposure are known to be harmful, but complex causal chains of events obscure whether manifest harms are associated with exposure. This further distinct form of uncertainty undermines, in other words, our ability to discern whether it is the emission of and subsequent exposure to a harmful substance, or some other cause entirely, that begets the harm we observe.

Consider, for instance, that we know radon is a "naturally occurring radioactive gas," which commonly seeps through foundation floors and into homes and is alleged to be the "second leading cause of lung cancer" in the United States.[42] Yet it is unclear whether exposure to radon alone induces lung cancer (because only a small fraction of radon-related cancers occur among nonsmokers[43]) or if another causal factor—like cigarette smoking—is actually what makes one susceptible to developing cancer from radon exposure.[44] Similarly, asbestos is known to be hazardous, and the inhalation of airborne asbestos fibers is known to cause asbestosis (a form of lung disease that hinders one's ability to breathe by restricting the lungs' capacity to "expand and contract" and which also "causes the heart to enlarge" by restricting blood flow to the lungs).[45] However, it is unclear whether different pathways of exposure cause similar health problems. It is unknown, for example, whether the ingestion of asbestos fibers—say, from drinking contaminated water or eating foods containing deposits of soil or dust—is harmful.[46] Buttressing the World Health Organization's claims that there is "no consistent, convincing evidence that ingested asbestos is hazardous to health,"[47] recent epidemiologic studies have found positive, albeit "weak" and statistically insignificant (i.e., inconclusive) associations between asbestos ingestion and common forms of gastrointestinal cancer.[48] These studies have also indicated that various "occupational and lifestyle risk factors," which confound the link between asbestos ingestion and adverse health effects, may be causally responsible for observable harms from asbestos exposure.[49] Both Browne et al. and Gamble, for instance, argue that "a history of cigarette smoking" is an extraneous (moderating) causal factor that may increase the likelihood of asbestos-related cancers,[50] which aligns with the Department of Human Health Services' analogous suggestion that smoking may make one more susceptible to developing lung cancer from exposure to (inhalation of) airborne asbestos fibers.[51]

Different exposure pathways (inhalation, ingestion, or absorption through the skin); diverse intervening factors; indirect and cumulative health effects; and the commonly deferred consequences of long-term, low-level exposure can independently and collectively obscure the causal influence that exposure to some environmental threat may have on human health. What is more, exposure across a given population is rarely uniform,[52] and consequently variation in the timing, duration, intensity, and frequency of exposure influences when injuries become observable. And because individual susceptibility (i.e., vulnerability or physiological predisposition) to being injured varies widely across populations, it is extremely difficult to causally associate any particular exposure with a demonstrable injury.[53] Perera notes that in addition to one's genetic makeup, among the "multiple susceptibility factors" that can amplify one's vulnerability to being harmed are "immunological impairment, pre-existing disease, and nutritional deficits."[54] For these reasons, some have not only underscored that "causal paths are extremely difficult to trace"[55] but also that our knowledge of these complex causal relationships often remains "indeterminate."[56]

Despite these different forms of uncertainty, as noted earlier, scholars and commentators have conventionally framed uncertainty in terms of "risk," which again is to say that they treat uncertainty narrowly as probability uncertainty.[57] In contrast, uncertainty is understood here as comprising *at least* outcome and probability uncertainty, or what some have indirectly referred to as "ignorance,"[58] or "incalculable uncertainty,"[59] or "unmeasurable uncertainty."[60] For the sake of clarity, the reader should note that throughout the rest of this book, unless otherwise specified, any reference to "uncertainty" or "conditions of uncertainty" is intended to denote this broader understanding of genuine uncertainty. And to avoid confusion with the prevalent language of *risk* and traditional "risk impositions," uncorroborated possibilities of environmental harm under conditions of (genuine) uncertainty are described here as "uncertain threats" or "uncertain environmental threats"—which are the product of what this book calls "endangering actions" as opposed to traditional "risky actions." This is all to say that the key difference between risk and uncertainty, between risk impositions and uncertain threats, is our knowledge or lack of knowledge of consequence: when we know the outcomes of our potentially harmful actions, we are in the domain of (probabilistic) risk (or "measurable risk"); when we lack this information, we are in the purview of (indeterminate) uncertainty (or "unmeasurable uncertainty").[61]

The chief reason for these deviations from convention is that the exercise of precaution is most clearly justified when our knowledge of the potential for harm to public health is so constrained that formal, quantitative risk assessments (QRAs) cannot be conducted and thus fail to prescribe reasonable safety measures. QRA, in other words, can successfully approximate thresholds of "acceptable" risk or "permissible exposure limits,"[62] and it can inform regulations that achieve adequate "margins of safety" for many threats of environmental harm[63]—provided the information exists to corroborate adverse health effects. Arsenic in drinking water,[64] particulate matter in the ambient air,[65] and methylmercury in foods[66] are but three examples that testify to the usefulness of this policy tool. Despite its own shortcomings,[67] QRA, as some have noted, which gained prominence in the late 1970s with marked improvements in toxicological studies and "detection capabilities," has become an integral (though nevertheless contentious) component of contemporary environmental risk management.[68] Consequently, in its defense of precautionary risk regulation, this book does not argue that formal risk assessments are unwarranted or that a precautionary approach is appropriate in all cases.[69] Indeed, the management of environmental threats should rest on no *one* policy approach.[70] What it *does* claim is that precautionary regulations are not only justified but are necessary when we lack the information required to substantiate inferences about the effects of exposure and/or the likelihood that harm will come to pass. This suggests that exercising precaution is justified either when outcome uncertainty prevails, or when *both* outcome and probability uncertainty are present, or when causal or scientific uncertainty undermines our ability to ascertain the effects of exposure or the probability that exposure will cause injury.

Yet in contrast to conventional defenses of precautionary risk regulation, it is not the lack of empirical evidence per se—it is not uncertainty—that demands that we implement precautionary measures to safeguard public health. Rather, it is the moral obligation we have to refrain from exposing others to potential and preventable injury: the right others have not to be exposed to unconsented to and undeserved possibilities of harm, which they do not surrender when uncertainty prevails. In addition to defending its normative foundations (Chapters 3 and 4), justifying this rights-based account of the precautionary principle requires demonstrating that it can avoid the charges commonly leveled against precautionary environmental risk regulation (Chapter 5)—objections to which the discussion now turns.

2.2 Contemporary Formulations and Common Objections

Several competing understandings of the precautionary principle have engendered widespread disagreement over the meaning and appropriate scope of the principle. Some have conceptualized the precautionary principle as strictly epistemic in nature, such that if we have *any* evidence—however cursory or thin—that some potential for harm exists, then this evidence should motivate us to accept the credibility of the risk.[71] In short, this implies that the evidentiary burden to corroborate the presence of a probable risk of nontrivial harm is quite weak and thus generally met with relative ease. Perhaps a more tempered version of this interpretation may consist in fostering a skeptical attitude toward "knowledge claims about the environment"[72] when the potential for harm to the public is unclear. This general skepticism would not motivate us to accept the credibility of some potential risk on weak evidentiary grounds (because this limited evidence should also be open to scrutiny), but it would commit us to deny the common assertion that the absence of corroborating *evidence* of a credible threat testifies to the absence of a credible *threat*. While a weak evidentiary burden or a general skepticism may inform our risk regulations, these epistemic understandings of the principle say nothing about how we should respond to a *prima facie* credible threat or the uncorroborated potential for harm to the public.

Accordingly, others have suggested that beyond the credibility of a given risk of environmental harm, the precautionary principle should more appropriately be understood as action guiding: understood, that is, as prescribing specific regulations to prevent *prima facie* credible threats of harm from materializing in actual injuries.[73] The language of the Rio Declaration certainly seems to connote this understanding, asserting that when faced with "threats of serious or irreversible environmental damage," prevailing uncertainties should not prevent us from instituting policies to safeguard against possible harm[74]—which is to say that *inaction* is unjustified. The widely recognized "Wingspread Statement" also lends credence to this interpretation of the precautionary principle, claiming that when human health or the environment is threatened, "precautionary measures should be taken even if some cause-and-effect relationships are not fully established scientifically."[75] Accordingly, Raffensperger (who, it should be noted, helped to convene the Wingspread Conference) and Tickner insist that "the precautionary principle has a dual trigger: if there is a potential for harm from an activity and if there is uncertainty about the magnitude of impacts or causality, then anticipatory action should be taken to avoid harm."[76] This means that unless we can confirm that an action is safe—that it entails *no* potential for harm (an idea many scholars reject[77])—precautionary measures are justified: for if we verify that an action is certain to cause harm, we should prevent it from coming to pass, and if we have *not* verified that an action is certain to be free of harm, we should preventatively strive to mitigate the potential for harm.

In a similar vein, it has been suggested that the precautionary principle foremost requires that the burden of proof be shifted from regulatory agencies to industry.[78] Proponents of this understanding insist that it should *not* be presumed that substances emitted into the environment are safe until regulatory agencies effectively demonstrate otherwise, but rather that industry should be prohibited from emitting potentially harmful substances until it corroborates the relative safety of its emissions to public health and welfare. Expressed differently, this interpretation requires that we assume that any given substance emitted into the environment is unsafe until industry provides us with adequate empirical evidence to the contrary—which, in effect, constitutes an interdiction against all risky behavior.

The less strict parallel of this interpretation claims that precaution entails "publicly examining a full range of alternatives to a potentially damaging human activity"[79] and then requiring that alternative policies or substitute technologies—whose environmental effects *are* known (or are less unclear) and can be mitigated—be implemented whenever possible. In response to uncorroborated public health threats, this interpretation of the principle may involve, for example, implementing best available control technologies (BACTs) to minimize the potential for adverse outcomes,[80] or working to safeguard the most vulnerable populations from potential harm,[81] or adopting broader or more ample margins of safety in establishing thresholds of acceptable risk.[82]

Conversely, some proponents of precaution have grounded their understanding of the purpose of and justification for the precautionary principle in the tenets of an ecocentric environmental ethics. By insisting that broader ecosystems—encompassing human beings and nonhuman sentient creatures, nonsentient living organisms, and nonliving features of the physical environment—enjoy a certain moral standing or intrinsic value that impose obligations on us to protect their interests and allow them to flourish,[83] some ecocentrists purport that these duties commit us to a "prevention-oriented conception of environmental protection."[84] The claim is that because anthropogenic changes to the environment alter the complex interactions, processes, and relationships that define an ecosystem and, therefore, force ecosystems to adapt to the changes imposed on them, precautionary environmental policies are necessary to allow ecosystems to exist and persist as they otherwise (naturally) would. In short, it is suggested that we must implement precautionary regulations to prevent human activities from undercutting the natural functions of ecosystems and their capacity to preserve and sustain themselves.[85]

Still others have conceived of the precautionary principle as less restrictive. Some maintain that precaution requires, more modestly, further scientific research on uncorroborated environmental threats in order to improve our understanding of actual risks to public health and the environment.[86] Others suggest that precaution also requires the "vigilant" monitoring of environmental and public health so as to identify early warning signs of potential environmental harms and to have the opportunity to prevent these harms from coming to pass.[87] It is argued that these measures not only are best advanced by or must consist in multidisciplinary efforts,[88] but that they also require a transparent auditing system. An enforcement system, that is, in which industry collaborates with regulators to ascertain credible threats to public health, fully and truthfully discloses its safety assessment data, keeps the public abreast of potential health hazards, and strives toward principles of corporate social responsibility in working with legislators and regulatory agencies to create viable environmental policies.[89]

Despite the lack of a "commonly accepted" definition of the principle or a settled "set of criteria to guide its implementation,"[90] critics have generally treated the precautionary principle as a policy prescription to mitigate exposure to uncertain threats of harm—the action-guiding formulation noted earlier. And one of the common objections to the logic of precaution, and the tenability of the precautionary approach toward risk regulation, is that by allowing for the regulation of unsubstantiated risks,

(1) the principle tolerates unfounded restrictions on actions that beget merely speculative risks.

Morris, for instance, charges that on precautionary accounts, the "mere *possibility*" for harm to human health is sufficient to prohibit or "severely" restrict the use of new technologies[91]—substantial constraints that warrant corroborating evidence, not mere speculation. In parallel fashion, scholars like Miller and Conko or Sunstein maintain that contrary to the objective nature of science-based risk management, which grounds policy recommendations in quantitative risk assessments and cost–benefit analyses,

(2) precautionary policies are commonly subjective and highly political.[92]

Tabling concerns with the assumptions that (science-based) quantitative risk assessments and risk–benefit analyses do, in fact, yield objective policy recommendations,[93] it is alleged that because the precautionary principle does not require corroboration of any actual or credible threat to public health, decisions whether or not to regulate threats of environmental harm are easily shaped by public (mis)perceptions of risk. Sunstein, for instance, argues at length that average citizens overstate the relevance of "worst-case" scenarios, personal observations, and sparse anecdotal evidence; that they generally are swayed by what *others* believe threatens public health; and that they base their appraisals of perceived risk on intuition or effect instead of on reliable probability assessments.[94] Amplifying concerns that ordinary people are poor judges of risk—ignoring statistical realities of actual threats to public health and entertaining instead irrational and inflated fears—others have argued that lay perceptions of risk are commonly influenced by sensationalist reporting on high-profile cases of environmental risk and harm.[95] Layzer notes that these extreme cases of environmental threats and harms receive more media coverage, which invariably skews the average person's belief in and understanding of the gravity of the threat.[96] The implication of these considerations is that the precautionary approach toward risk assessment and regulation is informed by this sort of unreliable and inaccurate "intuitive toxicology."[97]

Furthermore, because some level of risk pervades all human action and, hence, is inevitable with any regulatory alternative, others insist that

(3) the precautionary principle effectively "paralyzes" all policy making.[98]

Even precautionary regulations, which strive to prevent the actualization of potential harms to the public, run the risk of imposing (new) harms on those it aims to safeguard.[99] This is to say that what drives precautionary risk management is uncertainty about the possible harmful effects of nonregulation. Yet *all* policy decisions, including precautionary regulations, invariably entail some potential for harm. Accordingly, not only is it the case that what justifies precaution simultaneously undermines any effort to take precaution, but *any* policy response to environmental threats of harm is unfounded, given its own potential to cause subsequent harm.

For instance, suppose that David and Michael, senior members of a city council of a small Lake Erie town, are due to advise the city manager on policy alternatives to mitigate the dangerous algae blooms in the lake, which are polluting the town's primary source of drinking water. Let us say that David supports an alternative that involves releasing a new chemical substance into the waters along the shores of the town, which is designed to destroy the (cyano)bacteria responsible for the toxic blooms, whereas Michael supports an option that involves switching the source of the town's water back to a local river far enough inland that it is not vulnerable to being polluted by the algae. Knowing that the city manager is a proponent of precaution, Michael notes that David's plan is problematic because trace amounts of the chemical substance would remain in the city's treated tap water, the exposure to which is poorly understood and may put residents in the way of potential harm. Similarly, David raises concerns with Michael's plan because the low and corrosive pH levels of the town's river water are analogous to the pH levels found in the Flint River, which helped to cause the recent water crisis in Flint, Michigan—and so switching the city's source of drinking water to the local river might put residents at risk of lead poisoning. As a matter of precaution, the city manager rejects both plans and proposes a third alternative that involves distributing bottled water to residents until a more reliable, long-term solution can be found. Yet committed to their respective alternatives, David and Michael also appeal to precaution in noting that because the safety standards for bottled water are lax and cannot ensure the water's purity—for example, petroleum-based plastic bottles have been found to leach phthalates into the water, the levels of which are not regulated by the FDA—this alternative, too, could expose residents to possible harm.[100]

In this way, critics charge that precautionary risk regulation not only amounts to blanket bans of any risky behavior, but given the ubiquity of risk, a commitment to precaution absurdly leads to suspending all action—which itself poses some risk of harm and cannot be justified by the precautionary principle.[101] By invoking ostensibly problematic precautionary bans, including DDT and genetically modified organisms (GMOs), some critics also underscore that precautionary policies are unjustified because

(4) preventative measures may create more risk than they ameliorate.

In other words, these critics allege that exercising precaution is irrational, that the principle is "literally incoherent."[102] Some have alleged, for instance, that the banning of DDT was a clear catalyst for the resurgence of malaria in those lesser-developed countries that prohibited the use of the pesticide.[103] Consequently, this initiative is said to have produced greater malaria-related illness and death than any danger to human health that DDT posed. Likewise, it is argued that any possible harm that consuming genetically modified crops may pose to human health is starkly overshadowed by the malnutrition and starvation entailed by the ban of GMOs and subsequent prevailing food shortages in the developing world.[104] (And as Whiteside, a proponent of precaution, explains, it is "morally hard to urge caution in the face of such claims."[105]) The implication of this reasoning is that advocates of

(5) precautionary regulations "selectively" acknowledge certain costs of non-regulation while imprudently ignoring others.

That is, proponents justify the exercise of precaution by examining particular threats of harm in isolation from broader values, policy objectives, and costs and benefits of alternative policy options.[106] For instance, in critically examining the warrant for precautionary measures to ban DDT and GMOs and to aggressively curb the release of greenhouse gases, Goklany contends that crucial adverse consequences of these preventative measures have commonly been overlooked. And if we were to acknowledge these costs, the justification for exercising precaution would effectively be undermined.[107] This, too, is the case, says Goklany, with ignoring the *positive* consequences of *non*regulation, such as consuming less water and land and using fewer chemical fertilizers with the production of GMOs as opposed to conventional crops.[108] This approach to risk regulation, say Miller and Conko, which rejects the "careful balancing of risks and benefits . . . cost real lives due to forgone benefits."[109]

The precautionary principle is also censured for inherently failing to provide any substantive policy guidance. Skeptics posit that to exercise precaution, it is too general a concept to yield any substantive policy prescription and thus that

(6) the principle fails to be "action guiding"; it is, rather, vacuous.[110]

More specifically, it is said that the precautionary principle is "too vague to serve as a regulatory standard because it does not specify *how much* caution should be taken"[111] and, therefore, what it means to exercise precaution remains unclear. As Gardiner (a proponent of precaution) clarifies, conventionally, it has been unclear whether precautionary risk regulation should have us (merely) warn or educate others about the existence of an environmental threat, or to mitigate or prevent the potential effects of these threats of harm, or to eliminate the causes of these threats.[112] In a similar vein, even if the precautionary principle could provide substantive policy prescriptions, a precautionary approach to risk management lacks (quantifiable) measures that permit us to compare and rank policy alternatives and priorities. In short, there is no consistent way to determine what particular precautionary policy is better than alternative preventative initiatives.[113]

Alternatively, assuming that the precautionary principle *can* offer substantive policy recommendations, it has been widely suggested that the precautionary approach is overly demanding. This is to say that precautionary risk regulations unduly constrain the freedom and autonomy of emitters to perform actions that entail some potential for harm but whose outcomes may well prove to be benign.[114] The central concern here is that

(7) rigid precautionary standards fail to balance the benefits with the costs of regulation and, hence, unfairly burden industry.[115]

This criticism may be attributed to the austerity of early precautionary risk regulations, which established environmental standards strictly on the basis of potential dangers to public health and welfare. Consider the paradigmatic example of precautionary regulation, the so-called Delaney Clause: Section 409 of the 1958 Federal Food, Drug, and Cosmetics Act. This landmark initiative prohibited any food additive "found to induce cancer in man or animals" (Section 409(c)(3)(A)), "regardless of the magnitude of the dose"[116]—creating a highly stringent and economically burdensome standard for the food and cosmetic industries to meet.

Similarly, notable decisions upholding precautionary, health-based standards promulgated by the EPA include *Ethyl Corp. v. EPA* (1976), *Reserve Mining Company v. EPA* (1975), and *Chlorine Chemical Council v. EPA* (2000). The ruling in *Ethyl*[117] is one of clearest decisions championing the precautionary principle. In brief, this case concerns whether exposure to leaded gasoline poses a "significant" risk of harm—a case in which the U.S. Court of Appeals ruled that "significant" risk need not be precise and that to be threatened is to be endangered and, depending on the estimated probability and/or severity of harm, precautionary regulation demands that regulatory action precede and prevent the perceived threat. In short, *Ethyl* established a precedent that even in the absence of actual (or imminent) harm, regulation can be justified. Alternatively, *Reserve Mining*[118] led to an injunction against the release of taconite tailings that contain asbestos fibers, whose threat to public health remained scientifically unverified and did not seem to be imminent but which nevertheless involved a substance that shares certain characteristics of another known to cause harm: in this instance, asbestos fibers, which are known to be toxic. Lastly, in *Chlorine Chemical Council*[119] the EPA acknowledged that under certain levels, exposure to chloroform poses no risk of cancer, but in promulgating its Maximum Contaminant Level Goal (MCLG) for chloroform under the Safe Drinking Water Act, the EPA retained a zero standard based on the past assumption that there was no safe threshold. (Though the U.S. Court of Appeals ultimately ruled against the EPA's precautionary MCLG.)

Such efforts to institute precautionary standards have consistently been met with strong resistance—due in no small measure to the apparent inflexibility and impracticality of these standards. Prior to the relaxation of the foregoing food additives provision (per the 1996 Food Quality Protection Act), the Delaney Clause, arguably to its detriment, even prohibited what some might judge to be trivial or *de minimis* risks—risks, in other words, of such marginal nature, of such low probability of injuring those who are exposed or entailing such negligible harm, that their regulation seems dubious. This was reinforced, for example, in *Public Citizen v. Young* (1987), in which the U.S. Court of Appeals insisted that Congress did not recognize and thus did not allow for exceptions to *de minimis* risks and, accordingly, rejected the legitimacy of the FDA's relaxed, nonzero standard for pesticide residues in processed foods and cosmetics.[120] However, the court nevertheless declared that irrespective of Congress' intentions, the "failure to employ a *de minimis* doctrine may lead to regulation that not only is 'absurd or futile' in some general cost-benefit sense but also is directly contrary to the primary legislative goal."[121]

The unsympathetic attitude toward precautionary policies in *Public Citizen v. Young* followed such noteworthy cases as *Industrial Union Dept., AFL-CIO v. American Petroleum Institute* (1980) and *Corrosion Proof Fittings v. EPA* (1991), both of which also served to cement formal risk assessment and cost–benefit balancing in the United States' current approach toward environmental risk regulation, whereby the former redefined "safe" not as zero risk, but as "acceptable" risk and required efforts be made to quantify actual threats of harm (given the "best available evidence") and to weigh economic considerations in setting enforcement standards. Conversely, the latter, which regards the banning of products containing a substance known to cause harm to human health (in this case asbestos), reinforced the growing expectation that regulatory standards must be economically and technologically feasible by requiring that regulatory agencies adopt the "least burdensome" alternative in their efforts to safeguard public health. Similarly, the 1996 Food Quality Protection Act and its revision of the Delaney Clause discarded the strict and burdensome zero-risk, health-based standard and issued instead a relaxed requisite (for pesticide residue tolerance levels) of "reasonable certainty of no harm."

Finally, in concert with the objections in items 4, 5, and 7, whether the precautionary approach makes it too costly for industry to operate in compliance with precautionary standards or whether the approach ignores the negative upshots of regulation (or the positive consequences of *non*regulation) that would justify the preventative banning of relevant technologies,[122] critics also commonly alleged that

(8) the precautionary principle stifles technological innovation.[123]

Graham posits, for example, that a commitment to precaution would have prevented the discovery and development of beneficial technologies, such as "electricity, the internal combustion engine, plastics, pharmaceuticals, the computer, the Internet, the cellular phone, and so forth."[124] This is because the development and implementation of most new technologies require a period of implementation to reveal the actual effects they may have on the environment and the public, which may allow for improvements to be made to the technology or to regulations governing its use in order to mitigate the potential for harm. Yet this stage of experimentation, this process of trial and error, invariably creates some potential for unanticipated harm to the public—which is precisely what the precautionary principle aims to prevent. Thus, some suggest that the precautionary principle commits us to an implausible approach to risk management that either requires that regulations governing new technologies be implemented without error (where the public is never exposed to possibilities of irreparable harm) or that the research and development of new technologies be prevented from proceeding so as to safeguard the public from potential irreparable harm.[125] Whereas the former is wildly implausible, critics maintain that the latter is a peculiar claim, because innovation has been one of the principal drivers of mitigating risks to public health.[126]

2.3 Efforts to Answer Common Objections

Some scholars have attempted rejoinders to some of these charges by defending various reformulations of the precautionary principle. Sandin, for example, suggests that the principle should be understood more generally as a maxim that is rooted in our commonsense notions of precaution and what it means to engage in precautionary actions: namely, as striving to prevent something undesirable from transpiring. In this vein, Sandin claims that

> An action *a* is precautionary with respect to something undesirable *U*, if and only if:
>
> 1. *a* is performed with the intention of preventing *U*,
> 2. the agent does not believe it to be very likely that *U* will occur if *a* is not performed, and
> 3. the agent has externally good [objective] epistemic reasons for (a) believing that *U* might occur, (b) believing that *a* will in fact at least contribute to the prevention of *U*, and (c) not believing it to be certain or very likely that *U* will occur if *a* is not performed.[127]

This construal, however, similarly turns on whether we have adequate evidence—or are justified in believing—that some (undesirable) threat exists and whether we have adequate reason to believe that our taking precaution to prevent some undesirable state of affairs will be efficacious. Consequently, Sandin's account remains vulnerable at least to objections 3 and 6 earlier. Sandin does little more than to rephrase, albeit it quite vaguely, the action-guiding interpretation of the principle: where precautionary measures are responses to upshots that would be harmful in some way, and which we are concerned about coming to pass (his criterion 1), and about which we have some credible reason to be concerned about it coming to pass (his criteria 2 and 3)—such that if we want to try to prevent some such harmful outcome from actually occurring, we should act in a precautionary way.[128] Yet the absence of "externally good epistemic reasons"[129] is precisely the crux of the dilemma with regulating uncertain threats of environmental harm (because genuine uncertainty implies that such reasons are not readily available), which Sandin simply tables. Moreover, what that precaution would require—that is, what specific precautionary actions might prevent an undesirable consequence—remains unclear. In this way, Sandin's proposed maxim does not reframe the debate, as he suggests, but merely constitutes a way of retroactively cataloging whether an action was precautionary or not. And this certainly misses the commonsensical objective he attributes to the precautionary principle.

Of the numerous recent works that develop alternative normative justifications for precaution,[130] this section explores two landmark attempts to dismiss these objections and revive the stalled debate over the merits of precaution by developing—as this book project also strives to do—novel justificatory foundations for the precautionary principle, which are independent of what we can or cannot know about environmental health threats. The first is Gardiner's argument that we can ground precaution in a Rawlsian maximin principle, whose aim is to preventatively minimize the potential for harm. (Briefly discussed here is a related argument by Morgan-Knapp that a commitment to precaution requires redistributing some of the expected benefits of risk impositions so that no one who stands to be harmed would be made worse off.) The second is Whiteside's argument that we should understand precaution as a commitment to participatory and deliberative decision-making, which strives to improve our understanding of environmental risk and to achieve inclusive, practical responses to the environmental health threats we face. However, as the following discussion strives to demonstrate, the attempts by both Gardiner and Whiteside to vindicate a precautionary approach to risk regulation are problematic.

2.3.1 Precaution as Minimizing Harm

Like Sandin, Gardiner also endeavors to develop an intuitive account of the precautionary approach. In striving to identify the fundamental criteria that may justify precautionary risk regulation, Gardiner advances a unique interpretation of precaution that is couched in the normative conditions of Rawls's maximin principle. The reader may recall that this principle, detailed in Rawls's seminal contribution, *A Theory of Justice*, suggests that rational individuals—who suspend knowledge of various facts about themselves and their place in society so as to render unbiased decisions as to which foundational principles of justice should prevail,[131] would and should strive to maximize the position of the least well-off. Borrowed from this context, Gardiner envisages the maximin principle as analogously counseling us to strive toward the "least bad worst outcome."[132] In practice, this would mean that after considering different alternative responses to a given uncertain environmental threat, and after identifying the worst possible outcome for each possible alternative response, one should act in accordance with whatever policy alternative promises to yield the best of the bad consequences. One should choose the alternative, that is, which is most likely to cause the least amount of harm.

Employing this general principle, Gardiner propounds one possible account of the sufficient conditions for taking precaution, maintaining that (1) when a "genuine possibility" of severe harm exists, (2) when "decision-makers care relatively little for potential gains" associated with accepting (or having the public bear) the threat of harm, and (3) when "reliable" information is lacking about the likelihood or probability that the severe harm will occur or "about the size, distribution and timing of the costs," then we should, *ceteris paribus*, exercise precaution and try to prevent the potential harm.[133] More strongly, Gardiner claims that when these three conditions exist, failing to exercise precaution would be "foolhardy."[134]

The virtue of his formulation, claims Gardiner, is that it is capable of sidestepping some of the common objections to the precautionary principle. Namely, that the principle is vacuous and cannot "function as an independent decision-making principle" and "provide any practical guidance"[135] (objection 6 earlier). Moreover, Gardiner's account also seems to avoid objections 1, 3, and 4 earlier: that the action-guiding principle is implausibly "narrow" (exclusionary or myopic) and "decisive," requiring policy-makers to consider nothing more than the environmental threat in question, and thus to regulate activities that create potential harms even when other nonenvironmental or non–health-related considerations would have us refrain from restricting these activities.[136] However, it is unclear that Gardiner's "criterial approach"[137] toward understanding the precautionary principle actually accomplishes this.

Some have rejected procedural or criterial conceptions on the grounds that the precautionary principle "soon dissolves beyond recognition,"[138] because these interpretations admit a host of discrete, context-dependent precautionary rules. As Sunstein notes sarcastically, "[f]or every regulatory tool, there is a corresponding precautionary principle"—suggesting that there may well be a "Funding More Research Precautionary Principle," or an "Economic Incentives Precautionary Principle," or an "Information Disclosure Precautionary Principle," etc.[139] Hence, it is alleged that *the* precautionary principle is—or more precisely, its innumerable regulatory context–dependent versions are—largely devoid of any substance; that the principle really is no principle at all. We might anticipate Gardiner's rejection of this concern as a straw-man objection that misses the point: although Gardiner *does* admit that there may well be different salient criteria that establish the circumstances in which the precautionary principle applies, and thus that there may well be different versions of a "core" precautionary principle,[140] the aim of any such approach is to establish the conditions under which precaution should be exercised, irrespective of the particular details of the sundry contexts in which it may apply.

What is cause for greater concern with his criterial account, however, is that Gardiner, like many others, ignores the different forms of uncertainty that can undermine our knowledge of the actual dangers to public health—claiming instead that his reformulated precautionary principle applies only in instances when "probability information is [un]known."[141] Yet as Section 2.1 suggested, it is common for causal and scientific uncertainty to create outcome uncertainty: that is, for the different timing, intensities, and pathways of exposure, the different possible intervening causal factors, cumulative and deferred effects, inconsistent physiological dispositions, limited testing capabilities, disciplinary-specific testing standards, divergent subsequent interpretations of the findings of toxicological studies, and so forth, to obscure our understanding of the potential adverse health effects of exposure to many effluents. As such, by assuming that it is both possible to discern the different possible worst-case consequences of the various alternatives available to decision makers and to compare these consequences to identify the "least bad worst outcome,"[142] Gardiner's formulation will neglect to account for many environmental health threats, including all uncertain threats. Indeed, any substantive conclusions that may be drawn about potentially harmful outcomes, and any subsequent comparison between these outcomes, would require information about "the size, distribution and timing of the costs" of the outcome,[143] or the primary pathway(s) of exposure (inhalation, ingestion, absorption), or the physiological susceptibility of those exposed to the potentially harmful emissions to being injured by the exposure—details of the complex cause-and-effect relationships that uncertainty rules out and that Gardiner himself expressly denies is available to decision makers whenever the precautionary principle applies. Put plainly, Gardiner's position seems untenable, because criteria (a) and (c) are contradictory: one cannot *both* know she faces a "genuine possibility" of severe harm but simultaneously lack any reliable information about the threat of harm, such as the probability that it will come to pass.

The salience of this worry is amplified by Gardiner's qualification that only "reasonable" outcomes or credible threats (that is, probable threats of non-trivial harm) should be considered when deciding whether the precautionary principle should apply. Responding to critics who claim that any potential harm, even those that are wildly unlikely, can be used to justify precautionary policies,[144] Gardiner insists that we need

> some way of distinguishing a set of reasonable outcomes to contrast with those outcomes which are merely imaginable. This suggests that the three Rawlsian criteria mentioned so far must be supplemented with a further requirement: that the range of outcomes considered are in some appropriate sense "realistic," so that, for example, only credible threats are considered.[145]

However, this, too, seems contradictory. If we lack the knowledge necessary to ascertain the probability of some potentially harmful outcome, then it is unclear how we could feasibly discriminate between credible and unrealistic threats—a consideration that Gardiner does not acknowledge or expand on.

What is curious about Gardiner's account is that although it appeals to a central component of Rawls's moral theory about how a just society might be organized, Gardiner largely tables any discussion of the fundamentally normative nature of the precautionary principle. And yet it is by divorcing the principle from its usual narrow focus on epistemic standards and the warrant for regulating environmental threats in the absence of a preponderance of evidence confirming actual risks to public health, and by underscoring instead the principle's deontological motivation and the moral obligations we have to avoid putting others in the way of possible harm, that a defense for precautionary risk regulation can be made.

As an aside, in similar nonconsequentialist fashion, Morgan-Knapp argues that our choices not to regulate environmental risk are justified—our risky actions are permissible—just in case they would not make anyone worse off. Worse off, that is, than if precautionary regulations had been implemented.[146] More precisely, what forms the central tenet of this contractualist account of precaution is the requirement that we justify our actions to those who may be adversely affected, such that "If someone we affect does not have sufficient reason to consent, if we cannot give her a justification for our action that is acceptable from her point of view," then the risky action would be impermissible.[147] However, prevailing uncertainty means that we can only retroactively ascertain the effects of risky actions: in other words, it is only after the permitted risky action has been performed (and presumably performed for some time, because environmental harms are commonly deferred) that we can determine whether some have been adversely affected. Accordingly, because we can only predict or forecast the outcomes of our actions, our justification to others to perform our risky actions will be constrained by our limited knowledge, as will the reasons our fellows have to consent to our risky action or to withhold their consent.[148] Therefore, the contractualist defense of precaution that Morgan-Knapp espouses should have us ground the permissibility of risky actions or, conversely, the justifiability of precautionary measures that restrict or prohibit risk actions on *ex ante* consent. That is, consent that individuals give (or withhold) based on what knowledge of the potential for harm they have access to *before* the action is performed, given their subjective risk perceptions and tolerances.[149]

Concerned that this alternative may still be unfeasible—resulting in extensive prohibitions of actions that are risky but which we can foresee will have substantive social benefits—as individuals who perceive that they will be adversely affected by such risk impositions may still veto the permissibility of the risky activities, Morgan-Knapp suggests another avenue by which we can "protect these people from being wronged."[150] Instead of having regulators implement restrictive safety measures, we can hold actors responsible for safeguarding against unfair distributions of the benefits and burdens of their risky actions.[151] We can require, in other words, that "risk-imposers" safeguard against any and all negative "expected value[s]," which is to say that we can require that our regulatory decisions ensure that all those who we can foresee may be harmed by risk impositions receive benefits from risk imposers to offset foreseeable losses.[152] More specifically, Morgan-Knapp purports that "the expected winners must provide some benefit to the expected losers that outweighs the risks they will be subject to," which will be context dependent and may include monetary benefits, like direct payments or lower tax liability, or nonmonetary gains, like greater access to medical care.[153] In any event, the aim here is to make sure that no risk imposition makes anyone worse off than she otherwise would be.

The initial concern with Morgan-Knapp's analysis is that although he acknowledges the constraints of uncertainty, which necessitate his proposed standard of *ex ante* consent, his account still turns on what we can or cannot know about a given risk imposition and the potential for harm, and moreover his account still assumes we have access to greater knowledge than we actually do under uncertainty. Morgan-Knapp explains that establishing acceptable distributions of the burdens of benefits of a given risk imposition first requires identifying those who stand to lose the most and those who stand to gain the most and then conducting a "targeted cost-benefit analysis" on the subset of individuals who would likely bear the costs of the risky action so we may calculate what appropriate change to the distribution would be necessary to prevent them from experiencing any loss.[154] This seems to suggest that so long as we can discern the likely outcomes of the risk imposition, we can begin the process of amending the distributive scheme.

Yet this is a gross oversimplification of most environmental harms, even regarding those we have substantive knowledge about. Even if we grant that for any given risk imposition we can effectively narrow the likely consequences (which itself is a contentious assumption), outcome uncertainty is *but one* aspect of the complex causal story that defines many environmental harms. Mitigating outcome uncertainty, that is being able to estimate what the consequences may be, gives us no guidance about how the outcomes will come about, when they will occur, who will likely be harmed, or the degree of the harm. Morgan-Knapp seems to assume that from our knowledge of the likely consequences of a risk imposition we can reliably make these further inferences, not the least of which include discerning the different pathways of exposure (inhalation, ingestion, or absorption), durations of exposure, and timings of exposure (e.g., prenatal, infancy, adolescence, or in conjunction with an intervening causal factor), the plausible intervening causal factors, and the diversity of physiological predispositions to being harmed upon exposure (which often varies across individuals)[155]—all of which are prerequisites to identifying the subset of individuals who stand to lose if we permit the risk imposition (as exposure across a given population is rarely uniform[156]).

This assumption on its own is highly problematic, given the nature of environmental harms and the limitations of toxicological sciences, but Morgan-Knapp also assumes that those individuals who are identified as likely to absorb the costs of the risky action can discern "sufficient" reasons to offer or to withhold their consent to the risk imposition[157]—which also presupposes that average individuals have access to knowledge beyond the likely outcomes that inform their subjective risk perceptions and shape their tolerance or intolerance of a particular risk. For absent one's capacity to render an informed judgment about the acceptability of a given risk imposition, it is unclear what would constitute "sufficient reason" for one to consent to potential harm or what a justification for the risk imposition would be "acceptable from her point of view."[158] (In fact, prevailing uncertainty of our forecasts or predictions of the possibility for injury—that is, our incomplete knowledge of the potential for harm—is consistently treated by proponents of precaution as a compelling reason *not* to allow the risky activity. This would then suggest that all risk impositions are impermissible, which is an implausible conclusion that Morgan-Knapp expressly rejects.) Moreover, absent the capacity of individuals to judge the acceptability of the risk impositions they face, his contractualist account seems to collapse, because we then cannot generalize about what risks individuals can reasonably be expected to consent to. That is, unless we, as "risk imposers," project our own risk perceptions and tolerances on those populations that are likely to bear the costs of our risk impositions (which is precisely what Morgan-Knapp occasionally seems to do, as with his example of whether individuals would grant their *ex ante* consent "to the risks involved with allowing everyone in a household to go to sleep at the same," to which Morgan-Knapp concludes that "it would be unreasonable for any of us to object to people having this freedom"[159]).

Finally, given the complexities of environmental harms reiterated earlier, it is unclear that individuals could offer *ex ante* consent in the first place. Chapter 3.3 will explore this consideration in further detail, but the immediate problem with grounding the permissibility of risk impositions in consent is that it is unclear that under conditions of uncertainty one's consent can be informed. For a prerequisite of offering meaningful consent (whether expressly or tacitly) is that one must understand what she is consenting to. That is, one must comprehend the meaning and implications of the agreement. Yet given one's difficulty of judging whether a foreseeable consequence of a risky action is likely to materialize in some actual injury, it is doubtful that one can offer her consent in any meaningful way. And hypothetical consent, as Chapter 3.3, also discusses, cannot provide a solution to this problem, because hypothetical consent would entail assuming that our own risk perceptions and tolerances define those of others, which would beg the very question of their permissibility.

2.3.2 Precaution as Deliberative Policy Making

Concerned about barriers to "sustained, concerted action" that undermine our ability to respond promptly to environmental problems and to effectively "forestall [the] severe damage" that they create,[160] in concert with the European Environment Agency, Harding and Fisher, and others,[161] Whiteside argues that the precautionary principle should be understood in its "deliberative form."[162] It should be understood, that is, as a commitment to more inclusive, "participatory," "democratic" regulatory decision-making processes,[163] which are grounded in the conviction that new environmental risks are not only poorly understood, but they also "have the unprecedented potential to destroy life."[164] (Whiteside refers to "new" risks or "new technologies" as a catch-all for all novel sources of potential environmental health hazards.) Precaution, then, requires that we—regulators, policy-makers, industry, and citizens alike—scrutinize and publicly deliberate about our understanding of nature and the impact human activity can have on the natural environment, as well as "the values that are implicit in the scientific framing of environmental issues" that inform our conception of what is in the public's interest.[165] Briefly, this means that to exercise precaution is to acknowledge "our *inability* to master the world," which is a consequence of our inherent epistemic limitations: a consequence, in other words, of our "incomplete" knowledge about how human behavior adversely affects the natural environment. Further, exercising precaution entails striving toward "better science and more self-conscious [and deliberative] political judgments" about what preventative risk regulations, in any given circumstance, should consist of.[166] In this way, in response to the charge that precautionary prescriptions are vacuous (objection 6 earlier), Whiteside argues that the principle *can* recommend policies with definitive content. A precautionary approach may entail, for example, testing new technologies (e.g., genetically modified foods) in smaller, controlled settings before exposing the public to their potentially adverse effects, or eliminating policies (and the underlying politics) that constrain the capacity of regulatory agencies to effectively monitor and independently enforce risk regulations, or revising the current approach toward risk assessment to include the general public (the nonscientific community) in identifying which risks should be regulated and how.[167]

Moreover, by emphasizing that "participatory precaution" is intended to augment, not substitute, science-based (technocratic) risk management—namely, that a more inclusive, deliberative decision process, which is marked by "regularized forms of non-expert citizen participation and collective judgment," cannot abandon the counsel of scientific experts and policy-makers and leave regulatory decisions to the whims of a general public and its "untutored, unquantified intuitions"[168]—Whiteside acknowledges that the legitimacy of the precautionary principle depends on its practicality. In this vein, Whiteside rejects previous defenses of "precautionary deliberation"[169] for their principled, albeit implausible, claims and implications: that is, more specifically, for their severe skepticism of "technical expertise," their denial of the capacity of the scientific community and policy-makers "to know the common good better than anyone else," and their unfounded insistence that decision-making authority rests with citizens *especially* when much is unknown and administrators, who are accountable to the public and charged with championing the public's interests, lack "a firm factual foundation" on which to base any environmental risk regulation.[170] Not only does Whiteside argue that (his deliberative formulation of) the precautionary principle must temper the influence of lay perceptions of risk, which are commonly shaped by factors unrelated to public health and safety (for example, job security or distributions of risk and harm), but in maintaining that the principle must be efficacious, he also insists that any precautionary measure must take economic costs seriously.[171] Recognizing that the nontrivial costs of greater risk regulation must be borne somewhere and that ordinary citizens' judgments about how we should respond to threats of environmental harm are commonly informed by vague notions of cost-effectiveness, Whiteside makes plain that "precautionary policymaking [should not] be determined simply by counting noses."[172]

Worries of critics that the implementation of the precautionary principle countenances the regulation of speculative or unverified risks (objection 1) and that precautionary regulations are inherently subjective (objection 2) may be allayed by Whiteside's effort to reconcile—as opposed to replace—conventional approaches toward risk assessment and management with greater transparency and accountability via broader public participation in regulatory decisions. Similarly, in expressly grounding the legitimacy of the precautionary approach in its efficacy, Whiteside would not only deny that exercising precaution entails unqualified bans of potentially harmful behavior and thus paralyzes policy making (objection 3), but he would also deny that taking precaution would be justified if it were to create even greater public health risks (objection 4). His candid discussion on the costs of precautionary measures also underscores that economic feasibility is a requisite of any legitimate precautionary regulation, which undercuts the charges that the precautionary principle ignores the costs and inflates the benefits of regulation (objection 5). And it stands to reason that Whiteside's feasibility requirement would not only mitigate the burdens on industry that many proponents of precaution are prepared to accept (objection 7), but it would also *avoid* discouraging technological innovation (objection 8). In these ways, Whiteside anticipates and has answers to the common objections leveled against the precautionary principle.

The initial worry, however, with Whiteside's defense of the precautionary approach is that it focuses specifically on responding to *new* threats, which he says warrant preventative regulations because "ordinary assumptions about risk management do not hold," since the novelty of these risks amplifies our inability to foresee their potentially deleterious effects.[173] Whiteside notes, for example, that "sometimes a technology is so novel that there simply has not been the time to test its effects in the wide range of circumstances in which it will be used" and that the absence of reliable "long-term" scientific data about these effects clouds our understanding of the actual threat to public health.[174] Although this is a reasonable concern with novel sources of potential environmental health hazards, this narrow focus is problematic because it is not obvious why the justification for exercising precaution is limited to *new* risks and because it understates the potential for harm that *existing* threats may pose to public health and safety in ways that we do not adequately understand.

An illustrative example of this is the potential, pervasive, and *still* uncorroborated harm posed by the battery of more than 60,000 manufactured chemicals that were grandfathered under the Toxic Substances Control Act (TSCA) four decades ago—chemicals that were exempt from any prerequisite scientific testing to determine their relative safety to public health before their (continued) manufacture was permitted.[175] Beyond the concerns that only roughly 2 percent of these chemicals have undergone any toxicity testing, that they are assumed to be safe, and that they continue to be routinely and lawfully released into the environment,[176] roughly 3,000 of these substances are what the EPA terms "high production volume" chemicals.[177] Chemicals, in other words, whose annual rate of domestic production and/or importation exceed

1 million pounds.[178] Such rates of production and consumption make the emission of these substances into the environment more likely, and in turn make the public's exposure to the substances more likely. The fact that existing laws like TSCA aim specifically at regulating new threats of harm,[179] and the fact that there are policy gaps in the regulation of existing environmental threats, should amplify our concerns about previous or pre-existing as opposed to new threats of environmental harm to public health.

A further concern with Whiteside's analysis is that like many other proponents of precautionary risk regulation, he ostensibly treats uncertainty as probability uncertainty: where the outcomes of some threat of environmental harm are generally known or can be estimated, and what remains unclear is the likelihood that the harm will come to pass. Whiteside writes, for instance, that precaution entails engaging myriad relevant questions about risk management—from the efficacy of existing legal safeguards to public health, to the adequacy of industry's efforts to mitigate the risks to public health, to the capacity regulators have to identify the primary cause(s) of the environmental risk, to the public's ability to make informed decisions about what risks are reasonable—"with a care and thoroughness that is proportional to the seriousness of the potential dangers."[180] Elsewhere he writes that although the precautionary principle does *not* entail blanket prohibitions of risky behavior, it does require that our responses to potential environmental harms "be proportioned to the degree of uncertainty and gravity associated with the risk;" moreover, that it is in response to "serious and/or irreversible," "long-term, and uncertain threats" (where the "risks are poorly understood") that a precautionary approach is most clearly justified.[181] Consider also that for Whiteside, what should drive our commitment to precautionary risk regulation are (new) environmental risks "that are large scale and develop slowly, often with irreversible consequences."[182]

While it is true that not all threats of environmental harm are the same and that different kinds of uncertainty can obscure what risk regulations would effectively safeguard public health and safety, the foregoing passages illustrate that Whiteside assumes we have access to greater knowledge about threats of environmental harm than we commonly do. With many environmental threats—including Whiteside's chief focus on genetically modified foods, whose alleged health effects are hotly debated—the potential dangers cannot be ascertained in the manner he seems to suggest. In many cases, we know neither the likely harmful consequences of exposure (and thus whether these consequences will prove irreversible), nor the probability that exposure will entail these injuries, nor the scale of potential harm.

This assumption in Whiteside's analysis is rather curious, because he himself criticizes opponents of the precautionary principle who admit that there may be occasions when preventative measures are justified, yet who concurrently insist on various prerequisites to the exercise of precaution that presuppose knowledge about the effects of uncorroborated environmental threats. Whiteside chides Sunstein, for example, for suggesting that the precautionary principle "makes sense" when risks of harm are significant and when they can be mitigated[183]—because this position "effectively denies the existence of precautionary situations" by conceiving of all environmental risks as "calculable enough to be subject to cost-benefit analysis."[184] Similarly, Whiteside dismisses Goklany's proposed "precautionary framework," which requires regulators to demonstrate that any preventative effort to mitigate an environmental threat does not itself create graver threats or exacerbate other existing threats. Goklany suggests that by identifying the different environmental threats that a precautionary policy both intends to eliminate and also may create, and by assessing "the nature, magnitude, immediacy, uncertainty and persistence of each threat, and the extent to which it can be alleviated," the different environmental threats can be prioritized to determine whether exercising precaution is warranted.[185] (And, yet, when we are privy to this knowledge, as suggested in Section 2.1, the science of quantitative risk assessment may effectively inform our risk regulations. For instance, as some have argued, mitigating the release of, exposure to, and harm from asbestos and lead are among the noteworthy success stories of risk–benefit analysis.[186])

In any event, while Whiteside thoughtfully explores a unique justification for precaution—a commitment to more inclusive, transparent, and deliberative decision processes that empower average citizens to better protect themselves against potential environmental harms and which legitimize regulatory decisions by virtue of broad public participation—his analysis seems to perpetuate the stalled debate noted at this chapter's outset. For a central feature of his proposal is to have public debate and collective judgment determine what counts as credible threats of environmental harm: yet although Whiteside attempts to shift the debate from managing (probability) uncertainty to constructing decision procedures that yield justifiable risk regulations under conditions of (probability) uncertainty, the legitimacy of deliberative democratic precautionary measures still turns on whether participants believe that our lack of knowledge of the actual health risks justifies preventative regulation *or conversely* the absence of regulation. This is to say that critics of precaution may still deny the basis for exercising precaution on Whiteside's account even if they subscribe to his proposed participatory and deliberative decision procedures. At least, that is, when deliberative decisions to regulate potential environmental harms are reached in the absence of "a firm factual foundation" about the actual risks to public health.[187]

As already suggested, avoiding the impasse that marks current debates over the plausibility of the precautionary approach toward risk regulation requires a justification of precaution that is divorced from (independent of) the implications of our epistemic limitations on regulatory decisions.

2.4 Alternative Rights-Based Formulation

In contrast, then, to understanding the precautionary principle as "a reasoned effort to take account of the complexity of the processes through which environmental problems become known . . . and subject to regulation,"[188] or as a policy approach that "fashion[s] policy out of skepticism,"[189] this book denies that the precautionary principle is about managing (the diverse forms of) uncertainty, or that it is a policy approach grounded in scientific knowledge about environmental risk. Rather, this book recasts the precautionary principle as a normative principle and policy tool that safeguards against exposure to undeserved and preventable threats of harm. This book argues, in other words, that precautionary policies can be justified by appealing to our normative commitments: obligations we owe each other as moral equals, which are not shaped by and contingent on what we can or cannot know about threats of harm we author—notions of equality and reciprocity that translate into a duty to respect the right of others to not be put in potential harm's way without their consent or without first exercising due care (precaution).

Ironically, references to rights, albeit in passing, are made by both advocates and skeptics of the precautionary principle. Whiteside, for example, notes that among the "threshold[s] of significance" regarding the development of the principle was France's inclusion of precautionary language in its constitution in 2005, "alongside the 1789 Declaration of the Rights of Man and of the Citizen."[190] In arguing against the merit of contemporary applications of the precautionary principle, Goklany suggests that precautionary policy prescriptions may violate the rights of those they affect: the antithesis of what this book argues. In claiming, for example, that precautionary bans of genetically modified crops or preventative efforts to curb the concentration of greenhouse gases (GHGs) overlook the negative consequence of leaving more people without adequate nutrition,[191] Goklany implies[192] and elsewhere states explicitly (though in passing[193]) that these precautionary policies violate various human rights provisions. More specifically, he claims that they violate Article 25 of the Universal Declaration of Human Rights (UDHR), which states that "everyone has the right to a standard of living adequate for the health and well-being of himself and of his family, including food";[194] as well as Article 10 of the UDHR, which states "no one shall participate, by act or failure to act where required, in violating human rights and fundamental freedoms";[195] and the Universal Declaration on the Eradication of Hunger and Malnutrition, which states that "every man, woman, and child has the inalienable right to be free from hunger and malnutrition."[196]

Despite these occasional references, however, the plausibility of a rights-based formulation of the precautionary principle has not yet been explored in the contemporary debate over the merit of precautionary risk regulations. Although Chapter 3 develops in detail the defense of our moral obligation to exercise due care to safeguard against unconsented-to uncertain threats of environmental harm, the general idea is that if we take seriously the moral equality between persons (which undergirds their equal battery of rights), then it is necessary to consider what this equality demands of those standing in moral relation to each other. Briefly, in a broadly Kantian fashion, the reciprocity between moral equals obliges us to treat others with mutual respect, to regard them as ends in themselves, whereby to perform an action that begets an uncertain threat of harm is to fail to grant others due regard as autonomous agents—so long as their consent is not earned or reasonable measures are not taken to prevent their possible injury. Such actions can be said to gamble with their welfare and to undercut their capacity for self-authorship by ignoring the importance of consent and discounting the interests and ambitions of others, which may not include being placed in the way of possible harm.

Suppose, for instance, that after a couple unsuccessful seasons of organic gardening, Maria decides to mix a new synthetic fertilizer with the soil in her garden and to apply a synthetic pesticide to her vegetable plants and that she actually enjoys a substantial yield this year. And let us stipulate that the health effects of both the fertilizer and the pesticide are unknown. Also, suppose that Maria's housemates, Silvia and Gabi, have agreed to allow Maria pay less in rent so long as Silvia and Gabi would be free to eat vegetables from Maria's garden (in turn, reducing their monthly expenditures on food). Given that residues of both the fertilizer and the pesticide will remain on these vegetables and that the health effects of exposure to these substances remain uncorroborated, Maria's actions put not only herself but also Silvia and Gabi in potential harm's way.

Assuming that Silvia and Gabi are unaware of Maria's use of the synthetic fertilizer and pesticide (and thus that they have not granted their consent to being exposed to these substances) and that Silvia and Gabi are, accordingly, unaware of the uncorroborated threat they face, if Maria does not take certain reasonable preventative measures to mitigate the potential for harm to her housemates, she wrongfully gambles with their welfare. To respect their equal moral standing, in this context Maria may be obliged to investigate the actual risk of harm that the fertilizer or the pesticide entails: to contact the producer, the regional EPA office, or the Health Department, to inquire about what toxicity data are available on these substances. If her investigations reveal that exposure entails a probable risk of nontrivial harm to human health, Maria may be obliged to stop using the substances, discard the plants in her garden, and find an alternative, safer way to grow her vegetables. At the very least, Maria would be obliged to inform Silvia and Gabi of the confirmed risk of harm to allow them to make a more informed and consensual decision about consuming vegetables from the garden. Yet even if Maria's investigations fail to confirm that an actual risk exists—that is, if she confirms that we know neither the outcome of exposure nor the probability that exposure will beget harm—she would still be obliged to inform her housemates of the uncertain potential for harm. And if a feasible alternative fertilizer and pesticide are available for Maria to use whose effects *are* corroborated and which are subsequently judged to pose no adverse health risks to humans, then she would be obliged to switch to those alternatives.

Recognizing the equal moral standing of others and treating others as ends in themselves demand that we take strides to mitigate the possibility that our actions will cause them harm: that we acknowledge the right of our fellow moral equals not to be placed in the way of possible harm (especially when they are unaware of the potential dangers) and that we refrain from projecting our own risk perceptions on others and effectively deciding for them which threats of environmental harm are acceptable or reasonable. And as Chapter 3 explains, because it is implausible to expect actors to garner the (express, tacit, or hypothetical) consent of those who may be exposed to the uncertain threats we create, respecting the standing of others under uncertainty will require the exercise of due care (precaution).

This is to say that to perform a gamble, an "endangering action"—again, understood here as an action that entails an uncertain threat of harm to others—without first satisfying some reasonable standard of due care to mitigate the potential for injury is to commit a wrongdoing: that in the absence of due care, creating an uncertain possibility of harm is morally impermissible, rendering the actor liable to blame and punishment *even if* the action ultimately proves to be harmless (that is, if and when uncertainty is eliminated and we discover that there is no actual danger to public health). This does not mean, however, that the burdens of exercising due care are shouldered exclusively by authors of uncertain threats.

As both Chapters 4.4 and 5.4 explore in detail, because uncertain threats may prove to be harmless and because it is the public that benefits from a precautionary standard of due care, it would be unreasonable to expect emitters to bear all the costs of working to mitigate the potential for harm. However, equally unreasonable is the suggestion by critics of precaution that the public should bear all the costs of potential (and eventual) harm and of scientifically corroborating actual risks to public health before restrictions may be imposed on industry. A feasible principle of due care under outcome and probability uncertainty, which requires authors of uncertain threats to take reasonable preventative measures to try to avoid exposing others to possible harm, must be able to reconcile—as a matter of moral equality and reciprocity—the right of those who wish to exercise their autonomy and engage in endangering actions, with the freedom of those who may be exposed to the consequences of these actions to *not* have others place them in potential harm's way. Yet because what due care under uncertainty requires of us (how this duty can be discharged) varies from context to context, as Chapters 4 and 5 demonstrate, adjudication between the competing interests and rights of authors of uncertain threats and those of the public will also be context dependent. That said, when uncertainty prevails, our overarching aim should be to avoid treating endangering actions as decisively safe or unsafe—to avoid granting industry unqualified license to release effluents that may well prove to cause harm but to avoid imposing strict restrictions or blankets bans on the release of these effluents. Expressed differently, our overarching aim is to navigate between these extremes to achieve mutually acceptable compromises.

This is the central thread of the book, which will reappear in one form or another in each of the subsequent chapters. This chapter began with an explanation about how conventional arguments for and against precautionary environmental risk regulation have run roughshod over the multifaceted concept of uncertainty—that both proponents and opponents of precaution assume that we generally understand the causal complexities of environmental harms and that what remains unknown is simply the probability that exposure will result in known harmful outcomes (what was defined as "probability uncertainty"). After complicating this view by arguing that it is common for outcome, causal, and scientific uncertainty to also undermine our understanding of the actual dangers to public health, this chapter explained how one of the problems with the debate over the merits of precaution is that both advocates and critics appeal to our epistemic limitations to justify their antithetical conclusions. It was suggested that this impasse permits but one plausible alternative: that we seek an independent foundation for the precautionary principle that is divorced from what it is we can or cannot know about the potential dangers our actions impose on others. After detailing several enduring objections to existing arguments for precaution, this chapter explored two notable defenses of the precautionary principle that develop justifications for the exercise of precaution independent from our epistemic limitations and that seem to have answers for these objections. Yet it was shown that these arguments remain vulnerable to criticism in large measure because they, too, wrongly conceive of uncertainty as merely probability uncertainty. A brief sketch of the rights-based conception of the precautionary principle followed, which is capable of withstanding the series of objections discussed earlier against the plausibility of precautionary risk regulation.

However, before it is possible to demonstrate how this rights-based conception can avoid these charges, it is necessary both to defend the central normative claim that emitters do wrong by neglecting their duties of due care under conditions of uncertainty (which is the subject of Chapters 3 and 4) and to explain what a reasonable standard of due care consists of (which is explored in Chapter 5). Traditional accounts of moral culpability and theories of risk, as well as conventional arguments from moral luck, each deny (either explicitly or by implication) that individuals can be held culpable for the potential harms they create when uncertainty prevails and the effects of their actions cannot be foreseen. And if one cannot be culpable for exposing others to uncertain threats, then any requirement of due care, any implementation of preventative measures, is without foundation. As such, the defense of the proposed rights-based precautionary approach foremost requires demonstrating how various existing normative accounts of risk are incomplete and understate or dismiss (either explicitly or by implication) the moral problem that uncertain threats of environmental harm create. Accordingly, it is not until the final section of Chapter 5 that the discussion returns to the eight common objections noted earlier to bring this defense of precaution full circle by demonstrating how the proposed rights-based account is not only normatively justified, but it can avoid these charges against the feasibility of precautionary risk regulations.

Notes

1. An abridged version of this chapter appears in Levente Szentkirályi, "A Rights-Based Conception of the Precautionary Principle," in *Handbook of Philosophy and Public Policy*, David Boonin, ed. (New York: Palgrave Macmillan, 2018): 749–65.
2. Joel Tickner, "A Map toward Precautionary Decision Making," and Andrew Jordan and Timothy O'Riordan, "The Precautionary Principle in Contemporary Environmental Policy and Politics," in *Protecting Public Health and The Environment*, Carolyn Raffensperger and Joel Tickner, eds. (Washington, DC: Island Press, 1999).
3. What Kerry Whiteside refers to as "well developed" proof not only of the scientific evidence of harm but also of the policy-oriented benefits of regulation (*Precautionary Politics: Principle and Practice in Confronting Environmental Risk* (Cambridge: MIT Press, 2006): *viii*, 29).
4. Whiteside, *Precautionary Politics*, 29, 34.
5. Wildavsky, *But Is It True?*; Henry Miller and Gregory Conko, "Genetically Modified Fear and the International Regulation of Biotechnology," in *Rethinking Risk and the Precautionary Principle*, Julian Morris, ed. (Oxford: Butterworth-Heinemann, 2000); Henry Miller and Gregory Conko, "The Perils of Precaution: Why Regulators' 'Precautionary Principle' Is Doing More Harm than Good," *Policy Review* 107 (2001); Indur Goklany, *The Precautionary Principle: A Critical Appraisal of Environmental Risk Assessment* (Washington, DC: CATO Institute, 2001); Cass Sunstein, *Risk and Reason: Safety, Law, and the Environment* (Cambridge: Cambridge University Press, 2002); Cass Sunstein, *Laws of Fear* (Cambridge: Cambridge University Press, 2005); Whiteside, *Precautionary Politics*, 34.
6. Kristin Shrader-Frechette, *Taking Action, Saving Lives: Our Duties to Protect Environmental and Public Health* (Oxford: Oxford University Press, 2007): 5.
7. Sven Ove Hansson, "Decision Making under Great Uncertainty," *Philosophy of the Social Sciences* 26 (1996).
8. Hansson ("Decision Making Under Great Uncertainty") offers a helpful, nuanced discussion of different forms of uncertainty—which broadly include uncertainty of alternative policy choices, of the consequences of policy choices, of the reliability of information available to decision makers, and of the values of decision makers (which are not static)—and he astutely explores how the decision process with environmental policy issues is both shaped by and can overcome these different constraints.
9. Daniel Steel (*Philosophy and the Precautionary Principle: Science, Evidence, and Environmental Policy* (Cambridge: Cambridge University Press, 2015)) also tries to broaden our conception of uncertainty as involving substantively more than "ignorance of probability" (95), which is the narrower conception of uncertainty that is adopted by scholars of risk analysis. In this vein, Steel aptly notes that uncertainty can persist even when we can ascertain probabilities that particular outcomes will come to pass (96, 100) and that the precautionary principle is well suited to shape our decision-making when quantitative risk assessment fails to yield the information necessary to substantiate a particular course of action (96). Accordingly, Steel views the precautionary principle as "compatible" with risk analysis (108–11). And although Steel's definitions of uncertainty and risk in the philosophy of science diverge from those commonly employed in normative ethics, my own view parallels Steel's conclusion: as noted in Chapter 1, a precautionary approach can effectively augment our dominant risk assessment–based regulatory regime. However, contrary to Steel, who argues that these two decision procedures can operate simultaneously, because uncertainty is

just "an aspect of risk" (99, 100) and regards the capacity of a "well-confirmed" empirical model to achieve high degrees of "predictive validity" (103–4)—and so "should not be restricted to situations involving unquantifiable risks" (199)—my account does treat the precautionary approach as a mutually exclusive decision process: for I contend that a precautionary approach is only applicable when the uncertainty we face thwarts our ability to conduct reliable quantitative risk assessments. This is to say that the conception of uncertainty adopted here seems to more closely align with Hansson's notion of degrees of "uncertainty of consequences" (Hansson, "Decision Making Under Great Uncertainty," 376), whereby at some point what we know about foreseeable consequences is so constrained that it is not possible to meaningfully talk of statistical probability. Although this is *not* to deny that we can be uncertain about different aspects of our risk assessments (uncertainty about probabilities as one example), the complications and semantic differences within the philosophy of science that Steel engages are tabled here.

10. Shrader-Frechette's, *Taking Action, Saving Live*, 79; Whiteside, *Precautionary Politics*, 33.
11. Michael Alavanja, "Health Effects of Chronic Pesticide Exposure: Cancer and Neurotoxicity," *Annual Review of Public Health* 25 (2004): 156–8; John Wargo, *Our Children's Toxic Legacy: How Science and Law Fail to Protect Us from Pesticides*, 2nd ed. (New Haven: Yale University Press, 1998): x-xii, 262–3, 264–5, 274; Ken Sexton and Dale Hattis, "Assessing Cumulative Health Risks from Exposure to Environmental Mixtures: Three Fundamental Questions," *Environmental Health Perspectives* 115 (2007): 825–6.
12. Environmental Protection Agency, "Assessing Human Health Risk from Pesticides," http://epa.gov/pesticide-science-and-assessing-pesticide-risks/assessing-human-health-risk-pesticides, last updated September 30, 2015.
13. Environmental Protection Agency, "Assessing Human Health Risk from Pesticides."
14. Sunstein, *Risk and Reason*, 104, 109; Sunstein, *Laws of Fear*, 109, 117; Whiteside, *Precautionary Politics*, 38, 49–5; Environmental Protection Agency, "Assessing Human Health Risk from Pesticides."
15. United Nations Environment Programme, "Rio Declaration on Environment and Development," *Principle 15, U.N. Conference on Environment and Development*, Rio de Janeiro, Brazil, June 14, 1992.
16. Hansson ("Decision Making Under Great Uncertainty," 375–7) rightly notes that any form of uncertainty is a matter of degree, and in this vein he identifies four degrees of outcome uncertainty (or what he terms "uncertainty of consequences"), which include (1) knowing the probabilities that particular outcomes will come to pass, (2) having some knowledge—albeit incomplete knowledge—of these probabilities, (3) knowing *only* that these probabilities are nonzero, and finally (4) having no substantive knowledge of these probabilities at all. Hansson defines decision-making "under uncertainty" differently than I do: namely, as choosing a course of action with incomplete knowledge of the probability that a foreseeable consequence will come to pass [item (2) earlier], whereas acting under uncertainty is defined here (see below) as choosing a course of action when we know neither what the outcomes will be nor what the probabilities are that these outcomes will come to pass—which may be understood as a further degree of uncertainty, which I term "genuine" uncertainty (see later). Despite his distinct taxonomy, Hansson motivates precisely the sort of discussion about the meaning of uncertainty that is necessary before we can determine how to respond to the uncertainty. However, unlike Hansson, who maintains that normative values are but one component of the decision process, when it comes to genuine uncertainty of environmental harm, moral considerations are all we have to substantiate the decisions we make (see Section 2.2 below).

17. Alan Loeb, "Birth of the Kettering Doctrine: Fordism, Sloanism and Tetraethyl Lead," *Business and Economic History* 24 (1995); Bill Kovarik, "Charles F. Kettering and the 1921 Discovery of Tetraethyl Lead In the Context of Technological Alternatives" (working paper), *Presented to the Society of Automotive Engineers Fuels and Lubricants Conference*, Baltimore, MD, 1994 (revised in 1999); Jamie Lincoln Kitman, "The Secret History of Lead," *The Nation*, March 2, 2002: www.thenation.com/article/secret-history-lead; Gerald Markowitz and David Rosner, *Deceit and Denial: The Deadly Politics of Industrial Pollution* (Berkeley: University of California Press, 2002); Robert Percival et al., *Environmental Regulation: Law, Science, and Policy*, 6th ed. (New York: Aspen Publishers, 2009): 184, 191–2.
18. Carson, *Silent Spring*; Environmental Protection Agency, "DDT, a Review of Scientific and Economic Aspects of the Decision to Ban Its Use as a Pesticide," *Prepared for the Committee on Appropriations of the U.S. House of Representatives*, EPA-540/1-75-022, July 1975: www2.epa.gov/aboutepa/ddt-regulatory-history-brief-survey-1975; Environmental Protection Agency, "DDT: A Brief History and Status," http://epa.gov/ingredients-used-pesticide-products/ddt-brief-history-and-status, last updated November 5, 2015.
19. Centers for Disease Control and Prevention, "DES History," http://cdc.gov/des/consumers/about/history.html, last updated June 1, 2015.
20. Jun Sekizawa, "Low-Dose Effects of Bisphenol A: A Serious Threat to Human Health?" *Journal of Toxicological Sciences* 33 (2008): 389–403; Richard Sharpe, "Is It Time to End Concerns over the Estrogenic Effects of Bisphenol A?" *Toxicological Sciences* 114 (2010): 1–4; Beverly Rubin, "Bisphenol A: An Endocrine Disruptor with Widespread Exposure and Multiple Effects," *Journal of Steroid Biochemistry and Molecular Biology* 127 (2011): 27–34; Food and Drug Administration, "Food and Drug Administration Continues to Study BPA," March 2012: http://fda.gov/ForConsumers/ConsumerUpdates/ucm297954.htm, last updated January 29, 2015.
21. Sabrina Tavernise, "FDA Makes It Official: BPA Can't Be Used in Baby Bottles and Cups," *New York Times*, July 17, 2012: http://nytimes.com/2012/07/18/science/fda-bans-bpa-from-baby-bottles-and-sippy-cups.html?_r=0; Food and Drug Administration, "Food and Drug Administration Continues to Study BPA."
22. Sarah Vogel, "The Politics of Plastics: The Making and Unmaking of Bisphenol A Safety," *American Journal of Public Health* 99 (2009): 559–66.
23. Program on Breast Cancer and Environmental Risk Factors, Cornell University, "Consumer Concerns about Hormones in Food," June 2000: http://envirocancer.cornell.edu/factsheet/diet/fs37.hormones.cfm, last updated May 2, 2003; American Cancer Society, "Learn about Cancer: Recombinant Bovine Growth Hormone," http://cancer.org/cancer/cancercauses/othercarcinogens/athome/recombinant-bovine-growth-hormone, last updated September 10, 2014.
24. Food and Drug Administration, "Interim Guidance on the Voluntary Labeling of Milk and Milk Products from Cows That Have Not Been Treated with Recombinant Bovine Somatotropin," *Federal Register* 59 (February 10, 1994): https://gpo.gov/fdsys/pkg/FR-1994-02-10/html/94-3214.htm; Program on Breast Cancer and Environmental Risk Factors, "Consumer Concerns about Hormones in Food;" Food and Drug Administration, "Report on the FDA's Review of the Safety of Recombinant Bovine Somatotropin," April 23, 2009: http://fda.gov/AnimalVeterinary/SafetyHealth/ProductSafetyInformation/ucm130321.htm, last updated July 28, 2014.
25. Food and Drug Administration, "Interim Guidance on the Voluntary Labeling of Milk and Milk Products from Cows That Have Not Been Treated with Recombinant Bovine Somatotropin;" Rachel Schurman and William Munro, *Fighting for the Future of Food: Activists versus Agribusiness in the Struggle over Biotechnology* (Minneapolis: University of Minnesota Press, 2010): 217, fn. 35; Diane

Thue-Vasquez, "Genetic Engineering and Food Labeling: A Continuing Controversy," *San Joaquin Agricultural Law Review* 10 (2000).

26. *International Dairy Foods Association v. Boggs*, 622 F. 3d 628 (6th Cir. 2010); National Public Radio, "Court OKs Hormone-Free Label on Dairy Products In Ohio," October 1, 2010: http://npr.org/sections/health-shots/2010/10/01/130270131/court-give-hormone-free-label-on-dairy-products-an-ok-in-ohio; Libby Moulton, "Labeling Milk from Cows Not Treated with rBST: Legal in All 50 States as of September 29th, 2010," *Columbia Science and Technology Law Review*, October 28, 2010: http://stlr.org/2010/10/28/labeling-milk-from-cows-not-treated-with-rbst-legal-in-all-50-states-as-of-september-29th-2010/.
27. Food and Drug Administration, "Report on the FDA's Review of the Safety of Recombinant Bovine Somatotropin."
28. Program on Breast Cancer and Environmental Risk Factors, "Consumer Concerns about Hormones in Food."
29. American Cancer Society, "Learn about Cancer: Recombinant Bovine Growth Hormone."
30. Ibid.
31. Ibid.
32. Whiteside, *Precautionary Politics*, 33–4.
33. Finn Bro-Rasmussen, "Risk, Uncertainties, and Precautions in Chemical Legislation," in *Precaution: Environmental Science and Preventative Public Policy*, Joel Tickner, ed. (Washington, DC: Island Press, 2003): 94; Shrader-Frechette, *Taking Action, Saving Lives*, 99–100; Judith Layzer, "Love Canal: Hazardous Waste and the Politics of Fear," in *The Environmental Case: Translating Values into Policy*, 3rd ed. (Washington, DC: CQ Press, 2012): see, e.g., 69–70.
34. United Nations Millennium Ecosystem Assessment, "Living Beyond Our Means: Natural Assets and Human Well-being," *Statement of Millennium Assessment Board* (2005): 15; Whiteside, *Precautionary Politics*, 33.
35. Roger Pielke, Jr., *The Honest Broker: Making Sense of Science in Policy and Politics* (Cambridge: Cambridge University Press, 2007); Naomi Oreskes and Erik Conway, *Merchants of Doubt: How a Handful of Scientists Obscured the Truth on Issues from Tobacco Smoke to Global Warming* (New York: Bloomsbury Publishing, 2010).
36. Shrader-Frechette, *Taking Action, Saving Lives*, 11, 39–112, particularly 52–3, 68, 77–8.
37. Ibid.
38. Sunstein, *Risk and Reason*, 34–5, 53–77; Sunstein, *Laws of Fear*, 6–7, 126–8, 129; see also Sunstein, "Moral Heuristics and Risk," in *Risk: Philosophical Perspectives*, Tim Lewens, ed. (New York: Routledge, 2007).
39. Shrader-Frechette, *Taking Action, Saving Lives*, Chapters 2–3; Whiteside, *Precautionary Politics*, Chapter 2.
40. United Nations Millennium Ecosystem Assessment, "Living Beyond Our Means," 15; Whiteside, *Precautionary Politics*, 34.
41. Whiteside, *Precautionary Politics*, 34; Sunstein, *Risk and Reason*, 36.
42. Environmental Protection Agency, "Health Risks of Radon," http://epa.gov/radon/health-risk-radon, last updated October 22, 2015; National Cancer Institute, "Radon and Cancer," http://cancer.gov/about-cancer/causes-prevention/risk/substances/radon/radon-fact-sheet, last updated December 6, 2011.
43. Environmental Protection Agency, "Health Risks of Radon;" National Cancer Institute (NCI), "Radon and Cancer." The EPA and the NCI report, for instance, that of the roughly 21,000 radon-related lung cancer deaths, fewer than 3,000 (or roughly 10 to 15 percent) occurred among nonsmokers.
44. Thomas D. Luckey, *Radiation Hormesis* (Boca Raton: CRC Press, 1991): 136.
45. Agency for Toxic Substances and Disease Registry, "Toxicological Profile for Asbestos" (Atlanta: U.S. Department of Health and Human Services, 2001): 5.

46. World Health Organization, "Asbestos in Drinking Water: Background Document for Development of WHO Guidelines for Drinking Water Quality," in *Guidelines for Drinking-Water Quality*, 2nd ed., Vol. 2 (Geneva: World Health Organization, 1996), last updated 2003; John Gamble, "Risk of Gastrointestinal Cancers from Inhalation and Ingestion of Asbestos," *Regulatory Toxicology and Pharmacology* 52 (2008). See also Peter Toft et al., "Asbestos in Drinking-Water," *Critical Reviews in Environmental Control* 14 (1984); World Health Organization and International Programme on Chemical Safety, *Asbestos and Other Natural Mineral Fibres* (Geneva: World Health Organization, 1986); Department of Health and Human Services Working Group, "Report on Cancer Risks Associated with the Ingestion of Asbestos," *Environmental Health Perspectives* 72 (1987).
47. World Health Organization, "Asbestos in Drinking Water," 2–3.
48. Marilyn Browne et al., "Cancer Incidence and Asbestos in Drinking Water, Town of Woodstock, New York, 1980–1998," *Environmental Research* 98 (2005): 229, 231; Gamble, "Risk of Gastrointestinal Cancers from Inhalation and Ingestion of Asbestos," S125, S146–7, S148–9.
49. Browne et al., "Cancer Incidence and Asbestos in Drinking Water," 231–2; Gamble, "Risk of Gastrointestinal Cancers from Inhalation and Ingestion of Asbestos," S146, S148.
50. Ibid., 229 and S149, respectively. Gamble argues, e.g., that smokers experience "an 80% increased risk of stomach cancer" and that "colon and rectal cancer risks are increased about 2-fold among heavy current smokers."
51. Agency for Toxic Substances and Disease Registry, "Toxicological Profile for Asbestos," 6. See also the decision in *Jackson v. Johns-Manville Sales Corp.*, 781 F.2d 394 (5th Cir. 1986), which establishes employer liability for the (mere) *possibility* of future cancers in employees whose workplace exposure to airborne asbestos makes them more vulnerable.
52. Frederica Perera, "Environment and Cancer: Who Are Susceptible?," *Science* 278 (1997): 1072; Shrader-Frechette, *Taking Action, Saving Lives*, 80–1.
53. Perera, "Environment and Cancer: Who Are Susceptible?," 1071–2; Evangelia Samoli et al., "Estimating the Exposure: Response Relationships between Particulate Matter and Mortality within the APHEA Multicity Project," *Environmental Health Perspectives* 113 (2005): 88.
54. Perera, "Environment and Cancer: Who Are Susceptible?," 1072.
55. Whiteside, *Precautionary Politics*, 33.
56. Timothy O'Riordan and Andrew Jordan, "The Precautionary Principle in Contemporary Environmental Politics," *Environmental Values* 4 (1995): 199; Whiteside, *Precautionary Politics*, 34.
57. See Carolyn Raffensperger and Joel Tickner, eds., *Protecting Public Health and the Environment* (Washington, DC: Island Press, 1999); Sunstein, *Risk and Reason*; Sunstein, *Laws of Fear*; Whiteside, *Precautionary Politics*.
58. European Environment Agency, "Late Lessons from Early Warnings: The Precautionary Principle, 1896–2000," *Environmental Issue Report*, No. 22 (2001); Whiteside, *Precautionary Politics*, 49.
59. William Boyd, "Genealogies of Risk: Searching for Safety, 1930s–1970s," *Ecology Law Quarterly* 39 (2012): 986.
60. Frank Knight, *Risk, Uncertainty, and Profit* (Boston: Houghton Mifflin Co., 1921): 19–20, 233.
61. The distinction and significance between "measurable risk" and "unmeasurable uncertainty" (or that which we do not know) were made as early as the 1920s: see Frank Knight, *Risk, Uncertainty, and Profit* (Boston: Houghton Mifflin Co., 1921): 19–20, 233. See also John Maynard Keynes, "The General Theory of Employment," *Quarterly Journal of Economics* 51 (1937): 209, 214.
62. Robert V. Percival et al., *Environmental Regulation: Law, Science, and Policy*, 6th ed. (New York: Aspen Publishers, 2009): 204–5; William Lowrance,

Of Acceptable Risk: Science and the Determination of Safety (Los Altos: W. Kaufmann, 1976): 75.

63. Percival et al., *Environmental Regulation*, 288–9; *Industrial Union Dept., AFL-CIO v. American Petroleum Institute*, 448 U.S. 607 (1980); and *Corrosion Proof Fittings v. Environmental Protection Agency*, 947 F.2d 1201 (5th Cir. 1991). The former case, e.g., which regards exposure to benzene, and in which the Supreme Court insisted that efforts must be made to quantify the risk of harm given the "best available evidence," effectively cemented the plausibility of and need for QRA. The decision in the latter case similarly lent credence to the requirement of "substantial evidence" of the risks of harm to public health for any risk regulation to be justified.
64. National Research Council, *Arsenic in Drinking Water* (Washington, DC: National Academy Press, 1999); Environmental Protection Agency, "National Primary Drinking Water Regulations: Arsenic and Clarifications to Compliance and New Source Contaminants Monitoring," *Federal Register* 66, Nos. 14 and 78 (2001).
65. David Abbey et al., "Chronic Respiratory Symptoms Associated with Estimated Long-Term Ambient Concentrations of Fine Particulates Less Than 2.5 Microns in Aerodynamic Diameter (PM2.5) and Other Air Pollutants," *Journal of Exposure Analysis and Environmental Epidemiology* 5 (1995); Daniel Krewski et al., *Reanalysis of the Harvard Six Cities Study and the American Cancer Society Study of Particulate Air Pollution and Mortality* (Cambridge: Health Effects Institute, 2000); C. Arden Pope et al., "Lung Cancer, Cardiopulmonary Mortality, and Long-Term Exposure to Fine Particulate Air Pollution," *Journal of the American Medical Association* 287 (2002); Environmental Protection Agency, "Quantitative Health Risk Assessment for Particulate Matter," EPA-452/R-10-005 (June 2010): www3.epa.gov/ttn/naaqs/standards/pm/data/PM_RA_FINAL_June_2010.pdf.
66. Rita Schoeny, "Use of Genetic Toxicology Data in U.S. EPA Risk Assessment: The Mercury Study Report as an Example," *Environmental Health Perspectives* 104, Supplement 3 (1996); National Research Council, *Toxicological Effects of Methylmercury* (Washington, DC: National Academy Press, 2000); Daniel Axelrad et al., "Dose-Response Relationship of Prenatal Mercury Exposure and IQ," *Environmental Health Perspectives* 115 (2007); Environmental Protection Agency, "Regulatory Impact Analysis for the Final Mercury and Air Toxics Standards," EPA-452/R-11-011 (December 2011): www3.epa.gov/mats/pdfs/20111221MATSfinalRIA.pdf.
67. John Wargo, *Our Children's Toxic Legacy: How Science and Law Fail to Protect Us from Pesticides* (New Haven: Yale University Press, 1996): 111–2; Peter Wright et al., "Twenty-Five Years of Dioxin Cancer Risk Assessment," *Natural Resources and Environment* 19 (2005): 31, 35; National Research Council, *Science and Decisions: Advancing Risk Assessment* (Washington, DC: National Academies Press, 2009): ix, 3–4, 17, 113–9; Boyd, "Genealogies of Risk," 981–3.
68. Boyd, "Genealogies of Risk," 902, 904, 943–4, 964–6, 976, 978–9, 982–3, 986.
69. This is, however, precisely what the authors of the "Wingspread Statement" imprudently claim, insisting that we "must adopt a precautionary approach to *all* human endeavors" (emphasis added). See Global Development Research Center, "Wingspread Statement on the Precautionary Principle," January 1998: http://gdrc.org/u-gov/precaution-3.html.
70. See, e.g., National Research Council, *Understanding Risk: Informing Decisions in a Democratic Society* (Washington, DC: National Academy Press, 1996); National Research Council, *Risk and Decisions About Disposition of Transuranic and High-Level Radioactive Waste* (Washington, DC: National Academies Press, 2005); National Research Council, *Science and Decisions*.

71. John Harris and Søren Holm, "Extending Human Lifespan and the Precautionary Paradox," *Journal of Medicine and Philosophy* 27 (2002).
72. Whiteside, *Precautionary Politics*, 28.
73. Jeremy Leggett, *Global Warming: A Greenpeace Report* (Oxford: Oxford University Press, 1990); Tickner, "A Map toward Precautionary Decision Making;" Christopher Stone, "Is There a Precautionary Principle?," *Environmental Law Reporter* 31 (2001); Elizabeth Fisher, "Precaution, Precaution Everywhere: Developing a 'Common Understanding' of the Precautionary Principle in the European Community," *Maastricht Journal of European and Comparative Law* 9 (2002): 7–28; Whiteside, *Precautionary Politics*, 46, 49.
74. See, e.g., Robyn Eckersley, *Environmentalism and Political Theory: Toward an Ecocentric Approach* (Albany: State University of New York Press, 1992): 46.
75. Global Development Research Center, "Wingspread Statement on the Precautionary Principle."
76. Raffensperger and Tickner, *Protecting Public Health and the Environment*, 1.
77. Madeleine Hayenhjelm and Jonathan Wolff, "The Moral Problem of Risk Impositions: A Survey of the Literature," *European Journal of Philosophy* 20 (2012): e37; David McCarthy, "Rights, Explanation, and Risks," *Ethics* 107 (1997); Sven Hansson, "Ethical Criteria for Risk Acceptance," *Erkenntnis* 59 (2003).
78. Shifting the burden of proof is but one of the several requisites to successfully implementing the precautionary principle that Raffensperger and Tickner delineate (*Protecting Public Health and the Environment*); see also Fisher, "Precaution, Precaution Everywhere;" Steve Maguire and Jaye Ellis, "Redistributing the Burden of Scientific Uncertainty: Implications of the Precautionary Principle for State and Non-State Actors," *Global Governance* 11 (2005).
79. Mary O'Brien, Alternatives Assessment and the Precautionary Principle," in *Protecting Public Health and the Environment*, Carolyn Raffensperger and Joel Tickner, eds. (Washington, DC: Island Press, 1999): 208.
80. Daniel Bodansky, "The Precautionary Principle in U.S. Environmental Law," in *Interpreting the Precautionary Principle*, Tim O'Riordan and James Cameron, eds. (London: Earthscan, 1994): 217; O'Riordan and Jordan, "The Precautionary Principle in Contemporary Environmental Politics," 193; John Applegate, "The Precautionary Preference: An American Perspective on the Precautionary Principle," *Human and Ecological Risk Assessment* 6 (2000):436–7.
81. Robert Goodin, *Protecting the Vulnerable: A Re-Analysis of Our Social Responsibilities* (Chicago: University of Chicago Press, 1985); Whiteside, *Precautionary Politics*, 55.
82. Percival et al., *Environmental Regulation*, 266, 288–9.
83. Aldo Leopold, *A Sand County Almanac* (New York: Oxford University Press, 1949); Arne Næss, "The Shallow and the Deep, Long-Range Ecology Movement: A Summary," *Inquiry* 16, Nos. 1–4 (1973); Holmes Rolston, *Environmental Ethics: Duties to and Values in the Natural World* (Philadelphia: Temple University Press, 1988); Baird Callicott, *In Defense of the Land Ethic: Essays in Environmental Philosophy* (Albany: SUNY Press, 1989); Robyn Eckersley, *Environmentalism, and Political Theory: Toward an Ecocentric Approach* (Albany: SUNY Press, 1992); Leena Vilkka, *The Intrinsic Value of Nature* (Amsterdam: Rodopi, 1997); Andrew Dobson, *Green Political Thought*, 3rd ed. (New York: Routledge, 2000).
84. Whiteside, *Precautionary Politics*, 25.
85. See, for example, O'Riordan and Jordan, "The Precautionary Principle in Contemporary Environmental Politics," 196; Robyn Eckersley, "The Discourse Ethic and the Problem of Representing Nature," *Environmental Politics* 8 (1999): 26, 46; Robin Attfield, *Environmental Ethics* (Cambridge: Polity Press, 2003): 145.

Whiteside is quick to note, however, that this formulation of the precautionary principle ostensibly commits its proponents to untenable policy implications: requiring the unqualified prohibition of any activity that undermines the "self-realization" of natural ecosystems (*Precautionary Politics*, 26–7).

86. Whiteside, *Precautionary Politics*, 53.
87. European Environment Agency, "Late Lessons from Early Warnings," 170–3.
88. Ronnie Harding and Elizabeth Fisher, "The Precautionary Principle: Toward a Deliberative, Transdisciplinary Problem-Solving Process," in *Perspectives on the Precautionary Principle*, Ronnie Harding and Elizabeth Fisher, eds. (Annandale: Federation Press, 1999): 290–8; Joel Tickner, ed., *Precaution: Environmental Science and Preventive Public Policy* (Washington, DC: Island Press, 2003): 11.
89. See, e.g., Whiteside, *Precautionary Politics*, 16; Shrader-Frechette, *Taking Action, Saving Lives*, 11, 13, 39–112.
90. Jordan and O'Riordan, "The Precautionary Principle in Contemporary Environmental Policy and Politics," 22.
91. Julian Morris, "Defining the Precautionary Principle," in *Rethinking Risk and the Precautionary Principle*, Julian Morris, ed. (Oxford: Butterworth-Heinemann, 2000): 6.
92. Miller and Conko, "The Perils of Precaution," 26, 29, 36. Sunstein, *Risk and Reason*; Sunstein, *Laws of Fear*.
93. See, e.g., Mark Sagoff, *Economy of the Earth: Philosophy, Law, and the Environment* (Cambridge: Cambridge University Press, 1988): Chapters 2–4 (on the policy and normative shortcomings of cost-benefit analysis); Pielke, *The Honest Broker*, Chapters 8–9 (on "politicized" or policy-driven science); Shrader-Frechette, *Taking Action, Saving Lives*, Chapters 2–3 (on "private-interest" or industry-driven science); and Naomi Oreskes and Erik Conway, *Merchants of Doubt: How a Handful of Scientists Obscured the Truth on Issues from Tobacco Smoke to Global Warming* (New York: Bloomsbury Publishing, 2010): Chapters 1 and 5 (on the purposeful distortion of truth by industry scientists).
94. Sunstein, *Risk and Reason*, 37–8, 158; Sunstein, *Laws of Fear*, Chapters 3–4.
95. Layzer, "Love Canal," 56–7, 62–3, 76–7; Jane Brody, "Don't Lose Sight of Real, Everyday Risks," *New York Times*, October 9, 2001. Some might resist this conclusion and underscore that even poor judges of risk have the right to withhold their consent to being exposed to risks they (wrongly) believe are credible. That is, that pedestrian risk perceptions, although often mistaken, are still morally relevant. This objection against the precautionary approach is refuted in Chapter 5, but it should be noted that under conditions of uncertainty, as Chapter 3.3 explains, offering one's informed consent is far from straightforward.
96. Sunstein, *Risk and Reason*, 33; Sunstein, *Laws of Fear*, 5, 102–4, and Chapter 4; Layzer, "Love Canal: Hazardous Waste and the Politics of Fear," 57, 63.
97. Sunstein, *Risk and Reason*, 35; Sunstein, *Laws of Fear*, 83.
98. Edward Soule, "Assessing the Precautionary Principle," *Public Affairs Quarterly* 14 (2000); Sunstein, *Risk and Reason*; Sunstein, *Laws of Fear*; Martin Peterson, "The Precautionary Principle Is Incoherent," *Risk Analysis* 26 (2006); Per Sandin, "Commonsense Precaution and Varieties of the Precautionary Principle," in *Risk: Philosophical Perspectives*, Tim Lewens, ed. (New York: Routledge, 2007).
99. Sunstein, *Risk and Reason*, 100, 104; Sunstein, *Laws of Fear*, 5.
100. National Resource Defense Council, "The Truth about Tap," January 5, 2016: https://nrdc.org/stories/truth-about-tap.
101. Sunstein, *Risk and Reason*, 104.
102. Wildavsky, *But Is It True?*: 55–80; Frank Cross, "Paradoxical Perils of the Precautionary Principle," *Washington and Lee Law Review* 53 (1996); Indur Goklany, "Applying the Precautionary Principle in a Broader Context," in *Rethinking Risk and the Precautionary Principle*, Julian Morris, ed. (Oxford:

Butterworth-Heinemann, 2000); Morris, "Defining the Precautionary Principle;" Soule, "Assessing the Precautionary Principle," Stone, "Is There a Precautionary Principle?;" Sunstein, *Risk and Reason*, 104; Calum Turvey and Eliza Mojduszka, "The Precautionary Principle and the Law of Unintended Consequences," *Food Policy* 30 (2005); Sunstein 2005: 51, Whiteside, *Precautionary Politics*, 44; Tim Lewens, ed., *Risk: Philosophical Perspectives* (New York: Routledge, 2007).

103. Wildavsky, *But Is It True?*, 55–80; Goklany, "Applying the Precautionary Principle in a Broader Context," 191–2; Goklany, *The Precautionary Principle*.
104. Goklany, *The Precautionary Principle*.
105. Whiteside, *Precautionary Politics*, 36.
106. Goklany, "Applying the Precautionary Principle in a Broader Context," 221; Giandomenico Majone, "What Price Safety? The Precautionary Principle and Its Policy Implications," *Journal of Common Market Studies* 40 (2002); Whiteside, *Precautionary Politics*, 39–40.
107. Goklany, *The Precautionary Principle*, 26, 55, 86.
108. Ibid., 26, 55, 86.
109. Miller and Conko, "The Perils of Precaution," 26.
110. Daniel Bodansky "Scientific Uncertainty and the Precautionary Principle," *Environment* 33 (1991); Per Sandin, "Dimensions of the Precautionary Principle," *Human and Ecological Risk Assessment* 5 (1999); Soule, "Assessing the Precautionary Principle;" Harris and Holm, "Extending Human Lifespan and the Precautionary Paradox;" Per Sandin, "Commonsense Precaution and Varieties of the Precautionary Principle," in *Risk: Philosophical Perspectives*, Tim Lewens, ed. (New York: Routledge, 2007).
111. Bodansky, "Scientific Uncertainty and the Precautionary Principle," 5 (emphasis added).
112. Stephen Gardiner, "A Core Precautionary Principle," *Journal of Political Philosophy* 14 (2006): 36–7.
113. Whiteside, *Precautionary Politics*, 39–40; see also Austin Hill, "The Environment and Disease: Association or Causation?," *Proceedings of the Royal Society of Medicine* 58 (1965).
114 *Public Citizen v. Young*, 831 F. 2d 1108 (D.C. Circuit 1987); Carl Cranor and Kurt Nutting, "Scientific and Legal Standards of Statistical Evidence in Toxic Tort and Discrimination Suits," *Law and Philosophy* 9 (1990); Philip Howard, *The Death of Common Sense: How Law is Suffocating America* (New York: Random House, 1994); Government Publishing Office, Food Quality Protection Act, H.R.1627, 104th Congress Public Law 170 (August 3, 1996); see also Robert Nozick, *Anarchy, State, and Utopia* (New York: Basic Books, 1974).
115. Miller and Conko, "The Perils of Precaution;" Whiteside, *Precautionary Politics*, 39, 42.
116. Goklany, *The Precautionary Principle*, 4; see also Donna Vogt, *The Delaney Clause Effects on Pesticide Policy* (Washington, DC: Congressional Research Service, 1995); and Percival et al., *Environmental Regulation*, 244, 283–8.
117. *Ethyl Corp v. EPA*, 541 F. 2d 1 (D.C. Circuit 1976).
118. *Reserve Mining Company v. EPA*, 514 F.2d 492 (8th Circuit 1975).
119. *Chlorine Chemical Council v. EPA*, 206 F. 3d 1286 (D.C. Circuit 2000).
120. Percival et al., *Environmental Regulation*, 284–5.
121. *Public Citizen v. Young* (1987), majority opinion, §21.
122. Technologies that would include, for example, synthetic pesticides, GMOs, artificial sweeteners, compounds in plastics, medicines, and so forth.
123. Cross, "Paradoxical Perils of the Precautionary Principle;" Miller and Conko, "Genetically Modified Fear and the International Regulation of Biotechnology;" Morris, "Defining the Precautionary Principle;" Goklany, *The Precautionary Principle*; Stone, "Is There a Precautionary Principle?;" John Graham, "The Role of

Precaution in Risk Assessment and Management: An American's View," Remarks Prepared for "The US, Europe, Precaution and Risk Management: A Comparative Case Study Analysis of the Management of Risk in a Complex World" (January 11–12, 2002): http://whitehouse.gov/omb/inforeg/eu_speech.html.
124. Graham, "The Role of Precaution in Risk Assessment and Management: An American's View."
125. Aaron Wildavsky, "Trial and Error versus Trial without Error," in *Rethinking Risk and the Precautionary Principle*, Julian Morris, ed. (Oxford: Butterworth-Heinemann, 2000).
126. Morris, "Defining the Precautionary Principle," 12.
127. Sandin, "Commonsense Precaution and Varieties of the Precautionary Principle," 108.
128. Indeed, elsewhere Sandin writes even more generally that the precautionary principle commonsensically entails that "If there is (1) a threat, which is (2) uncertain, then (3) some kind of action (4) is mandatory" ("Dimensions of the Precautionary Principle," 889–91).
129. Sandin, "Commonsense Precaution and Varieties of the Precautionary Principle," 108.
130. See, e.g., Christian Munthe, *The Price of Precaution and the Ethics of Risk* (New York: Springer 2011); Catriona McKinnon, *Climate Change and Future Justice: Precaution, Compensation, and Triage* (New York: Routledge, 2012); Christopher Morgan-Knapp, "Non-Consequentialist Precaution," *Ethical Theory and Moral Practice* 18 (2015); and Lauren Hartzell-Nichols, *A Climate of Risk: Precautionary Principles, Catastrophes, and Climate Change* (New York: Routledge, 2017).
131. John Rawls, *A Theory of Justice* (Cambridge: Harvard University Press, 1971): 402.
132. Gardiner, "A Core Precautionary Principle," 45.
133. Ibid., 47, 49, 55.
134. Ibid.
135. Gardiner, "A Core Precautionary Principle," 43–5, 53.
136. Ibid.
137. Ibid., 48.
138. Sandin, "Commonsense Precaution and Varieties of the Precautionary Principle," 104–5.
139. Sunstein, *Laws of Fear*, 120.
140. Gardiner, "A Core Precautionary Principle," 48.
141. Ibid., 50.
142. Ibid., 45, 50.
143. Ibid., 55.
144. See, e.g., Neil Manson, "Formulating the Precautionary Principle," *Environmental Ethics* 24 (2002).
145. Gardiner, "A Core Precautionary Principle," 51.
146. Morgan-Knapp, "Non-Consequentialist Precaution"
147. Ibid., 787.
148. Ibid., 786.
149. Ibid., 788.
150. Ibid., 791, 793.
151. Ibid., 786, 791.
152. Ibid., 793.
153. Ibid.
154. Ibid., 792.
155. Bro-Rasmussen, "Risk, Uncertainties, and Precautions in Chemical Legislation," 94; Shrader-Frechette, *Taking Action, Saving Lives*, 80–1, 99–100; Layzer, "Love Canal," 69–70; Boyd, "Genealogies of Risk," 914.

156. Perera, "Environment and Cancer," 1072.
157. Morgan-Knapp, "Non-Consequentialist Precaution," 787–9.
158. Ibid., 787.
159. Ibid., 788.
160. Kerry Whiteside, *Precautionary Politics: Principle and Practice in Confronting Environmental Risk* (Cambridge: MIT Press, 2006): 38.
161. European Environment Agency, "Late Lessons from Early Warnings," 169; Harding and Fisher, "The Precautionary Principle;" Global Development Research Center, "Wingspread Statement on the Precautionary Principle;" Shrader-Frechette, *Taking Action, Saving Lives*.
162. Whiteside, *Precautionary Politics*, ix.
163. Ibid., 23, 28, 117–8.
164. Ibid., xii.
165. Ibid., 27, also Chapter 5.
166. Ibid., xi, xiii.
167. Ibid., 27–8, 30.
168. Ibid., 118–20.
169. Ibid., 122. Whiteside's criticisms of earlier accounts of deliberative democratic understandings of the precautionary principle focus on Harding and Fisher, "The Precautionary Principle;" and Ulrich Beck, *Risk Society: Towards a New Modernity* (London: Sage Publications, 1996).
170. Whiteside, *Precautionary Politics*, 122–3.
171. Ibid., 120.
172. Ibid., 120, 122–3.
173. Ibid., 30–7.
174. Ibid., 33.
175. Percival et al., *Environmental Regulation*, 243–9; Office of the Inspector General, "The EPA's Fiscal Year 2014 Management Challenges" (Washington, DC: U.S. Environmental Protection Agency, May 28, 2014).
176. With many of these chemicals falling out of production for various reasons since TSCA's enactment, Dr. Steve DeVito, senior scientist and advisor with the EPA in Washington, DC (who has been with the agency since 1988), suggests that the number of chemicals currently being manufactured, processed, or imported for commerce in the United States is closer to 10,000 (personal correspondence, February 15, 2017). However, this figure is highly speculative, since the EPA has no central, comprehensive, and accurate list of the chemical substances in current production, including those pre-1976 substances that were exempt from mandatory testing under TSCA: the Agency for Toxic Substances and Disease Registry, the Toxic Release Inventory Program, the TSCA Hotline, and the Office on Chemical Data Reporting have not only been unable to confirm which grandfathered chemical substances are still being produced and at which volumes, but they have also failed to confirm what toxicity data exist or are lacking for these pre-existing substances.
177. Percival et al., *Environmental Regulation*, 213.
178. Ibid.
179. Percival et al., *Environmental Regulation*, 244–5; Robert V. Percival and Christopher H. Schroeder, *Environmental Law: Statutory and Case Supplement 2012–2013* (New York: Wolters Kluwer Law and Business, 2012): 81. TSCA, for instance, regulates the manufacture of new chemicals (§5(a)(1)) and new, substantively different uses of existing chemicals (§5(a)(2)).
180. Whiteside, *Precautionary Politics*, 12.
181. Ibid., 30, 38, 46, 49, 53, 68, 123.
182. Ibid., 30.
183. Sunstein, *Risk and Reason*, 104, 109; Sunstein, *Laws of Fear*, 18, 23, 24, 109.

184. Whiteside, *Precautionary Politics*, 49.
185. Goklany, *The Precautionary Principle,* 9, 89; Whiteside, *Precautionary Politics*, 44–5.
186. Sunstein, *Risk and Reason*, 27.
187. Whiteside, *Precautionary Politics*, 122–3.
188. Ibid., xi.
189. Ibid., x.
190. Whiteside, *Precautionary Politics*, viii.
191. Goklany (*The Precautionary Principle*, 85) alleges that restrictions on GHG emissions constrain economic development and growth, which in turn reduce affluence and also lead to "greater hunger, poorer health, and higher mortality."
192. Goklany, *The Precautionary Principle*, 8, 86.
193. Ibid., 56.
194. United Nations, *Universal Declaration of Human Rights*, General Assembly Resolution 217A (III), December 10, 1948.
195. Ibid.
196. United Nations, *Universal Declaration on the Eradication of Hunger and Malnutrition*, General Assembly Resolution 3348 (XXIX), December 17, 1974.

References

Abbey, David, et al. "Chronic Respiratory Symptoms Associated with Estimated Long-Term Ambient Concentrations of Fine Particulates Less Than 2.5 Microns in Aerodynamic Diameter (PM2.5) and Other Air Pollutants." *Journal of Exposure Analysis and Environmental Epidemiology* 5 (1995): 137–59.

———. "Toxicological Profile for Asbestos." Atlanta: Department of Health and Human Services, 2001.

Alavanja, Michael. "Health Effects of Chronic Pesticide Exposure: Cancer and Neurotoxicity." *Annual Review of Public Health* 25 (2004): 155–97.

American Cancer Society. "Learn about Cancer: Recombinant Bovine Growth Hormone." Last updated September 10, 2014. http://cancer.org/cancer/cancercauses/othercarcinogens/athome/recombinant-bovine-growth-hormone.

Applegate, John. "The Precautionary Preference: An American Perspective on the Precautionary Principle." *Human and Ecological Risk Assessment* 6 (2000): 413–43.

Attfield, Robin. *Environmental Ethics*. Cambridge: Polity Press, 2003.

Axelrad, Daniel, et al. "Dose-Response Relationship of Prenatal Mercury Exposure and IQ." *Environmental Health Perspectives* 115 (2007): 609–15.

Bodansky, Daniel. "Scientific Uncertainty and the Precautionary Principle." *Environment* 33 (1991): 4–44.

———. "The Precautionary Principle in U.S. Environmental Law." In *Interpreting the Precautionary Principle*, edited by Tim O'Riordan and James Cameron. London: Earthscan, 1994.

Boyd, William. "Genealogies of Risk: Searching for Safety, 1930s–1970s." *Ecological Law Quarterly* 39 (2012): 895–988.

Brody, Jane. "Don't Lose Sight of Real, Everyday Risks." *New York Times*, October 9, 2001.

Bro-Rasmussen, Finn. "Risk, Uncertainties, and Precautions in Chemical Legislation." In *Precaution: Environmental Science and Preventative Public Policy*, edited by Joel Tickner, 87–102. Washington: Island Press, 2003.

Browne, Marilyn, et al., "Cancer Incidence and Asbestos in Drinking Water, Town of Woodstock, New York, 1980–1998." *Environmental Research* 98 (2005): 224–32.

Callicott, Baird. *In Defense of the Land Ethic: Essays in Environmental Philosophy*. Albany: SUNY Press, 1989.

Carson, Rachel. *Silent Spring*. Boston: Houghton Mifflin, 1962.

Centers for Disease Control and Prevention. "DES History." Last updated June 1, 2015. www.cdc.gov/des/consumers/about/history.html.

Chlorine Chemical Council v. Environmental Protection Agency, 206 F.3d 1286 (D.C. Circuit 2000).

Cranor, Carl and Kurt Nutting. "Scientific and Legal Standards of Statistical Evidence in Toxic Tort and Discrimination Suits." *Law and Philosophy* 9 (1990): 115–56.

Cross, Frank. "Paradoxical Perils of the Precautionary Principle." *Washington and Lee Law Review* 53 (1996): 851–925.

Department of Health and Human Services Working Group. "Report on Cancer Risks Associated with the Ingestion of Asbestos." *Environmental Health Perspectives* 72 (1987): 253–65.

Eckersley, Robyn. *Environmentalism and Political Theory: Toward an Ecocentric Approach*. Albany: State University of New York Press, 1992.

Environmental Protection Agency. "DDT, a Review of Scientific and Economic Aspects of the Decision to Ban Its Use as a Pesticide." Prepared for the Committee on Appropriations of the U.S. House of Representatives. EPA-540/1-75-022, July 1975. www2.epa.gov/aboutepa/ddt-regulatory-history-brief-survey-1975.

———. "National Primary Drinking Water Regulations: Arsenic and Clarifications to Compliance and New Source Contaminants Monitoring." *Federal Register* 66, nos. 14 and 78 (2001).

———. "Quantitative Health Risk Assessment for Particulate Matter." EPA-452/R-10-005, June 2010. www3.epa.gov/ttn/naaqs/standards/pm/data/PM_RA_FINAL_June_2010.pdf.

———. "Regulatory Impact Analysis for the Final Mercury and Air Toxics Standards." EPA-452/R-11-011, December 2011. www3.epa.gov/mats/pdfs/20111221MATSfinalRIA.pdf.

———. "Assessing Human Health Risk from Pesticides." Last updated September 30, 2015. http://epa.gov/pesticide-science-and-assessing-pesticide-risks/assessing-human-health-risk-pesticides.

———. "Health Risks of Radon." Last updated October 22, 2015. http://epa.gov/radon/health-risk-radon.

———. "DDT: A Brief History and Status." Last updated November 5, 2015. http://epa.gov/ingredients-used-pesticide-products/ddt-brief-history-and-status.

Ethyl Corp. v. EPA, 541 F. 2d 1 (D.C. Circuit 1976).

European Environment Agency. "Late Lessons from Early Warnings: The Precautionary Principle, 1896–2000." *Environmental Issue Report*, No. 22 (2001).

Fisher, Elizabeth. "Precaution, Precaution Everywhere: Developing a 'Common Understanding' of the Precautionary Principle in the European Community." *Maastricht Journal of European and Comparative Law* 9 (2002): 7–28.

Food and Drug Administration. "Interim Guidance on the Voluntary Labeling of Milk and Milk Products from Cows That Have Not Been Treated with Recombinant Bovine Somatotropin." *Federal Register* 59 (February 10, 1994). https://gpo.gov/fdsys/pkg/FR-1994-02-10/html/94-3214.htm.

———. "Report on the FDA's Review of the Safety of Recombinant Bovine Somatotropin." April 2009. Last updated July 28, 2014. http://fda.gov/AnimalVeterinary/SafetyHealth/ProductSafetyInformation/ucm130321.htm.

———. "Food and Drug Administration Continues to Study BPA." March 2012. Last updated January 29, 2015. http://fda.gov/ForConsumers/ConsumerUpdates/ucm297954.htm.

Gamble, John. "Risk of Gastrointestinal Cancers from Inhalation and Ingestion of Asbestos." *Regulatory Toxicology and Pharmacology* 52 (2008): S124–53.

Gardiner, Stephen. "A Core Precautionary Principle." *Journal of Political Philosophy* 14 (2006): 33–60.

Global Development Research Center. "Wingspread Statement on the Precautionary Principle." January 1998. http://gdrc.org/u-gov/precaution-3.html.

Goklany, Indur. "Applying the Precautionary Principle in a Broader Context." In *Rethinking Risk and the Precautionary Principle*, edited by Julian Morris. Oxford: Butterworth-Heinemann, 2000.

———. *The Precautionary Principle: A Critical Appraisal of Environmental Risk Assessment*. Washington: Cato Institute, 2001.

Goodin, Robert. *Protecting the Vulnerable: A Re-Analysis of Our Social Responsibilities*. Chicago: University of Chicago Press, 1985.

Government Publishing Office. "Food Quality Protection Act, H.R.1627." *104th Congress Public Law 170*, August 3, 1996. https://congress.gov/bill/104th-congress/house-bill/1627/text.

Graham, John. "The Role of Precaution in Risk Assessment and Management: An American's View." Prepared for The US, Europe, Precaution and Risk Management: A Comparative Case Study Analysis of the Management of Risk in a Complex World. January 11–12, 2002. http://whitehouse.gov/omb/inforeg/eu_speech.html.

Hansson, Sven. "Decision Making Under Great Uncertainty." *Philosophy of the Social Sciences* 26 (1996): 369–86.

———. "Ethical Criteria for Risk Acceptance." *Erkenntnis* 59 (2003): 291–309.

Harding, Ronnie and Elizabeth Fisher. "The Precautionary Principle: Toward a Deliberative, Transdisciplinary Problem-Solving Process." In *Perspectives on the Precautionary Principle*, edited by Ronnie Harding and Elizabeth Fisher. Annandale: Federation Press, 1999.

Harris, John and Søren Holm. "Extending Human Lifespan and the Precautionary Paradox." *Journal of Medicine and Philosophy* 27 (2002): 355–68.

Hartzell-Nichols, Lauren. *A Climate of Risk: Precautionary Principles, Catastrophes, and Climate Change*. New York: Routledge, 2017.

Hayenhjelm, Madeleine and Jonathan Wolff. "The Moral Problem of Risk Impositions: A Survey of the Literature." *European Journal of Philosophy* 20 (2012): E26–51.

Hill, Austin. "The Environment and Disease: Association or Causation?" *Proceedings of the Royal Society of Medicine* 58 (1965): 295–300.

Howard, Philip. *The Death of Common Sense: How Law Is Suffocating America*. New York: Random House, 1994.

International Dairy Foods Association v. Boggs, 622 F. 3d 628 (6th Circuit 2010).

Jackson v. Johns-Manville Sales Corp., 781 F.2d 394 (5th Circuit 1986).

Jordan, Andrew and Timothy O'Riordan. "The Precautionary Principle in Contemporary Environmental Policy and Politics." In *Protecting Public Health and The Environment*, edited by Carolyn Raffensperger and Joel Tickner. Washington: Island Press, 1999.

Keynes, John Maynard. "The General Theory of Employment." *Quarterly Journal of Economics* 51 (1937): 209–23.

Kitman, Jamie Lincoln. "The Secret History of Lead." *The Nation*, March 2, 2002. http://thenation.com/article/secret-history-lead.

Knight, Frank. *Risk, Uncertainty, and Profit*. Boston: Houghton Mifflin Co., 1921.

Kovarik, Bill. "Charles F. Kettering and the 1921 Discovery of Tetraethyl Lead in the Context of Technological Alternatives." Presented to the *Society of Automotive Engineers Fuels and Lubricants Conference*, Baltimore, Maryland, 1994.

Krewski, Daniel, et al. *Reanalysis of the Harvard Six Cities Study and the American Cancer Society Study of Particulate Air Pollution and Mortality*. Cambridge: Health Effects Institute, 2000.

Layzer, Judith. *The Environmental Case: Translating Values Into Policy*, 3rd edition. Washington: CQ Press, 2012.

Leggett, Jeremy. *Global Warming: A Greenpeace Report*. Oxford: Oxford University Press, 1990.

Leopold, Aldo. *A Sand County Almanac*. New York: Oxford University Press, 1949.

Lewens, Tim, ed. *Risk: Philosophical Perspectives*. New York: Routledge, 2007.

Loeb, Alan. "Birth of the Kettering Doctrine: Fordism, Sloanism and the Discovery of Tetraethyl Lead." *Business and Economic History* 24 (1995): 72–87.

Lowrance, William. *Of Acceptable Risk: Science and the Determination of Safety*. Los Altos: W. Kaufmann, 1976.

Luckey, Thomas. *Radiation Hormesis*. Boca Raton: CRC Press, 1991.

Maguire, Steve and Jaye Ellis. "Redistributing the Burden of Scientific Uncertainty: Implications of the Precautionary Principle for State and Non-State Actors." *Global Governance* 11 (2005): 505–26.

Majone, Giandomenico. "What Price Safety? The Precautionary Principle and Its Policy Implications." *Journal of Common Market Studies* 40 (2002): 89–109.

Manson, Neil. "Formulating the Precautionary Principle." *Environmental Ethics* 24 (2002): 263–74.

Markoitz, Gerald and David Rosner. *Deceit and Denial: The Deadly Politics of Industrial Pollution*. Berkeley: University of California Press, 2002.

McCarthy, David. "Rights, Explanation, and Risks." *Ethics* 107 (1997): 205–25.

McKinnon, Catriona. *Climate Change and Future Justice: Precaution, Compensation, and Triage*. New York: Routledge, 2012.

Miller, Henry and Gregory Conko. "Genetically Modified Fear and the International Regulation of Biotechnology." In *Rethinking Risk and the Precautionary Principle*, edited by Julian Morris. Oxford: Butterworth-Heinemann, 2000.

———. "The Perils of Precaution: Why Regulators' 'Precautionary Principle' Is Doing More Harm Than Good." *Policy Review* 107 (2001): 25–39.

Morgan-Knapp, Christopher. "Non-Consequentialist Precaution." *Ethical Theory and Moral Practice* 18 (2015): 785–97.

Morris, Julian. "Defining the Precautionary Principle." In *Rethinking Risk and the Precautionary Principle*, edited by Julian Morris. Oxford: Butterworth-Heinemann, 2000.

Moulton, Libby. "Labeling Milk from Cows Not Treated with rBST: Legal in All 50 States as of September 29th, 2010." *Columbia Science and Technology Law Review*, October 28, 2010. http://stlr.org/2010/10/28/labeling-milk-from-cows-not-treated-with-rbst-legal-in-all-50-states-as-of-september-29th-2010/.

Munthe, Christian. *The Price of Precaution and the Ethics of Risk*. New York: Springer, 2011.

Næss, Arne. "The Shallow and the Deep, Long-Range Ecology Movement: A Summary." *Inquiry* 16 (1973): 95–100.

National Cancer Institute. "Radon and Cancer." Last updated December 6, 2011. http://cancer.gov/about-cancer/causes-prevention/risk/substances/radon/radon-fact-sheet.

National Public Radio. "Court OKs Hormone-Free Label on Dairy Products in Ohio." October 1, 2010. http://npr.org/sections/health-shots/2010/10/01/130270131/court-give-hormone-free-label-on-dairy-products-an-ok-in-ohio.

National Research Council. *Understanding Risk: Informing Decisions in a Democratic Society*. Washington: National Academy Press, 1996.

———. *Arsenic in Drinking Water*. Washington: National Academy Press, 1999.

———. *Toxicological Effects of Methylmercury*. Washington: National Academy Press, 2000.

———. *Risk and Decisions about Disposition of Transuranic and High-Level Radioactive Waste*. Washington: National Academies Press, 2005.

———. *Science and Decisions: Advancing Risk Assessment*. Washington: National Academies Press, 2009.

National Resource Defense Council. "The Truth about Tap." Last updated January 5, 2016. https://nrdc.org/stories/truth-about-tap.

Nozick, Robert. *Anarchy, State, and Utopia*. New York: Basic Books, 1974.

O'Brien, Mary. "Alternatives Assessment and the Precautionary Principle." In *Protecting Public Health and the Environment*, edited by Carolyn Raffensperger and Joel Tickner. Washington: Island Press, 1999.

Office of the Inspector General. "The EPA's Fiscal Year 2014 Management Challenges." Washington: Environmental Protection Agency, May 28, 2014.

Oreskes, Naomi and Erik Conway. *Merchants of Doubt: How a Handful of Scientists Obscured the Truth on Issues from Tobacco Smoke to Global Warming*. New York: Bloomsbury Publishing, 2010.

O'Riordan, Timothy and Andrew Jordan. "The Precautionary Principle in Contemporary Environmental Politics." *Environmental Values* 4 (1995): 191–212.

Percival, Robert and Christopher Schroeder. *Environmental Law: Statutory and Case Supplement 2012–2013*. New York: Wolters Kluwer Law and Business, 2012.

Percival, Robert, et al. *Environmental Regulation: Law, Science, and Policy*, 6th edition. New York: Aspen Publishers, 2009.

Perera, Frederica. "Environment and Cancer: Who Are Susceptible?" *Science* 278 (1997): 1068–73.

Peterson, Martin. "The Precautionary Principle Is Incoherent." *Risk Analysis* 26 (2006): 595–601.

Pielke, Roger, Jr. *The Honest Broker: Making Sense of Science in Policy and Politics*. Cambridge: Cambridge University Press, 2007.

Pope, C. Arden, et al. "Lung Cancer, Cardiopulmonary Mortality, and Long-Term Exposure to Fine Particulate Air Pollution." *Journal of the American Medical Association* 287 (2002): 1132–41.

Program on Breast Cancer and Environmental Risk Factors, Cornell University. "Consumer Concerns about Hormones in Food." June 2000. Last updated May 2, 2003. http://envirocancer.cornell.edu/factsheet/diet/fs37.hormones.cfm.

Public Citizen Health Research Group v. Young, 831 F.2d 1108 (D.C. Circuit 1987).

Raffensperger, Carolyn and Joel Tickner, eds. *Protecting Public Health and the Environment*. Washington: Island Press, 1999.

Rawls, John. *A Theory of Justice*. Cambridge: Harvard University Press, 1971.

Reserve Mining Company v. EPA, 514 F. 2d 492 (8th Circuit 1975).

Rolston, Holmes. *Environmental Ethics: Duties to and Values in the Natural World*. Philadelphia: Temple University Press, 1988.

Rubin, Beverly. "Bisphenol A: An Endocrine Disruptor with Widespread Exposure and Multiple Effects." *Journal of Steroid Biochemistry and Molecular Biology* 127 (2011): 27–34.

Sagoff, Mark. *Economy of the Earth: Philosophy, Law, and the Environment*. Cambridge: Cambridge University Press, 1988.

Samoli, Evangelia, et al. "Estimating the Exposure: Response Relationships between Particulate Matter and Mortality within the APHEA Multicity Project." *Environmental Health Perspectives* 113 (2005): 88–95.

Sandin, Per. "Dimensions of the Precautionary Principle." *Human and Ecological Risk Assessment* 5 (1999): 889–907.

———. "Commonsense Precaution and Varieties of the Precautionary Principle." In *Risk: Philosophical Perspectives*, edited by Tim Lewens. New York: Routledge, 2007.

Schoeny, Rita. "Use of Genetic Toxicology Data in U.S. EPA Risk Assessment: The Mercury Study Report as an Example." *Environmental Health Perspectives* 104, no. 3 (1996): 663–73.

Schurman, Rachel and William Munro. *Fighting for the Future of Food: Activists versus Agribusiness in the Struggle over Biotechnology*. Minneapolis: University of Minnesota Press, 2010.

Sekizawa, Jun. "Low-Dose Effects of Bisphenol A: A Serious Threat to Human Health?" *Journal of Toxicological Sciences* 33 (2008): 389–403.

Sexton, Ken and Dale Hattis. "Assessing Cumulative Health Risks from Exposure to Environmental Mixtures: Three Fundamental Questions." *Environmental Health Perspectives* 115 (2007): 825–32.

Sharpe, Richard. "Is It Time to End Concerns over the Estrogenic Effects of Bisphenol A?" *Toxicological Sciences* 114 (2010): 1–4.

Shrader-Frechette, Kristin. *Taking Action, Saving Lives: Our Duties to Protect Environmental and Public Health*. Oxford: Oxford University Press, 2007.

Soule, Edward. "Assessing the Precautionary Principle." *Public Affairs Quarterly* 14 (2000): 309–28.

Steel, Daniel. *Philosophy and the Precautionary Principle: Science, Evidence, and Environmental Policy*. Cambridge: Cambridge University Press, 2015.

Stone, Christopher. "Is There a Precautionary Principle?" *Environmental Law Reporter* 31 (2001): 10790–9.

Sunstein, Cass. *Risk and Reason: Safety, Law, and the Environment*. Cambridge: Cambridge University Press, 2002.

———. *Laws of Fear: Beyond the Precautionary Principle*. Cambridge: Cambridge University Press, 2005.

———. "Moral Heuristics and Risk." In *Risk: Philosophical Perspectives*, edited by Tim Lewens. New York: Routledge, 2007.

Szentkirályi, Levente. "A Rights-Based Conception of the Precautionary Principle." In *Handbook of Philosophy and Public Policy*, edited by David Boonin. New York: Palgrave Macmillan, 2018.

Tavernise, Sabrina. "FDA Makes It Official: BPA Can't Be Used in Baby Bottles and Cups." *New York Times*, July 17, 2012. http://nytimes.com/2012/07/18/science/fda-bans-bpa-from-baby-bottles-and-sippy-cups.html?_r=0.

Thue-Vasquez, Diane. "Genetic Engineering and Food Labeling: A Continuing Controversy." *San Joaquin Agricultural Law Review* 10 (2000): 77–119.

Tickner, Joel. "A Map Toward Precautionary Decision Making." In *Protecting Public Health and the Environment*, edited by Carolyn Raffensperger and Joel Tickner. Washington: Island Press, 1999.

———, ed. *Precaution, Environmental Science, and Preventive Public Policy*. Washington: Island Press, 2003.

Toft, Peter, et al. "Asbestos in Drinking-Water." *Critical Reviews in Environmental Control* 14 (1984): 151–97.

Turvey, Calum and Eliza Mojduszka. "The Precautionary Principle and the Law of Unintended Consequences." *Food Policy* 30 (2005): 145–61.

United Nations. *Universal Declaration of Human Rights*. General Assembly Resolution 217A (III), December 10, 1948.

———. *Universal Declaration on the Eradication of Hunger and Malnutrition*. General Assembly Resolution 3348 (XXIX), December 17, 1974.

United Nations Environment Programme. *Rio Declaration on Environment and Development*, Principle 15, UN Conference on Environment and Development, Rio de Janeiro, Brazil, June 14, 1992.

United Nations Millennium Ecosystem Assessment. "Living Beyond Our Means: Natural Assets and Human Well-being." Statement of Millennium Assessment Board, 2005.

Vilkka, Leena. *The Intrinsic Value of Nature*. Amsterdam: Rodopi, 1997.

Vogel, Sarah. "The Politics of Plastics: The Making and Unmaking of Bisphenol A Safety." *American Journal of Public Health* 99 (2009): S559–66.

Vogt, Donna. *The Delaney Clause Effects on Pesticide Policy*. Washington: Congressional Research Service, 1995.

Wargo, John. *Our Children's Toxic Legacy: How Science and Law Fail to Protect Us from Pesticides*, 2nd edition. New Haven: Yale University Press, 1998.

Whiteside, Kerry. *Precautionary Politics: Principle and Practice in Confronting Environmental Risk*. Cambridge: MIT Press, 2006.

Wildavsky, Aaron. *But Is It True? A Citizen's Guide to Environmental Health and Safety Issues*. Cambridge: Harvard University Press, 1995.

———. "Trial and Error versus Trial without Error." In *Rethinking Risk and the Precautionary Principle*, edited by Julian Morris. Oxford: Butterworth-Heinemann, 2000.

World Health Organization. "Asbestos in Drinking Water: Background Document for Development of WHO Guidelines for Drinking Water Quality." In *Guidelines for Drinking-Water Quality*, 2nd edition, Vol. 2. Geneva: World Health Organization, 1996 [2003].

World Health Organization and International Programme on Chemical Safety. *Asbestos and Other Natural Mineral Fibres*. Geneva: World Health Organization, 1986.

Wright, Peter, et al. "Twenty-Five Years of Dioxin Cancer Risk Assessment." *Natural Resources and Environment* 19 (2005): 31–4.

3 Uncertain Environmental Threats as Objective Wrongs

A plausible rights-based defense of the precautionary principle requires a firm normative foundation. But what is the justification for constraining the rights of emitters to expose others to uncertain threats of environmental harm—what can justify their duty to take reasonable preventative measures to mitigate the possibility for avoidable and undeserved[1] harm when outcome and probability uncertainty prevail, and thus when their emissions may prove in the end to be harmless? Chapter 3 begins to construct the argument that it is the disregard of the moral status of those who are put in potential harm's way, and thus flouting the demands of reciprocity, that renders one's failure to exercise due care objectionable and makes one liable to both blame and punishment.

Section 3.1 reconciles the difference between assigning responsibility for neglecting to exercise due care, which inherently is backward-looking (concerns retroactive appraisals of one's actions), with the duty to exercise due care, which is inherently forward-looking (aims to alter one's future actions). The aim of this section is to stipulate that although this book consistently shifts between talk of duties and responsibility under conditions of uncertainty, this should not be understood as conflating these discrete claims and concepts. It is consistent to speak simultaneously of one's duty to strive to mitigate the potential for uncorroborated harm to others and of one's culpability for being derelict in discharging this duty. Section 3.2 introduces the deontological argument for exercising precaution and explores its Kantian foundation, claiming that for many uncertain environmental threats, our failure to strive to prevent putting others in the way of possible harm constitutes wrongdoing. This is because to neglect to exercise due care, even when the consequences of our actions and the probability that these consequences may injure others is there, is to disregard the equal moral standing of others by gambling with their welfare and projecting one's own perceptions of risk and risk tolerance on others by deciding oneself whether the threat is acceptable (and, thus, whether exposing others to the threat is permissible). Section 3.3, then, defends one of the controversial premises of this argument, namely that exposing others to uncertain possibilities of harm violates their autonomy. Finally, Section 3.4 alludes to the context-dependent nature of our duties of due care under uncertainty (which is the focus of Chapter 5) by noting that not all uncertain threats of harm are alike. This acknowledgement requires distinguishing between having reasons to exercise precaution and having an obligation to do so—which presupposes that we have *compelling* reasons to strive to mitigate the potential for harm. And while Section 3.4 explores how we can reasonably infer or intuit morally relevant considerations about the potential, albeit uncertain, danger to others that our actions entail—reasons that can then cement or attenuate our duty to strive to avoid exposing others to these threats—it also underscores that such subjective inferences are tenuous at best and cannot absolve us of the universal obligation to exercise due care.

3.1 On the Association Between Obligation and Culpability

It should be clarified at the outset to avoid confusion that although the aim here is to justify one's duty to take reasonable precautionary measures to strive to prevent exposing others to possible harm (that is, to exercise precaution with what Nagel terms "decision[s] under uncertainty"[2]), the following discussion makes consistent reference to one's moral responsibility (or culpability) for failing to exercise this mandatory due care.[3] Having a duty to avoid putting others in potential harm's way is forward-looking or proactive, intended to shape one's future behavior, whereas moral responsibility is inherently backward-looking, or retroactive, consisting of the appraisal of one's past actions and the assignment of blame for past wrongdoings—which may then entail subsequent obligations of liability to make right these wrongs (e.g., compensating those whom one has wronged). Having a duty and being responsible are substantively different normative claims.[4] However, switching from talk of the former to talk of the latter should not be understood as conflating these claims. For moral culpability follows from doing wrong by others (assuming there are no conditions that excuse one's wrongful action), and that which is wrong or worthy of reproach is behavior we should generally refrain from engaging in.

There are salient exceptions to this. For instance, one may act with the best of intentions and with the interests of another in mind, but may unintentionally cause harm to those she aims to help. In such cases, although a person may commit a wrong, she may deserve being excused of culpability. Consider the Good Samaritan but poor swimmer, who wades into the shallow pond with the intention of rescuing the drowning child and whose efforts, however noble, inadvertently lead to the child's death.[5] Similarly, consider the Good Samaritan who mistakes the interests of a person he aims to help—for example, forcefully preventing a passerby from crossing a faulty bridge, only to learn upon knocking him firmly to the ground that the passerby had knowingly intended to cross the bridge.[6] In the first example, one causes another lethal harm, while in the second example, one thwarts the autonomy of another. Let us suppose that in both cases the Good Samaritan could have and should have known better: our weak swimmer perhaps should have heeded his limitations and tried to assist the child by extending a large branch for her to grab hold of, and our tackler perhaps should have taken the bridge walker's arm to warn him of the danger instead of physically restraining him. Yet even if we grant that it was reasonable to expect our Good Samaritans to have known better and to have acted in ways that did not harm or violate the rights of others, in both scenarios, the harmful actions, the wrongs committed, seem excusable, given the well-placed intentions.

Analogously, it is possible for one to be blameworthy without committing a wrong. Consider, for instance, one's decision to drive his car while inebriated or one's failure to properly maintain and service his car (say, failing to ensure that the brakes of the vehicle are in good repair). Even if the actions of the drunk driver and the negligent driver never injure others, because they put innocent pedestrians and other drivers at greater and avoidable risk of harm, their actions are worthy of blame: they *are* still culpable. Similarly, consider the individual who deliberately tries to harm another but fails to do so in the process. We might envision the disillusioned, radical environmental activist, for instance, hammering spikes into trees destined for logging with the intention of damaging the logging company's machinery or the sawmill's processing equipment and of physically injuring the loggers in an attempt to draw media attention to the destruction of wilderness. Yet let us suppose that our activist is a novice and mistakes how to properly position the spikes, such that none of the rods she hammers into the trees are struck during the felling of the trees and the processing of the lumber. Thus, the activist causes no physical injury or property damage. But her malicious intent still warrants holding her culpable.[7] Now the drunk driver, the negligent driver, and the activist are not culpable for the *outcomes* of their respective actions: for in each scenario, the consequences prove harmless. However, they are culpable for maliciously or negligently ignoring the welfare and interests of others, failing to discharge their obligations to take reasonable measure to prevent causing others harm.

Exceptions notwithstanding, I take it to be uncontroversial to claim that if one were culpable for some harmful outcome, then she should have acted otherwise—implying that she *had* a (*pro tanto*) obligation *to act otherwise* and that she retains the duty to refrain from performing this blameworthy action in the future. In short, if one would be blameworthy for performing some action, *A*, then one has an obligation *not* to do *A*,[8] and this forward-looking duty takes shape before culpability may retroactively be assigned by considering the likely consequences of doing *A* before performing the action. And yet in the case of creating uncertain threats, as is argued in Section 3.3, even when the *de facto* consequences of these threats remain scientifically indeterminate and may prove to be benign, one would be culpable for failing to exercise due care in performing a potentially harmful action. This means that one has a duty *not* to fail to exercise due care—an obligation, that is, to take reasonable measures to prevent exposing others to potential harm. Hence, it is plausible to speak concurrently of a forward-looking moral obligation (of due care) and a backward-looking moral responsibility (for failing to act in accord with this duty).[9]

In developing a comprehensive theory of moral responsibility as answerability,[10] Scanlon makes a similar acknowledgement, noting the simultaneous prospective and retroactive nature of moral permissibility. While we usually think of permissibility as regarding the justification one may have to perform an action—that is, as "a precursor to a decision" establishing how an individual should act—Scanlon suggests that the question whether some action or another is morally permissible "can also be asked retrospectively, or hypothetically, about the way a person behaved on some past, or imagined, occasion."[11] And in framing the question of permissibility in this backward-looking way, as whether a person's past act was permissible—that is, whether the person acted permissibly (given the details of the circumstance in which the action was performed)—our examination *both* confirms forward-looking duties required by what we estimate to be morally impermissible and gestures toward judgments of blame or culpability insofar as our examination yields reasons why the action in question was or was not permissible. In this way, questions of permissibility at once both shape our deliberations about (the acceptability of) future actions and inform the standards by which we appraise (the acceptability of) past actions.[12]

3.2 From Moral Equality to Duties of Due Care

Existing theories of moral responsibility either claim that uncertain threats are morally permissible or they hold that uncertain threats are not permissible but then do not offer a sufficient explanation of why actors who create uncertain threats may be held culpable. Arguments from moral luck, on the other hand, would have us believe that although the consequences of uncertain threats may be morally wrong, actors should not be held culpable for these threats or harms they create, given the unavoidable ignorance that prevailing uncertainty entails. To the contrary, theories in the ethics of risk imply that uncertain threats are trivial (i.e., highly improbable or would result in only negligible harm) or that these unquantifiable threats should be presumed to be safe (i.e., treated as reasonable risks)—concluding in either case that causing these threats is morally permissible. Concerned with these analyses and their treatments of uncertainty, this section argues that for many uncertain threats of environmental harm, failure to take reasonable preventative measures to mitigate the potential for harm to public health—failure, that is, to exercise due care under conditions of uncertainty—constitutes wrongdoing.

The argument that emitters do wrong by performing endangering actions and exposing others to uncertain threats of environmental harm without first taking reasonable precautionary measures to try to safeguard others from possible harm is founded on two central and broadly Kantian assumptions:

P_1: All persons (*ceteris paribus*) have equal moral standing.

P_2: This equal moral standing requires that we respect the autonomy of others.

The first assumption is uncontroversial and is treated as axiomatic. The second assumption deserves some explanation. And while a thorough exploration of Kant's complex and nuanced deontology—which is rooted in his teleological theories of human nature and history, his epistemological account of moral truth and enlightenment, and his metaethical and normative theories about moral agency—exceeds the scope of this discussion, several tangential clarifications are in order to bear out the premium Kant places on moral equality and reciprocity.

3.2.1 A Kantian Commitment to Equality

There are various ways to understand the complex notion of autonomy. Some maintain that autonomy depends on the capacity to create and act on one's volitions.[13] Tabling the significance of acting from higher-order interests, others stress that autonomy requires no more than the absence of external interference to one's choices and actions.[14] Still others insist that the capacity for autonomous action is defined by a robust and meaningful set of alternatives.[15] The conception of autonomy we glean from Kant, which is the notion of autonomy this argument adopts, emphasizes the capacities for self-determination and moral enlightenment.[16]

The requisite of self-authorship assumes the capacity to formulate and to act on (higher-order) volitions and, thus, also assumes the absence of unjustified external interference.[17] This is evident from the importance Kantian deontology places on exercising the ability to choose to act as morality demands and the idea that one's choice to act *from* moral duty must be self-determined and purposeful.[18]

This is a key requisite for Kant, because he views human beings as inherently self-interested and impulse driven; we are, says Kant, beings of original sin, inherently "warped,"[19] and born into the world with the capacity to do evil (or, more precisely, with the capacity to *choose* to do evil). And while this is the source of the moral problems that afflict us and encumber our interactions with others, this capacity is also what permits us to improve ourselves and to seek moral enlightenment.[20] For we have the choice *not* to do evil. Kant emphasizes that one's moral maturation is dependent on one's having the choice to promote her rationality, to pursue moral enlightenment, to act *from* her moral duty[21] and that these choices must come from within and cannot be coerced from without.[22] Accordingly, he claims that the authority of the categorical imperative and one's moral obligations "can only be imposed by practical reason, acting without any external constraint"[23]—made plain by his exhortation that we should "Dare to be wise!" (*Sapere aude!*), by which Kant means that we should all have the "courage to use [our] *own* understanding"[24] (employ our freedom of conscience). In this way, we must internalize, so to speak, the demands of the categorical imperative and must voluntarily hold ourselves to these universal moral laws.

We cannot be coerced to act morally (though coercive laws do prove necessary) because to act morally means to act for the proper reasons, which for Kant is but one: namely, because morality requires it.[25] This notion of acting *from* or *for the sake of* duty[26] implies that one acts morally only when he complies with the moral laws because he recognizes that it is his moral responsibility to do so. Kant is decisive on this point because moral laws are only universal, and thus only law-like if they provide everyone the same objective motivation to comply with their demands.[27] Conversely, with "subjective conditions of choice"—whereby individuals are motivated by their discrete, subjective "faculties of desire," their diverse and subjective desires and interests—moral laws have no such objective grounding.[28] That is, if grounded in subjective necessity, the demands of morality will be subject to "endless" exceptions whenever moral laws (invariably) fail to satisfy the personal inclinations of some.[29] Yet if such exceptions are granted, there can be no universal law, since the very concept of law would, then, suffer contradiction. Convinced that we can improve upon our imperfect human nature, Kant insists that if we heed the counsel of our rationality, we will not only comprehend but also voluntarily embrace the demands of the categorical imperative, freely and conscientiously choosing not to bring evil upon others—a process of moral enlightenment that is grounded in Kant's teleology.

Briefly, according to Kant, humanity's purpose, and hence the purpose of (human) history, is to allow human beings to learn from and gain the wisdom of previous generations so as to make progress toward achieving their full natural capacities: to become, in a word, rational.[30] More specifically, our *telos* is to champion freedom: to overcome the brute impulses, instincts, and desires that constrain us and incite antagonism toward our fellows, and to act instead from reason and with subsequent regard for the moral standing of others. Accordingly, this is why Kant insists that as we become more rational, and thus as we progress toward the implementation of the universal principle of right—that is, the universal rule of law that recognizes the intrinsic worth, freedom, equality, and self-determination of all human beings[31]—our *telos* also entails instituting a constitutional republic.[32] For it is only when we achieve true enlightenment that we are genuinely free; it is only then, in recognizing the warrant for and espousing the demands of the categorical imperative and voluntarily willing universal moral law, that everything we do, *we do freely*.[33] This is the essence of the self-authorship or autonomy that Kant prizes and that is the cornerstone of the constitutional republic he envisions: where moral law is voluntarily and deliberately obeyed by enlightened and morally mature citizens, who comply with the rule of law because they recognize that it is both rational and thus morally compulsory for them to do so.

Paralleling the requisite of self-authorship, our capacity for moral enlightenment is also central to the conception of autonomy we glean from Kant, as it enables us to discern what moral obligations we have toward others. Treating as axiomatic the belief that all individuals have the capacity to reason,[34] Kant maintains that what morality demands of us can be discerned via rational reflection, which reveals objective *a priori* moral truths on which our rationality should compel us to act. And among the universal moral laws that we learn in this way is that all individuals are morally equal and that this equality requires that all be afforded the same rights that prevent others from transgressing against them. However, Kant is equally explicit elsewhere that our *a priori* truths are judged to be objectively true through our direct interactions with the external world—including in no small measure our corporeal interactions and relations with our fellows—and our subsequent achievement of morally relevant *a posteriori* knowledge.[35] Our subjective interactions with others would reveal to us, for instance, that individuals often make great sacrifices to achieve their interests and ends, whose pursuit can be undermined by the self-interested actions of others. Our awareness of this, coupled with our *a priori* knowledge, demands that we take the interests and equal rights of others seriously and that we refrain from violating their capacity for self-determination.[36]

And to respect one's capacity for self-determination requires that in my outward behavior toward another person and in my reflective deliberations about the reasons I have to perform or to refrain from performing a given action, I regard him as an end in himself and show him mutual respect. Put differently, it is to "honor his status as an independent center of value [and] as an originator of projects that demand my respect"[37]—"to see the situation of others from their point of view, from the perspective of their conception of their good; and in our being prepared to give [sound] reasons for our actions whenever the interests of others [may be] materially affected."[38] Accordingly, within the context of uncertain threats of environmental harm, to treat others as ends demands that we exercise due care to try to prevent putting them in the way of possible injury. (More on this below.)

3.2.2 Argument for Due Care in Brief

With P_1 and P_2 as our starting assumptions—that all persons have equal moral standing and that this equal moral standing demands that we respect their autonomy—the plausibility of the thesis that *to fail to exercise due care to prevent exposing others to uncertain threats of environmental harm is to commit a wrongdoing* rests on the following considerations:

P_3: To expose others to uncertain possibilities of harm (that is, to gamble with their welfare) is to fail to treat them as ends in themselves.

P_4: To fail to exercise due care to prevent exposing others to uncertain threats of environmental harm is to gamble with their welfare.

P_5: Hence, to fail to exercise due care to prevent exposing others to uncertain threats of environmental harm is to fail to treat them as ends in themselves.

P_6: To knowingly fail to treat others as ends in themselves is to commit wrongdoing, rendering the actor liable to blame and punishment.[39]

P_7: That it is unknown whether uncertain environmental threats will injure others or expose them to unreasonable risks neither excuses one of culpability nor justifies one's endangering action.

Thus, to fail to exercise due care to prevent exposing others to uncertain threats of environmental harm is to commit wrongdoing.

Thus, to fail to exercise due care under uncertainty is to be liable to blame and punishment.

Therefore, we have a *pro tanto* duty to exercise due care under conditions of uncertainty.[40]

This argument turns on P_3 and P_7, and the remainder of this chapter clarifies the former, whereas Chapter 4 engages the latter. However, a few initial clarifications are in order.

As an aside on P_5, the reader should note that precautionary measures that would satisfy one's obligations of due care are context dependent and are thus diverse. They may range, for instance, from informing the public about the uncertain threats they create and disclosing pertinent information about the possibility for harm, to proactively striving to prevent exposing traditionally vulnerable populations to uncertain threats (as with industry's proactive decision to pull plastic baby bottles and baby food packaging products containing bisphenol A (BPA) and altering their manufacturing processes to offer BPA-free versions of many of their consumer goods[41]), to conducting basic toxicity tests to try to discern the actual health effects of exposure and disclosing this information to the public, to taking alternative courses of action that do not entail indeterminate threats (for example, substituting substances whose potential for harm is scientifically uncorroborated with those whose effects of exposure have been verified[42]). This will be the focus of Chapter 5, which explores what a reasonable standard of due care under uncertainty may consist in and which demonstrates how the flexibility of the proposed standard of due care is one of the key virtues of this book's defense of precautionary risk regulation.

With regard to P_6, an adequate discussion of what punishment would consist of exceeds the scope of this book. Scholarship in normative ethics conventionally dismisses unquantifiable and uncorroborated threats of harm as morally innocuous, and the purpose of this project is to demonstrate that we can make sense of imposing restrictions on actions whose effects we cannot foresee and whose probability of causing harm we cannot estimate. Once this argument is substantiated, subsequent arguments can be made about how to hold emitters culpable for neglecting to exercise due care. It is important to note, however, as Chapter 4.4 and Chapter 5 explain, what these emitters are liable to will vary across different contexts and actors: because the strength of one's duty of due care is contextual, so, too, will be the strength of the violation of this duty. That said, as the purpose of this book is to provide a normative argument that may justify tangible environmental policy reform, forms of punishment that we might envisage cannot be limited to moral sanction; legal punishments would be central to responding to and deterring future violations of our duties of due care.

Finally, as an aside on P_7, excuses are reasons we invoke in our defense to deny responsibility while acknowledging that the consequences in question are morally bad—and they serve to diminish, if not pardon, one's culpability for some *prima facie* wrongdoing, by demonstrating that the actor could not have helped bringing about some injury to another. Conversely, justifications amount to reasons one may invoke in her defense to deny that the consequences of her actions are morally bad (that one's action was right or at least permissible), while admitting to her responsibility for bringing them about.[43] These are important considerations that Chapter 4 will return to in its rejection of the "epistemic limitation" excuse (that ignorance absolves emitters of culpability), which will comprise a key part of its defense of P_7.

3.3 Uncertain Threats and Autonomous Standing

The plausibility of P_3—that to expose others to uncertain possibilities of harm, which involves gambling with their welfare, is to fail to treat others as ends—does not foremost depend on the presence of some indeterminate possibility for harm. This is because under conditions of uncertainty, we are unable to verify whether the threat will actually materialize in any harm and there are no grounds for claiming that the (unquantifiable) threat poses a probable (or imminent) risk of nontrivial (or substantive) harm to others, which is generally how scholars of moral responsibility and the ethics of risk delimit unreasonable, and thus wrongful, risk impositions.[44] As Chapter 2.1 clarified, the difference between risk and uncertainty, between risk impositions and uncertain threats, is our knowledge of or our lack of knowledge of consequence: when we know the outcomes of our potentially harmful actions, we are in the domain of (probabilistic) risk (or "measurable risk"); when we lack this information, we are in the purview of (indeterminate) uncertainty (or "unmeasurable uncertainty").[45] Indeed, it may well retroactively prove to be the case that an action that entails an uncertain threat actually yields a benign or even beneficial consequence to those who are exposed to the threat.[46] Thus, it is not tenable to claim that the threat itself is what violates the autonomous standing of those who are exposed. Rather, autonomy is violated because of what the creation of the threat implies about the moral relationship between the author of the threat and those he puts in the way of potential harm.

Like Scanlon's interpersonal theory of moral responsibility (as answerability), which claims that one can mar her moral relationships with others by failing to show them the reciprocal concern or due regard that their particular moral relationships demand of each other,[47] P_3 suggests that those who create uncertain threats disrespect the autonomy of others by neglecting to heed their equal moral standing. Instead of treating the act of blaming, of assigning culpability, as the punitive issuance of sanctions for an actor's morally faulty conduct,[48] or as a negative assessment of an actor's moral character given some moral failing,[49] or as adopting "reactive attitudes" (emotive judgments) about the permissibility or wrongfulness of the actor's behavior,[50] Scanlon uniquely argues that to blame a person one judges to have acted wrongfully is to modify one's moral relationship with the actor in ways that appropriately reflect *both* this judgment of wrongdoing and the recognition that the conduct in question has "impaired" the relationship.[51] More precisely, to blame another is to acknowledge that the blameworthy individual has failed to show those whom she wrongs the reciprocal concern or due regard that their particular moral relationships demand of each other, which implies that the individual failed to show concern for the unjustifiability of her reasons for acting as she did.[52] With this acknowledgement, to blame the blameworthy person is to adopt a revised attitude toward her in accord with the altered, impaired relationship that her disregard creates—such that one is culpable just in case it is appropriate to demand that she justify her action.[53]

And in parallel fashion, P_3 and P_4 underscore that when one performs an endangering action that may potentially harm others without first exercising due care—the indeterminacy of this potential notwithstanding—her behavior manifests a dismissive attitude toward fellow moral agents who will bear the harms that may materialize. Yet beyond imposing unconsented-to costs of potentially harmful consequences on others, one demonstrates her moral indifference toward her fellows by deciding for them that the potential for harm they now face is tolerable. In other words, taking the gamble disregards the autonomy of others by impeding their ability to decide for themselves, from their own risk perceptions, what constitutes an acceptable threat of harm.

Respect for the intrinsic value of others and their autonomy, however, does *not* require that one refrain from performing actions that entail indeterminate possibilities of harm: such an implication would be wildly implausible, consisting in a near-wholesale prohibition on all action taking, since all actions have some potential to injure others.[54] Rather, to show regard for others as equals, to respect others as ends, requires that in performing the potentially harmful action, we exercise due care to try to mitigate the possibility for injury to others.

One might object that soliciting the consent of those who may be exposed to possible harm is sufficient to respect their moral standing.[55] After all, the capacity for self-determination implies rendering voluntary decisions about matters that affect one's interests, including decisions about what possibilities of harm to bear. Suppose that Jeff wishes to spray a pesticide on some trees in his yard and that the chemical substance is one whose health effects are uncertain. Because Jeff's trees stand adjacent to Adam's neighboring property where he happens to be gardening, if Jeff applies the pesticide to his trees, Adam may inhale some of the spray, and some of the pesticide is likely to land on the vegetables in his garden, which Adam may then ingest. Should Jeff peer over his fence and ask Adam if he minds that he apply the pesticide, Jeff demonstrates his regard for Adam's interests and his capacity for self-determination, and he further demonstrates his respect for his neighbor's autonomy by heeding Adam's response and refraining from spraying Jeff's trees if Adam withholds his consent. A principle of consent in this context would mean that authors of uncertain threats cannot treat others as ends without their agreeing to being exposed to possible harm (necessary). Further, with this consent there is no additional expectation for one to exercise due care (sufficient), because consent eliminates any possible wrongfulness of creating an uncertain threat: responsibility for the threat is then shared.[56]

The immediate problem, however, with soliciting consent when both outcome and probability uncertainty are present is that it is unclear that consent can be informed. A prerequisite of offering meaningful consent (whether expressly or tacitly) is that one must understand what she is consenting to. That is, one must comprehend the meaning and implications of the agreement. Yet when knowledge of the consequences of granting consent is impaired—when it is unclear what the health effects of exposure to the threat may be and what the probability that some (undefined) harm will come to pass—it is doubtful that one can offer consent in any meaningful way. Mere knowledge of an uncorroborated potential for harm is insufficient to render an informed decision. Thus, any principle of express or tacit consent would be a nonstarter.

One might resist this conclusion, however, and insist that uncertainty need not preclude the capacity to offer consent. Consider, for example, a scenario in which a physician offers to administer to a pregnant woman, who is likely to have a miscarriage without intervention, a drug that is known to help prevent miscarriages but whose health effects remain uncertain.[57] Let us also stipulate that while the effects remain scientifically uncorroborated, in objectively counseling her patient, the physician explains that no known adverse side effects are currently associated with this drug. It would seem reasonable to conclude, at least in some circumstances, that the decision to take the drug, which promises an expected benefit at the cost of a "merely possible" harm, would not only be a choice the pregnant woman would "rationally favor" but would be an option to which she could offer meaningful, express consent. After all, consent generally requires that one is informed about what she is consenting to and that she is not coerced in any way (and that she has feasible alternatives available to her, but this consideration is tabled here). And certainly we can grant that the pregnant woman understands the nature and difficulty of her situation better than anyone else, that she clearly has a vested interest in making a responsible decision that promotes her health and the health of her unborn child, and therefore, all things considered, that she seems well positioned to determine whether accepting the potential for harm is justified by the potential benefits of taking the drug. Moreover, the physician, as described, is not purposefully misleading or coercing her patient but rather presenting a possible treatment option. Consequently, it seems misguided to suggest that reasonable people like our pregnant woman, making decisions with limited knowledge—which is inherent in most all choices we make—cannot consent to using the proposed drug.

Although this explanation seems intuitive and reasonable, it begs the question to assume that the pregnant woman understands the nature of the situation. If the pregnant woman is told that she can enjoy the immediate benefits of the drug but that aside from preventing a miscarriage the effects of the drug remain unknown to her, we should conclude that the patient's understanding of the situation is actually significantly incomplete. For the physician can only speak to the benefits, which is but half of the scenario. Indeed, many pregnant women learned decades after being administered diethylstilbestrol (DES), a synthetic estrogen commonly prescribed to prevent miscarriages before the 1970s, that DES was associated with significant deferred harms in their children who were exposed to it in utero, including certain cancers.[58] Even if the physician in the example exercised due care and explained that the potentially adverse health effects of the drug were uncorroborated and disclosed what information she had on the possibility for harm, it is still unclear how the pregnant woman could meaningfully offer her consent without corroboration of the relative safety or danger of taking the drug: she may rationally decide to have the physician administer the drug, but the prevailing uncertainty nevertheless means that her decision is still uninformed. In this vein, we might reasonably expect that knowledge of DES-like deferred harm to her unborn child would significantly influence the pregnant woman's decision.

And, in fact, our intuition in this example, and the implied risk–benefit calculus that we might share with the pregnant woman and that undergirds this intuition, may well be shaped by (1) the urgency with which a decision to take a drug to prevent a miscarriage may be made—such that the pregnant woman may well significantly discount the unknown possibility of future harm for the prospect of immediate benefit—and (2) the fact that the recommendation for taking the drug is coming from a physician: an epistemic authority to which we often defer our decision-making.

Alternatively, a principle of hypothetical consent would suggest that authoring an uncertain threat of environmental harm is *prima facie* morally permissible just in case everyone who is or could be exposed to the threat could have expressly consented to it if they would have had the opportunity to do so.[59] As a heuristic, such a principle might yield a rule permitting emitters to release substances into the environment whose effects to public health are unknown *so long as* no individual or group of individuals would have a reasonable grievance against it[60]—a rule, for example, that would strive toward environmental justice and would ensure that no class of citizens would shoulder an inequitable distribution of uncertain threats of environmental harm.[61] Yet even if we were able to derive this sort of rule, hypothetical consent still effectively substitutes another person's judgment and exercise of self-authorship for one's own. If we take seriously the Kantian notion of autonomy as "as the capacity to bind one's own will by normative insights" one makes *herself*,[62] it is objectionable to project another person's risk perceptions and risk tolerance on others in determining whether exposure is acceptable and the endangering action is justified: doing so would ostensibly contradict a commitment to equality and self-determination.[63]

Moreover, in a Kantian account, it is not obvious that granting consent would absolve an actor of wrongdoing, since consent does not make permissible what is otherwise impermissible. For instance, granting your informed consent to slavery or torture or murder does not diminish the duties of others not to enslave, torture, or murder you: one still does wrong by those who willingly accept the consequences of morally objectionable actions. In other words, soliciting consent for Kant presumably is neither necessary nor sufficient to avoid wrongdoing, and doing wrong by others would preclude respecting them as ends. Given these diverse problems with consent as a necessary or sufficient condition for respecting the equal moral standing and autonomy of others, its plausibility as a component of the argument against the permissibility of uncertain threats of environmental harm must be tabled here.

The other key premise of the argument for due care under uncertainty that this chapter has begun to develop is P_7: that it is immaterial to assigning culpability, and immaterial to our corresponding duty to exercise due care, that it remains unknown whether uncertain environmental threats will cause harm or unreasonable risks of injury. And because an adequate defense of these subsequent claims requires a detailed examination of seminal arguments from moral responsibility, the ethics of risk, and moral luck—each of which should have us deny the plausibility of P_7—Chapter 4 is dedicated to explaining how each of these arguments and their conventional treatments of uncertainty are ultimately mistaken. Yet before turning to this discussion, the closing section draws an important distinction between having a reason to exercise precaution and having a duty to do so in order to clarify that although the reasons we may have to satisfy this obligation are context dependent and partially informed by our subjective judgments about the potential for harm, our duty to exercise due care is universal and cannot be mitigated by our subjective judgments that our actions pose nominal danger to others.

3.4 From Reasons to Duties

Some might be willing to accept that considerations of moral equality and autonomy substantiate a *reason* to exercise due care under conditions of uncertainty, but not a *duty* of due care (as duties presuppose much stronger reasons). After all, not all uncertain threats of environmental harm are alike: even as we lack scientific corroboration of the actual health effects of exposure so long as outcome and probability uncertainty persist, we can still deduce or intuit certain relevant facts about the potential for harm. And because the reasons we may have to believe that an uncertain threat will cause harm will vary, so, too, will the reasons we have to refrain from putting others in the way of indeterminate possibilities of harm. Consequently, the fewer the reasons we can deduce to believe that an uncertain threat will produce some (indeterminate) harm—that is, the closer we come to complete uncertainty—the less compelling our reasons become to refrain from authoring the uncertain threat: our reasons may not cement a duty to take reasonable precautionary measures to mitigate the potential for harm. This deserves unpacking.

Individuals bring their imperfect knowledge of "prior probabilities"[64] of harm and their preconceptions of and intuitions about environmental risks to bear on their judgments of the credibility of uncertain threats—on their judgments, that is, that exposure will cause adverse health effects. For example, while the health effects of consuming genetically modified (GM) foods remain scientifically uncorroborated (and thus, for our purposes, pose an uncertain threat of harm), we do not observe people falling dead from the consumption of GM crops or foodstuffs containing GM ingredients. Hence, regarding at least the short-term effects, one might tentatively infer that exposure to GM foods is not toxic; and with some studies claiming that no substantial difference exists between conventional and GM foods, coupled with the Food and Drug Administration's public statements to this effect, one might also tentatively infer that consuming GM foods poses no credible threat to public health: that is, that no prior probability of a risk of substantive harm to human health exists. It is inevitable that such inference drawing occurs under conditions of uncertainty when corroborating evidence is lacking. But how do our observations and intuitions shape whether we have reasons for or a duty to exercise due care with the uncertain threats of environmental harm we ourselves may create?

For example, consider that when I presume to pour the contents of a plastic container into a storm drain, which seems to me to resemble milk judging by the liquid's off-white color, opacity, consistency, dull odor, and perhaps even its sweet taste, my reasons are few for believing that the substance—whose effects, we can stipulate, remain scientifically uncorroborated—is harmful. In fact, the five characteristics listed earlier may equate to five reasons to believe that the substance may well be milk and, hence, will be harmless. Thus, I have *pro tanto* reason to avoid emptying the contents into the storm drain without first exercising due care to try to prevent exposing others to undeserved harm. After all, while I do not know what the substance is or what the effects of exposure might be, I can be expected to know the historical association between the discharge of substances into the environment and harm to public health. (In other words, even under conditions of outcome and probability uncertainty, we can be expected to be aware of our shared environmental history and the countless examples of how the emission of substances into the environment has harmed public health—not the least of which include such high-profile cases as the Cuyahoga River fire, the Love Canal tragedy, the banning of dichlorodiphenyltrichloroethane (DDT), the Three Mile Island nuclear accident, the phase-out of leaded gasoline, and the Deepwater Horizon oil spill.) Moreover, I am aware that in emptying the contents, I put my fellow moral equals in potential harm's way. However, it is not obvious that these reasons translate into a *duty* to take reasonable preventative measures. Consequently, my neglecting to act on these reasons, that is, my failure to exercise due care, constitutes no wrongdoing: there is no moral justification for assigning culpability.

In contrast, if I were to judge that the liquid that pours from the container resembles spent motor oil—given its dark color, sheen, viscosity, pungent odor, and perhaps displeasing taste—I have stronger reasons for believing that exposure to the substance would cause adverse health effects. Although we know milk is harmless (so should it enter into our shared water shed, there should be no substantive moral concern about exposure), the same cannot be said for the spent motor oil, which we know to be harmful, consisting of toxic heavy metals and petroleum-based substances. Accordingly, coupled with the historical association between the release of effluents into the environment and harm to public health, which we can reasonably expect emitters to know, given the substance's resemblance to spent motor oil, my *pro tanto* reasons to exercise due care translate into a *pro tanto duty* of due care—such that I do wrong by failing to take reasonable strides to mitigate the potential for harm: the uncertain threat I create does warrant the assignment of culpability.[65]

This reasoning would suggest that the clearest instances in which we have a duty, as opposed to mere reasons, to exercise due care is when two criteria are met. First, one recognizes her ignorance of the potential for harm to others that her actions beget, knows the demands of reciprocity and moral equality, and draws the historically substantiated inference that the release of substances whose effects are unverified will eventually cause some material harm to some people—each of which we can reasonably expect actors to know. (That is, one cannot be excusably ignorant of these three factors.) Second, the effluent in question either shares an observable likeness to other substances whose adverse health effects *have* been scientifically verified and *are* known to cause material harm or unreasonable risks of harm, or the effluent is produced and/or emitted through processes commonly associated with the emission of known pollutants (i.e., processes that have in the past produced harmful substances).[66]

But this reasoning—and justificatory appeals to what some have termed "intuitive toxicology," which inform our "lay" perceptions of risk[67]—needs to proceed with caution. For the crux of the problem of uncertain environmental threats is that we do *not* know: we cannot draw definitive conclusions about the potential for harm. And to do so—to suggest, for example, that the release of a substance that resembles milk is itself, then, harmless—is to wrongly assume access to knowledge that uncertainty precludes. Even when it comes to ostensibly harmless substances with which we may be quite familiar, our reasonable preconceptions and intuitions can be misleading, and the conclusions we draw about the potential for harm can be misguided. A paradigmatic example of this, relating back to the example provided earlier, is the growing concern about long-term exposure to trace levels of antibiotics and growth hormones in milk.

What is more, scholars like Shrader-Frechette or Oreskes and Conway have effectively demonstrated that the science of public health risks is vulnerable to misrepresentation, since environmental policy is commonly informed by industry-led studies, that evidence corroborating adverse health effects has often been withheld from the public domain, and that "private interest science"[68] has even been known to fabricate data and engage in false public relations campaigns to convince average citizens and policy-makers of the absence of environmental threats to public health. Further, scholars like Sunstein and Layzer have convincingly shown that public perceptions of environmental risks are easily manipulated, widely inconsistent, highly subjective, and fickle.

Thus, although we can infer morally relevant information about uncertain environmental threats by bringing our pre-existing beliefs, lay observations, and intuitions to bear on our judgments about the potential for harm, it is important to reiterate that our knowledge of prior probabilities and our capacity to appraise the likelihood of harm are quite tenuous.

It is also important to note that acknowledging the salience of our subjective preconceptions and intuitions to forming our judgments about the potential for harm does not amount to suggesting that these prior beliefs about the potential for harm determine the moral permissibility of the uncertain threat. The permissibility of exposing others to uncertain threats is not a matter of subjective justification. As the defense of P_7 in the following chapter demonstrates, having a reasonable belief—given the absence of corroborating evidence to the contrary—that an uncertain threat that one authors will cause no harm does *not* justify one's action or absolve her of wrongdoing. Paralleling Kant's notion that moral laws are only universal and only law-like if they provide everyone the same objective motivation to comply with their demands[69] (see Section 3.2 earlier), our duty to exercise due care is universal, and the moral permissibility of the uncertain threats we create turns on whether we respect the moral standing of others and exercise due care accordingly. This is to say that although the strength of one's moral obligation and the ways in which one may discharge her duty must vary with context (see Chapter 5), our duty of due care under uncertainty permits no exceptions.

Notes

1. Undeserved implies innocence or having done nothing to merit this exposure to potential harm. Following Anscombe, the innocent engage in no "objectively unjust proceeding" and thus forfeit no right against being harmed (G.E.M. Anscombe, "War and Murder," in *The Collected Philosophical Papers of G.E.M. Anscombe*, Vol. 3 (Minneapolis: University of Minnesota Press, 1981): 51–61. Similarly, following Thomson, the innocent are "free of fault" (Judith Jarvis Thomson, "Self-Defense," *Philosophy and Public Affairs* 20 (1991): 284, fn.1). (Though Thomson does maintain in her final analysis that neither fault nor agency is necessary to violate another's right to not be substantively harmed (ibid: 301–2).)
2. Thomas Nagel, "Moral Luck," in *Mortal Questions* (Cambridge: Cambridge University Press, 1979): 31.
3. Following scholars like Gideon Rosen ("Skepticism About Moral Responsibility," *Philosophical Perspectives* 18 (2004): 296), moral responsibility, culpability, and blameworthiness are understood here as synonymous: where responsibility (or culpability) for some injury denotes *fault* for begetting the harm and where one's *being at fault* warrants (*ceteris paribus*) blaming or condemning the actor for not acting otherwise—thus equating his action to a wrongdoing. Similarly, Jonathan Bennett ("Accountability," in *Philosophical Subjects: Essays Presented to P.F. Strawson*, Van Straaten, ed. (Oxford: Clarendon Press, 1980): 15) clarifies that accountability is to be deserving of praise or blame, where "someone is 'accountable' for an action . . . if a blame- or praise-related response to the action would not be inappropriate." For similar conceptions, see John L. Austin, "A Plea for Excuses: The Presidential Address," *Proceedings of the Aristotelian Society* 57 (1956): 7 fn. 2;

Thomas Reid, *Essays on the Active Powers of the Human Mind* (Cambridge: MIT Press, 1969 [1788]): 262, 315; and Gerald Dworkin, "Intention, Foreseeability, and Responsibility," in *Responsibility, Character, and the Emotions*, Ferdinand Schoeman, ed. (Cambridge: Cambridge University Press, 1987): 351.

4. Michael Zimmerman, "Taking Luck Seriously," *Journal of Philosophy* 99 (2002): 554.
5. Example is drawn from Peter Singer, "Famine, Affluence, and Morality," *Philosophy and Public Affairs* 1 (1972): 231.
6. Example is drawn from John Stuart Mill, *On Liberty*, Elizabeth Rapaport, ed. (Indianapolis: Hackett Publishing Co., Inc., 1978): 95.
7. Thomas Reid ("Of the Notion of Duty, Rectitude, Moral Obligation," in *Essays on the Active Powers of the Human Mind* (Cambridge: MIT Press, 1969): 230) expressly acknowledges this consideration—insisting that "if a man should give to his neighbor a potion which he really believes will poison him, but which, in the event, proves salutary, and does much good; in moral estimation, he is a poisoner, not a benefactor."
8. This overlooks the relevance of excuses and justifications that mitigate one's blameworthiness; considerations that are addressed in Sections 4.1–4.3.
9. Henry Richardson ("Institutionally Divided Moral Responsibility," *Social Philosophy and Policy* 16 (1999); and "Beyond Good and Right," *Philosophy and Public Affairs* 24 (1995)) makes unique reference to the notion of "forward-looking" or "prospective" moral responsibility (1999: 221). He argues that it is shortsighted of deontologists to suggest that moral principles can or should apply similarly for all people in all contexts and that their justifiable failure to obtain in a given instance—e.g., lying to a friend to spare him unnecessary grief—merely constitute exceptions to otherwise universal or absolute principles (1999: 226). Stressing that the circumstances in which we discharge our moral duties are often contingent and changing and unforeseeable, that "the future always surprises us [and] rules end up clashing and harmonizing in ever-novel ways," Richardson maintains that it is necessary to acknowledge the practical, "future-oriented" nature of responsibility in order to allow agents to adjust to unpredictable and morally relevant changes in context (1999: 221, 235). This requires us to conscientiously "bend or revise preexisting rules," and thus to refine our understanding of those rules, in reasonable and limited ways (1999: 221–2, 224, 234, 236)—offering substantive justification for any such revision to avoid the mistake of treating "logically flexible" principles and their prescriptions as mere *recommendations* for action (as opposed to being properly action guiding) and thus of undermining their normative force and "relatively fixed" nature (1999: 226; 1995: 128–30). Despite Richardson's unique reference to "forward-looking" responsibility, his analysis does not help to illuminate the interdependence between forward-looking duties and retroactive assignments of culpability (Angela Smith, "On Being Responsible and Holding Responsible," *Journal of Ethics* 11 (2007): 468, fn.7). For he problematically conflates responsibility with duty or obligation, such that (forward-looking) responsibility consists of critically examining the merit or applicability of extant moral rules to discern *what one ought to do*, given the unique conditions of her particular "moral situation," and then to act in accordance with these considered judgments about one's duties (1999: 221, 229, 236). This conflation is most clearly manifest in his assertion that "someone on whom a duty is incumbent has a responsibility that extends both to looking out for the concern that provides the duty its point [such as the welfare or interests of those to whom we make promises] and to revising the initially understood terms of the duty, if necessary" (1999: 229). Although these concepts *are* related and interdependent, as the foregoing has suggested, they are substantively different and deserve more careful treatment.

10. Thomas M. Scanlon, *Moral Dimensions: Permissibility, Meaning, and Blame* (Cambridge: Belknap Press, 2008).
11. Ibid., 9, 218 fn. 9.
12. Ibid., 22, 24, 27.
13. Reid, *Essays On the Active Powers of the Human Mind*; Charles Campbell, *In Defense of Free Will with Other Philosophical Essays* (London: Allen and Unwin, 1967); Gary Watson, "Responsibility and the Limits of Evil," in *Responsibility, Character, and the Emotions*, Ferdinand Schoeman, ed. (Cambridge: Cambridge University Press, 1987); Susan Wolf, *Freedom Within Reason* (Oxford: Oxford University Press, 1990); Harry Frankfurt, *The Importance of What We Care About* (Cambridge: Cambridge University Press, 2007); Angela Smith, "Control, Responsibility, and Moral Assessment," *Philosophical Studies* 138 (2008).
14. Robert Nozick, *Anarchy, State, and Utopia* (New York: Basic Books, 1974), Chapter 3 on side constraints, and 169–72 on forced labor.
15. Joseph Raz, *The Morality of Freedom* (Oxford: Oxford University Press, 1986); Gerald Cohen, *Self-Ownership, Freedom, and Equality* (Cambridge: Cambridge University Press, 1995).
16. Immanuel Kant, "Theory and Practice" (22, 25, 55–6, 74–5, 77, 79, 84) and "Perpetual Peace" (99f) and "Idea for a Universal History" and "What is Enlightenment?," in *Kant's Political Writings*, Hans Reiss, ed., H.B. Nisbet, trans. (Cambridge: Cambridge University Press, 1970).
17. Kant, "Theory and Practice," 74.
18. Immanuel Kant, "Groundwork of the Metaphysics of Morals" and "Critique of Practical Reason," in *Practical Philosophy*, Mary Gregor, ed. and trans. (Cambridge: Cambridge University Press, 1996).
19. Immanuel Kant, "Idea for a Universal History with a Cosmopolitan Purpose" and "What Is Enlightenment?" in *Kant Political Writings*, Hans S. Reiss, ed. (Cambridge: Cambridge University Press, 1970): 4.
20. Kant, "Idea for a Universal History with a Cosmopolitan Purpose," 44: this regards Kant's notion of human beings' "unsocial sociability," whereby individuals are "constantly attracted to and repelled by others." That is, while we inherently are social and political beings, we are competitive and antagonistic toward each other, and no matter how enlightened we become, this antagonism persists.
21. A crucial distinction Kant draws regards acting *from* versus *in accord with* moral duty. Acting *from* duty implies satisfying the demands of morality *because* it is right, whereas acting *in accord with* duty implies acting in such a way that it turns out to be what morality requires but where one's motive is something other than this because it is right. Good actions are done *from* duty, where acknowledging that it is the right thing to do is one's *only* motive.
22. Kant makes a clear distinction between coercion and omission, or the difference between having the development of one's rationality impeded from without (coercion) and when one chooses not to develop his skills to think for himself and achieve greater rationality (omission).
23. Kant's, "Perpetual Peace," 112–3.
24. Kant's, "What is Enlightenment," 54.
25. Immanuel Kant, "Critique of Practical Reason" and "The Metaphysics of Morals," in *Practical Philosophy*, Mary Gregor, ed. and trans. (Cambridge: Cambridge University Press, 1996): 45–6, 158, 159, 161, 165–6, 523, 527–30, 566–7, respectively; see also Immanuel Kant, *Groundwork of the Metaphysics of Morals*, H.J. Paton, trans. (New York: Harper and Row Publishers, 1964): 67–9; and Kant, "Idea for a Universal History with a Cosmopolitan Purpose," 25. See *supra* note 84.
26. Kant, "Critique of Practical Reason," 45–6.
27. Ibid., 158–9.
28. Ibid., 158–9; "Theory and Practice," 73–4.

29. Kant's, "Critique of Practical Reason," 160–2; "Perpetual Peace," 116.
30. Kant, "Idea for a Universal History with a Cosmopolitan Purpose," 43, 49, 52–3; Kant, "Theory and Practice," 88–9; Immanuel Kant, "The Contest of Faculties," in *Kant's Political Writings*, Hans S. Reiss, ed. (Cambridge: Cambridge University Press, 1970): 181. See also Reiss's introductory remarks, 36–7. For Kant, history is a progress toward rationality. If human history is not purposive, then neither is human nature, and if human nature is not purposive, if it has no *telos*, then human beings are no different from lower animals: driven by impulse and instinct, on the order of "small material particles" randomly colliding with one another in an arbitrary and meaningless existence (48: Kant's analogy concerning states).
31. Kant, "Theory and Practice," 74.
32. Kant, "Idea for a Universal History," 47.
33. When all individuals behave in this manner (having internalized, so to speak, the demands of the categorical imperative), history's *telos* would be realized.
34. Kant, "Idea for a Universal History," 44.
35. Kant, "Groundwork of the Metaphysics of Morals" and "Critique of Practical Reason;" also John Rawls, *A Theory of Justice* (Cambridge: Belknap Press, 1971): 515–6.
36. Kant, "Theory and Practice," 74.
37. Cohen, *Self-Ownership, Freedom, and Equality*, 239.
38. Rawls, *A Theory of Justice*, 337–8; Bernard Williams, "The Idea of Equality," in *Philosophy, Politics, and Society*, Peter Laslett and W.G. Runciman, eds. (Oxford: Basil Blackwell, 1962): 118f.
39. As Chapter 4.3 on moral luck notes, committing a wrongdoing does not necessarily mean that one is blameworthy. The very notion of the "epistemic limitation excuse," e.g., assumes that although a person can do wrong by others, her "reasonable ignorance" can absolve her of blame. Suppose I violently swing my arm, assuming that I am alone in the room, but as it turns out, unbeknownst to me, you had just entered the room, and suppose that I strike and break your nose. If my ignorance of your presence or of the potential danger that arm swinging entails were reasonable, although I committed a wrongdoing by injuring you, I can hardly be held blameworthy for a consequence that I could not have reasonably foreseen. A consequence, moreover, that I would have tried to avoid had I known.
40. Some might deny that we have a duty of due care, but may accept that we have a *pro tanto* reason to exercise due care: this idea is explored in Section 3.4 below.
41. Sarah Vogel, "The Politics of Plastics: The Making and Unmaking of Bisphenol A Safety," *American Journal of Public Health* 99 (2009): 559–66. Though, as noted in the introduction, the example of BPA is contentious, for it is unclear that we would judge these proactive measures as precautionary in nature, that is, as intending to mitigate the potential for harm to public health.
42. Among the possible objections to these criteria that comprehensive defense of this rights-based conception of the precautionary principle would have to address is the concern that these substitutions may well entail greater risk impositions—as clarified, e.g., in *Public Citizen v. Young* (1987): "As a result, makers of drugs and cosmetics who are barred from using a carcinogenic dye carrying a one-in-20-million lifetime risk may use instead a noncarcinogenic, but toxic, dye carrying, say, a one-in-10-million lifetime risk. The substitution appears to be a clear loss for safety."
43. For details see Watson, "Responsibility and the Limits of Evil" or Austin, "A Plea for Excuses."
44. Ernest Weinrib, "Toward a Moral Theory of Negligence Law," *Law and Philosophy* 2 (1983): 37; Joel Feinberg, *Harm to Others: The Moral Limits of the Criminal Law*, Vol. 1 (Oxford: Oxford University Press, 1984): 190–2; Thomson, "Imposing Risks," 126, 131; Robinson, "Risk, Causation, and Harm," 320–1; Stephen

Perry, "Risk, Harm, Interests, and Rights," in *Risk: Philosophical Perspectives*, Tim Lewens, ed. (New York: Routledge, 2007): 190–210.

45. The distinction and significance between "measurable risk" and "unmeasurable uncertainty" (or that which we do not know) were made as early as the 1920s: see Frank Knight, *Risk, Uncertainty, and Profit* (Boston: Houghton Mifflin Co., 1921): 19–20, 233. See also John Maynard Keynes, "The General Theory of Employment," *Quarterly Journal of Economics* 51 (1937): 209, 214.
46. One might interject here that because this sort of action may yield a benign or harmless outcome, it is not obvious that any "threat" exists. However, the notion of "threat" in the context of outcome and probability uncertainty is simply intended to convey an uncorroborated potential for harm. Thus, to say that there is no "threat" is to either assume that the consequence *will* be harmless—which would be a false assumption, because the point is that we cannot know when uncertainty prevails—or to assume that "threat" equates to "risk"—which would ignore the purpose of distinguishing uncorroborated possibilities of harm from conventional language of probabilistic risks of harm (where the harmful outcomes are known). For more on the differences between these concepts, see Chapter 2.1.
47. Scanlon, *Moral Dimensions*, 6, 122–4, 128, 130, 141, 145.
48. See Chapter 4.1–4.3.
49. See Thomas Reid, *Essays On the Active Powers of the Human Mind* (Cambridge: MIT Press, 1969 [1788]); Angela Smith, "Responsibility for Attitudes: Activity and Passivity in Mental Life," *Ethics* 115 (2005); Angel Smith, "On Being Responsible and Holding Responsible," *Journal of Ethics* 11 (2007); and Angela Smith, "Control, Responsibility, and Moral Assessment," *Philosophical Studies* 138 (2008).
50. See Peter Strawson, "Freedom and Resentment," in *Freedom and Resentment and Other Essays* (London: Methuen and Co., 1974 [1962]); Jonathan Bennett, "Accountability," in *Philosophical Subjects: Essays Presented to P.F. Strawson*, Van Straaten, ed. (Oxford: Clarendon Press, 1980); Watson, "Responsibility and the Limits of Evil;" and R. Jay Wallace, *Responsibility and the Moral Sentiments* (Cambridge: Harvard University Press, 1996).
51. Scanlon, *Moral Dimensions*, 6, 122–4, 128, 130, 141, 145.
52. Ibid., 124, 127, 141–2, 189.
53. Ibid., 128–9, 137, 145.
54. David McCarthy, "Rights, Explanation, and Risks," *Ethics* 107 (1997); Madeleine Hayenhjelm and Jonathan Wolff, "Moral Problem of Risk Impositions," *European Journal of Philosophy* 20 (2012): e37.
55. Shrader-Frechette (*Taking Action, Saving Lives*, 58) maintains that "all legitimate risk impositions . . . rest on the consent of subjects." See also Nozick, *Anarchy, State, and Utopia*, 31.
56. Though consenting to being exposed to a threat of harm is distinct from consenting to being harmed, so consent here would not necessarily absolve an author of an uncertain threat of culpability for any ensuing harm.
57. My thanks to an anonymous reviewer for this example and pressing me to better clarify my reasoning here.
58. Centers for Disease Control and Prevention, "DES History," www.cdc.gov/des/consumers/about/history.html, last updated June 1, 2015.
59. Kant, "Theory and Practice," 77–80. Cohen (*Self-Ownership, Freedom, and Equality*, 241–2) interprets Kant's notion of hypothetical consent differently: viz., as what is or what is not "normatively possible," whereby there are certain arrangements to which one could not possibly consent without contradicting or rendering incoherent our broader moral system. For instance, one could not possibly consent to being enslaved—even if one actually gives his consent—for pain of contradiction of Kant's categorical imperative.
60. Kant, "Theory and Practice," 79; Rawls, *Theory of Justice*, 518–9.

61. Shrader-Frechette, *Taking Action, Saving Lives*, 13, 31; also Robert Bullard, "Unequal Environmental Protection," in *Worst Things First?*, Adam Finkel and Dominic Golding, eds. (Washington, DC: Resources for the Future, 1994); Robert Kuehn, "Environmental Justice Implications of Quantitative Risk Assessment," *University of Illinois Law Review* 103 (1996); Kristin Shrader-Frechette, *Environmental Justice* (Oxford: Oxford University Press, 2002).
62. Rawls, *Theory of Justice*, 518–9.
63. Reiss, *Kant's Political Writings*, 19. For a contrasting perspective, see Kant, "Theory and Practice," 85; Rawls, *Theory of Justice*, 518.
64. This notion is drawn from Bayesian theory, but the more general concept is motivated by Hume's writing in epistemology and his perspectives on induction.
65. The same may be said of the varying completeness of basic toxicity profiles. There are commonly six different toxicity measures that are tested for and that establish a substance's estimable threat to human health: (1) acute toxicity, (2) chronic toxicity, (3) developmental and reproductive toxicity, (4) mutagenicity, (5) ecotoxicity, and (6) environmental fate (Office of Pollution Prevention and Toxics, "High Production Volume Chemical Hazard Data Availability Study" (Washington, DC: EPA, 1998, last updated August 2, 2010): 2). We approximate genuine uncertainty when we lack all toxicity profiles for a given substance, and our reasons for exercising due care with regard to the release of this substance correspondingly become weaker and less compelling.
66. For instance, when substances that pose uncertain health effects are produced via standard industrial, commercial, and agricultural manufacturing processes that are commonly known to generate and to entail the discharge of harmful substances into the environment, emitters have a *pro tanto* duty to exercise due care. For this likeness gives emitters strong reason to believe that exposure to the substances they release into the environment will cause injury.
67. Cass Sunstein, *Risk and Reason: Safety, Law, and the Environment* (Cambridge: Cambridge University Press, 2002): 35; Sunstein, *Laws of Fear*, 83.
68. Shrader-Frechette, *Taking Action, Saving Lives*, 109.
69. Kant, "Critique of Practical Reason," 158–9.

References

Anscombe, G.E.M. "War and Murder." In *The Collected Philosophical Papers of G.E.M. Anscombe*, Vol. 3. Minneapolis: University of Minnesota Press, 1981.

Austin, John L. "A Plea for Excuses: The Presidential Address." *Proceedings of the Aristotelian Society* 57 (1956): 1–30.

Bennett, Jonathan. "Accountability." In *Philosophical Subjects: Essays Presented to P.F. Strawson*, edited by Zak van Straaten. Oxford: Clarendon Press, 1980.

Bullard, Robert. "Unequal Environmental Protection." In *Worst Things First? The Debate over Risk-Based National Environmental Priorities*, edited by Adam Finkel and Dominic Golding. Washington: Resources for the Future, 1994.

Centers for Disease Control and Prevention. "DES History." Last updated June 1, 2015. www.cdc.gov/des/consumers/about/history.html.

Cohen, Gerald. *Self-Ownership, Freedom, and Equality*. Cambridge: Cambridge University Press, 1995.

Dworkin, Gerald. "Intention, Foreseeability, and Responsibility." In *Responsibility, Character, and the Emotions*, edited by Ferdinand Schoeman. Cambridge: Cambridge University Press, 1987.

Feinberg, Joel. *Harm to Others: The Moral Limits of the Criminal Law*, Vol. 1. Oxford: Oxford University Press, 1984.

Frankfurt, Harry. *The Importance of What We Care about*. Cambridge: Cambridge University Press, 2007.

Hayenhjelm, Madeleine and Jonathan Wolff. "The Moral Problem of Risk Impositions: A Survey of the Literature." *European Journal of Philosophy* 20 (2012): E26–51.

Kant, Immanuel. "Idea for a Universal History." In *Kant's Political Writings*, edited by Hans Reiss, translated by H.B. Nisbet. Cambridge: Cambridge University Press, 1970 [1784].

———. "What Is Enlightenment?" In *Kant's Political Writings*, edited by Hans Reiss, translated by H.B. Nisbet. Cambridge: Cambridge University Press, 1970 [1784].

———. "Groundwork of the Metaphysics of Morals." In *Practical Philosophy*, edited and translated by Mary Gregor. Cambridge: Cambridge University Press, 1996 [1785].

———. "Critique of Practical Reason." In *Practical Philosophy*, edited and translated by Mary Gregor. Cambridge: Cambridge University Press, 1996 [1788].

———. "Theory and Practice." In *Kant's Political Writings*, edited by Hans Reiss, translated by H.B. Nisbet. Cambridge: Cambridge University Press, 1970 [1793].

———. "Perpetual Peace." In *Kant's Political Writings*, edited by Hans Reiss, translated by H.B. Nisbet. Cambridge: Cambridge University Press, 1970 [1795].

———. "The Contest of Faculties." In *Kant's Political Writings*, edited by Hans S. Reiss, translated by H.B. Nisbet. Cambridge: Cambridge University Press, 1970 [1798].

Keynes, John Maynard. "The General Theory of Employment." *Quarterly Journal of Economics* 51 (1937): 209–23.

Knight, Frank. *Risk, Uncertainty, and Profit*. Boston: Houghton Mifflin Co., 1921.

Kuehn, Robert. "Environmental Justice Implications of Quantitative Risk Assessment." *University of Illinois Law Review* 103 (1996): 1–67.

McCarthy, David. "Rights, Explanation, and Risks." *Ethics* 107 (1997): 205–25.

Mill, John Stuart. *On Liberty*, edited by Elizabeth Rapaport. Indianapolis: Hackett Publishing Co., Inc., 1978.

Nagel, Thomas. *Mortal Questions*. Cambridge: Cambridge University Press, 1979.

Nozick, Robert. *Anarchy, State, and Utopia*. New York: Basic Books, 1974.

Office of Pollution Prevention and Toxics. "High Production Volume Chemical Hazard Data Availability Study." Washington: EPA, 1998. Last updated August 2, 2010.

Perry, Stephen. "Risk, Harm, Interests, and Rights." In *Risk: Philosophical Perspectives*, edited by Tim Lewens. New York: Routledge, 2007.

Public Citizen Health Research Group v. Young, 831 F.2d 1108 (D.C. Circuit 1987).

Rawls, John. *A Theory of Justice*. Cambridge: Harvard University Press, 1971.

Raz, Joseph. *The Morality of Freedom*. Oxford: Oxford University Press, 1986.

Reid, Thomas. *Essays on the Active Powers of the Human Mind*. Cambridge: MIT Press, 1969 [1788].

Reiss, Hans, ed. *Kant's Political Writings*. Cambridge: Cambridge University Press, 1970.

Richardson, Henry. "Beyond Good and Right." *Philosophy and Public Affairs* 24 (1995): 108–41.

———. "Institutionally Divided Moral Responsibility." *Social Philosophy and Policy* 16 (1999): 218–49.

Robinson, Glen. "Risk, Causation, and Harm." In *Liability and Responsibility: Essays in Law and Morals*, edited by Raymond Frey and Christopher Morris. Cambridge: Cambridge University Press, 1991.

Rosen, Gideon. "Skepticism about Moral Responsibility." *Philosophical Perspectives* 18 (2004): 295–313.

Scanlon, Thomas M. *Moral Dimensions: Permissibility, Meaning, and Blame*. Cambridge: Belknap Press, 2008.

Shrader-Frechette, Kristin. *Environmental Justice: Creating Equality, Reclaiming Democracy*. Oxford: Oxford University Press, 2002.

———. *Taking Action, Saving Lives: Our Duties to Protect Environmental and Public Health*. Oxford: Oxford University Press, 2007.

Singer, Peter. "Famine, Affluence, and Morality." *Philosophy and Public Affairs* 1 (1972): 229–43.

Smith, Angela. "Responsibility for Attitudes: Activity and Passivity in Mental Life." *Ethics* 115 (2005): 236–71.

———. "On Being Responsible and Holding Responsible." *Journal of Ethics* 11 (2007): 465–84.

———. "Control, Responsibility, and Moral Assessment." *Philosophical Studies* 138 (2008): 367–92.

Strawson, Peter. *Freedom and Resentment and Other Essays*. London: Methuen and Co., 1974 [1962].

Sunstein, Cass. *Risk and Reason: Safety, Law, and the Environment*. Cambridge: Cambridge University Press, 2002.

———. *Laws of Fear: Beyond the Precautionary Principle*. Cambridge: Cambridge University Press, 2005.

Thomson, Judith Jarvis. "Imposing Risks." In *To Breathe Freely: Risk, Consent, and Air*, edited by Mary Gibson. Totowa: Rowman and Allenheld, 1985.

———. "Self-Defense." *Philosophy and Public Affairs* 20 (1991): 283–310.

Vogel, Sarah. "The Politics of Plastics: The Making and Unmaking of Bisphenol A Safety." *American Journal of Public Health* 99 (2009): S559–66.

Wallace, R. Jay. *Responsibility and the Moral Sentiments*. Cambridge: Harvard University Press, 1996.

Watson, Gary. "Responsibility and the Limits of Evil." In *Responsibility, Character, and the Emotions*, edited by Ferdinand Schoeman. Cambridge: Cambridge University Press, 1987.

Weinrib, Ernest. "Toward a Moral Theory of Negligence Law." *Law and Philosophy* 2 (1983): 37–62.

Williams, Bernard. "The Idea of Equality." In *Philosophy, Politics, and Society*, edited by Peter Laslett and W.G. Runciman. Oxford: Basil Blackwell, 1962.

Wolf, Susan. *Freedom within Reason*. Oxford: Oxford University Press, 1990.

Zimmerman, Michael. "Taking Luck Seriously." *Journal of Philosophy* 99 (2002): 553–76.

4 Uncertain but Culpable

Conventional scholarship in moral responsibility, the ethics of risk, and moral luck insists that prevailing uncertainty—when it is not possible to estimate the *de facto* consequences of one's actions or the probability that actual harm will come to pass—is a significant mitigating factor that should absolve actors of any culpability for their potentially harmful actions and thus denies (explicitly or by implication) that uncertain threats are morally problematic and warrant regulation in the first place. As the broadly Kantian argument introduced in Chapter 3 resists these conclusions—maintaining, instead, that it is immaterial to assigning culpability and immaterial to defining our corresponding duty of due care, that it remains unknown whether uncertain environmental threats will cause harm or unreasonable risks of injury (P_7)—a normative defense of exercising precaution requires demonstrating that these conventional accounts do not adequately justify the permissibility of uncertain threats of environmental harm.

To this end, Section 4.1 critically engages traditional theories of moral responsibility, which claim that we cannot be held culpable unless it can be shown that we are causally responsible for begetting an actual injury or an unreasonable risk of injury. Section 4.2, then, rejects arguments in the ethics of risk that contend that only imminent threats of serious harm are morally objectionable and therefore that uncertain threats are trivial and therefore permissible. This section also shows, on the other hand, that arguments in the ethics of risk that *are* favorable to regulating potentially harmful actions mistakenly treat uncertain threats as probabilistic risks and therefore neglect to acknowledge that the combination of outcome and probability uncertainty engenders a substantively different moral problem. Finally, Section 4.3 denies arguments from moral luck, which claim that because we are reasonably ignorant of the effects of our actions when outcome and probability uncertainty are present, culpability should be excused. More precisely, this section argues that the epistemic limitation excuse does not apply: that even in our ignorance we are privy to information that establishes a *pro tanto* duty to exercise due care.[1] As these three sections, taken together, vindicate P_7 (the remaining controversial premise of the argument for due care detailed in Chapter 3), Section 4.4 here explores several possible objections to this book's normative defense of precaution. And in refuting these charges, this concluding section aims to establish the practical feasibility of a normative standard that requires emitters to try to prevent putting the public in potential harm's way—considerations that preface the discussion in Chapter 5 on how this duty of due care, which varies across contexts and actors, can be satisfied.

4.1 Moral Responsibility and Causal Responsibility

Traditionally, the assignment of blame or culpability, which is grounded in a judgment that an action constitutes a wrongdoing that warrants sanctioning,[2] depends on corroborating one's role in bringing about an actual injury or an unreasonable risk of injury—where the extent to which one can be blameworthy depends on the extent to which one causes the wrongdoing.[3] Feinberg insists, for instance, that moral responsibility turns crucially on contributing in some "substantial" way to the harm coming to pass.[4] Postema echoes this consideration, suggesting that one may be held culpable only for those harms for which she is directly (and at least partially) causally responsible, such that her contribution is either a necessary or sufficient condition of the harm coming to pass. This means that if some harm would have precipitated regardless of one's contributing action, then one cannot be held morally responsible[5] (and thus she cannot be held liable[6]).

So, for instance, when coworkers Clayton and Monica tire of commuting by bus and decide to drive Monica's car to work instead, which adds to the congestion on the roads and the concentration of toxic heavy metals and particulates in the ambient air, they causally contribute to the diverse respiratory problems that residents in the communities along their daily commute may experience. That said, because it is Monica's car and Monica who drives, she can be said to be more causally responsible, and thus more morally responsible, for the ensuing harm to residents than Clayton is. As a bystander, we might even absolve Clayton of any causal or moral responsibility. Yet because any one vehicle on the road only marginally contributes to a broader collective harm that residents may experience along our busy thruways—that is, because the exhaust from Monica's car is, for the sake of argument, neither a necessary nor a sufficient condition for the harm to residents—Monica would not be morally responsible on this account.

When substantial causal responsibility *can* be established, however, then actors are morally responsible just in case factors that could excuse, justify, or exempt[7] one's contribution to a wrongdoing are absent. Such factors may include, for example, unintentionally causing harm, causing harm while striving toward some greater good,[8] acting under duress, being unaware of the consequences of one's actions, or acting from a diminished capacity for "morally responsible agency,"[9] and so forth. (The significance of certain mitigating factors to the assignment of responsibility for uncertain threats of harm is discussed below.) In the absence of these considerations, we can assign culpability to causally responsible actors: that is, we can judge them as morally at fault for acting or failing to act, where this "faulty conduct" is what begets the harm.[10]

Admittedly, this brief account ignores certain morally significant complicating factors, such as unexpected causal turns, overdetermination, doing versus allowing, accidents, and diverting "causal sequence[s] . . . that [are] already in existence" (as opposed to initiating a new causal chain of events),[11] which can confound our moral assessments. With causal turns, for example, or what Dworkin terms "unforeseen causal routes,"[12] someone may intend to achieve some wrongful end, but her action may fail to bring about her desired consequences—prompting, instead, the start of an unforeseen causal chain that does achieve the (ill-intentioned) end she desires. And this speaks to the consideration of overdetermination: where some harmful outcome can be caused through a number of different avenues or where different harmful outcomes can follow from a given action.[13] In such instances, it is unclear how a person's culpability should change (if at all) when one's action causes an intended harmful outcome but via an unforeseen and unintended causal path, or when one's ill-intentioned action causes a desired but unforeseen harmful outcome.

Nevertheless, the strong intuition behind the priority of causal responsibility is that if it cannot be established that one had a demonstrable influence over the course of events that adversely affected others, then assigning culpability would be arbitrary and capricious, and thus unfair and unjustified.[14] Williams expressly acknowledges this custom of assigning culpability "on the ultimately fair basis of the agent's own contribution, no more and no less."[15] Indeed, because the assignment of culpability can entail substantive burdens to the accused—forfeiture of rights, public shaming, or the imposition of other sanctions; compensatory claims of liability; etc.—requiring sufficient corroborating evidence of a person's causal contribution to some wrongdoing is a minimum standard to protect against imposing undue costs on those implicated in inflicting some harm.

Yet any account of moral responsibility that requires clear causal chains of events that permit us to identify the injury, the injured, and the injurer—and which presupposes that some material harm is a necessary condition of culpability—cannot account for, and cannot speak intelligibly about assigning moral responsibility for, most environmental harms. As noted earlier in Chapter 2, many environmental harms entail deferred, indirect, and cumulative effects, which vary according to physiological vulnerabilities and different pathways of exposure and are caused by long-term, low-level exposure to effluents, many of which are "tasteless, odorless, and unseen," and therefore "undetectable—until it is too late."[16] And this is to say nothing of the fact that the adverse health effects of exposure to effluents in the environment are commonly obscured by various forms of uncertainty that complicate, if not impede, our ability to establish causal responsibility. In this way, some have characterized environmental effluents as "slow-acting 'invisible bullets,' harming people who often cannot even prove they were 'shot.'"[17]

Consider those environmental harms that constitute cumulative side effects or externalities of otherwise morally permissible actions, such that any one particular action "could occur without ill consequence," but when numerous such actions are aggregated, they create a cumulative effect that does beget some injury—but only indirectly.[18] For instance, as with the example of Clayton and Monica earlier, no one person's drive to work, and this action's inevitable by-product of emitting various pollutants into the atmosphere, has the capacity to cause adverse health effects to those living in proximity to the commuter's route. However, when tens and hundreds of thousands of commuters take to the highways and byways, the aggregated side effects of their individual commutes do have the capacity to degrade local air quality and create short- and long-term respiratory problems (e.g., asthma, chronic bronchitis, and lung cancer) among those living near high-traffic areas.[19] Does this, then, mean that in causing no harm independently, albeit contributing to some collective harm, such an action is at one and the same time morally permissible and impermissible? Would this, then, mean that one is simultaneously blameworthy and also faultless? How might these judgments be reconciled?

In such cases, because no individual contribution is a necessary condition of the harm coming to pass, the absence of one's contributing action would do nothing to prevent the injury from materializing and thus would be causally irrelevant—*prima facie* relieving one of culpability. Intervening factors[20] pose similar problems for conventional theories of moral responsibility: for when some action causes some outcome_a, which then intervenes on the outcome_b of some other action to produce a harmful outcome

$$a \rightarrow b \rightarrow \text{harm}$$

neither *a* nor *b* (or either corresponding action) is sufficient to bring about the harmful consequence, but both are necessary conditions. For instance, the production of large volumes of gasoline and fuel additives by oil and chemical companies results in gas stations and related industries throughout the United States filling their underground storage tanks (UST) with known toxic and carcinogenic substances.[21] In turn, the storage of these materials invariably causes the contamination of municipal sources of drinking water, as UST commonly leach their contents into surrounding soils and groundwater systems: for example, since UST came under federal regulation in the early 1980s, more than 500,000 leaks have been reported.[22] When an intervening relationship is simple—permitting a clear causal connection between *a* causing *b* and *b* causing the harm—conventional theories of moral responsibility would suggest that an actor who causes *b* is more culpable, because her contribution to the harm is more direct. However, with greater numbers of the intervening variables and more complex causal chains, the appropriate distribution of moral responsibility becomes obscure. This is also in large measure because the passing of time between an action and some manifest harm confounds our moral assessments: "the lapse in time between the action of an agent and the time at which the effect takes place"[23] and imposes some harm to others, which can obscure the extent to which the agent should be held culpable. For the more time that passes, the more likely it is that some other causal event or actor intervenes on the causal chain and alters the course of events or contributes to the eventual harm.

The same can be said of moderating causal factors: for when some action$_a$ causes a harmful outcome whose severity or likelihood is influenced by some other action$_b$

$$\begin{array}{c} b \\ \downarrow \\ a \rightarrow \text{harm} \end{array}$$

neither *a* nor *b* is sufficient to bring about the harm that the interaction of the causal factors begets, but both again are necessary conditions for the harm to materialize. Some have argued, for instance, that the probability that workplace exposure to airborne asbestos fibers will cause cancer depends on whether those who are exposed have a history of smoking, whereby smoking is an extraneous (moderating) causal factor whose absence diminishes the likelihood and severity of asbestos-related cancers.[24] If inhalation of asbestos fibers do not on their own tend cause demonstrable adverse health effects, can employers be said to be causally responsible for the harm to their workers? To what degree is their moral responsibility attenuated by the lifestyle choices of workers that facilitate the injuries? While proponents of traditional accounts of moral responsibility may have straightforward remedies for these simplified examples, environmental public health threats are commonly much more complicated.

This implies that conventional theories of responsibility, which center on causal responsibility, are ill equipped to handle uncertain environmental threats, since the cause-and-effect judgments that their appraisals of culpability are grounded in are precluded by the uncertainty inherent to these threats of harm. As such, these accounts would dismiss uncertain threats as morally innocuous or permissible. However, this conclusion would commit us to countenancing innumerable potentially harmful actions that involve the emission of substances whose health effects are unverified and whose permissibility thus remains unclear.[25] It would commit us, in other words, to the controversial and implausible conclusion that uncertainty amounts to relative safety (that uncertain threats are safe), and it would also have us posit that the agency or moral standing of those who aim to perform endangering actions should take priority over the agency or standing of potential victims. That is, at least until the burden of proof is met by potential victims and a preponderance of evidence can confirm that the emissions in question do entail some actual harm or some unreasonable risk of harm. (That is, at least until uncertainty is overcome and knowledge of the consequences and the probability of harm is achieved.)

One might insist that this reasoning is contradictory, since proponents of the idea that we have duties of due care under uncertainty *are* prepared to restrict the agency of emitters and prioritize the standing of potential victims by requiring emitters to bear the costs of exercising precaution. Further, since restricting the agency of emitters is intended to mitigate a *merely* speculative restriction of the agency of members of the public (should exposure to the emissions actually prove harmful), expecting the public to bear the burden of proof and confirm the presence of an actual public health risk is, in fact, justified. This objection is slightly off the mark, however. The aim here is to reconcile the two parties' competing interests and standing, not to privilege one at the expense of the other. As such, the intention is to avoid giving emitters license under uncertainty to perform actions that may cause preventable harm to others, while also neglecting to impose unreasonable restrictions on the agency of emitters for the sake of insulating the public from effluents that may in the end cause no harm. As Chapter 5 explains in detail, when exploring how emitters can satisfy their duties of due care under uncertainty, it is the same commitment to equality and reciprocity that justifies precautionary measures to protect public health that also justifies protecting emitters from undue constraints and requiring that the public bear some of the burden of the costs of these safeguards.

4.2 Ethics of Risk and Unreasonable Risk Impositions

In broadening the purview from actual harms to mere risks of harm, scholarship in the ethics of risk suggests that the problem of uncertain threats can be explained away, that the moral permissibility of actions that entail indeterminate possibilities of harm can be validated, by demonstrating the trivial nature of uncertain threats.

With traditional risk impositions what remains unknown is only the probability that harm will come to pass, for it is generally assumed that the outcomes of risky actions can be foreseen. Moreover, it is presumed that probability uncertainty notwithstanding, we *can* still estimate the likelihood that some risky action will injure others: for it is presupposed that we are privy to certain knowledge about the possible harm, including but not limited to the actors and potential victims involved, the causal chain from the action to its effects, the influence of likely extraneous causal factors, the ways in which potential victims are exposed to the risk, and the severity of the foreseeable harms.[26] And with this knowledge, it is possible to delineate which risk impositions are wrongful.

Delimiting morally objectionable risk, however, is not just a matter of the probability that some action will cause harm (though Feinberg states that "we should rarely, if ever, tolerate a probability of more than half").[27] Rather, wrongful risks are defined along sliding scales of probability and magnitude (or severity) of anticipated harm—such that neither high probability nor lethal consequence is a sufficient condition of a wrongful imposition of risk. Rather, the greater the probability for injury, the lower the severity of the injury needs to be for the risk to constitute a moral wrong (and thus to justify restricting or prohibiting the risky action). Conversely, the lower the probability of harm, the more severe the (less likely) injury must be for the risk imposition to be objectionable.[28]

A somewhat exaggerated example of this is the wrongful risk created by playing Russian roulette on unsuspecting passersby.[29] Thomson maintains that even if no harm is caused (i.e., "no bullet was under the firing pin when [the gun was] fired"), and even if the target of the potential harm was unaware of the possibility for injury (and thus would not have experienced any psychological damage, for example), the fact that an avoidable, unprovoked, or undeserved "risk of death" is imposed on someone makes the risky action wrongful.[30] In exploring the possibility that existing tort law can address the normative and legal problems of risk (or "probabilistic indeterminacy"), Robinson echoes Thomson's claim that there are instances of "wrongful risk creation" and that individuals who impose "unreasonable risk[s] of harm" on others can be held culpable in much the same way that we hold perpetrators of actual harm responsible.[31]

Appealing to precedent-setting tort cases like *Summers v. Tice* (1948),[32] *Sindell v. Abbott Labs* (1980),[33] and *Jackson v. Johns-Manville Sales Corp.* (1986),[34] Robinson both clarifies that "victims now recover not simply for presently manifested harm but for estimated future harms that may or may not materialize," and he also explains that conventional tort law does *not* require the injured to demonstrate that the harm that is borne is the "certain product" of some action or omission of the injurer. Rather, among Robinson's central claims is that causation (and any proof thereof) is "inherently probabilistic"[35] and thus that causal responsibility may well be indeterminate[36]—as occurred in both *Summers v. Tice* and *Sindell v. Abbott Labs.*

In the former case, the California Supreme Court ruled against the defendants, two hunters, both of whom had discharged bird shots during a quail hunt, but neither of whom could be proven to have caused the gunshot injury to the plaintiff.[37] Similarly, in the latter case, the California Supreme Court ruled in favor of the plaintiff, who had contracted cancer as an adult from receiving diethylstilbestrol, or DES (a synthetic estrogen), while in utero, but was unable to identify the manufacturer of the particular drugs her mother had taken during the pregnancy and which had caused the injury.[38] And the *Jackson* case is especially germane here since it specifically concerns the potential for future environmental harm. The U.S. Court of Appeals found that although the plaintiff had been harmed by workplace exposure to airborne asbestos fibers (having developed asbestosis), this exposure made him susceptible to developing cancer in the future—a risk of harm for which the court ruled the plaintiff must be compensated. Robinson insists that cases like *Jackson v. Johns-Manville Sales Corp.* illustrate the plausibility of assigning moral responsibility (and legal liability) for mere risk impositions.[39]

Accordingly, proponents of this account might argue that they already provide a plausible expectation of due care to mitigate the possibility for harm to public health, undermining the need for a subsequent standard of due care, whereby the greater the probability that a risky action will cause some harm and/or the graver the anticipated harm becomes, the stronger one's obligation becomes to strive to prevent the adverse consequences from coming to pass. This would accord with Thomson's claim that it is those risk impositions that carry a "high risk of death" that are most clearly wrongful and blameworthy and aligns closely with Feinberg's analysis about when it is justified to coercively restrict one's right to engage in risky conduct.[40] Such a duty would at base require a person not engage in the risky action in the first place whenever some substantive (nontrivial) harm is highly probable—which would then become an epistemic question that turns on whether or not we know the anticipated consequence(s) to be substantive or trivia, and whether or not we know that the probability this substantive or trivial harm will occur is strong or weak. Whether concerning the possible dangers of color additives in foods and cosmetics,[41] of exposure to asbestos in various consumer products,[42] of ingestion of chloroform in public drinking water,[43] and so forth, decisions to protect public health from risks of environmental harm commonly take this approach: with legislators, regulators, and the courts striving to establish a standard for what an illegitimate or unreasonable risk consists of.

Despite controversy over what distinguishes "safe" or "acceptable" risks from "unreasonable" risks of environmental harm,[44] the inclination in the ethics of risk is to establish a general principle of tolerable risk, which identifies some lower threshold of *de minimis* (or trivial) risk, below which no risk imposition can be wrongful, and some upper threshold of grave risk, above which no probability, however slight, is acceptable.[45] These extremes are typically regarded as uncontroversial, with the enduring normative debates centering on demarcating wrongful risks between the peripheries—debates that have given shape to the guiding principle that *nothing less than* a clear and present danger, an imminent (highly probable) and substantive (nontrivial) risk of harm, is necessary to justify restricting actions that beget these credible risks.[46] Like actual harms, credible risks are regarded as impermissible—galvanizing our duty *not* to act in ways that expose others to these risks and our blameworthiness whenever we fail to satisfy this obligation. (Though one would be more blameworthy if the risk causes harm than if the risk never materializes in any actual injury.) In contrast, risks that fail to meet this benchmark may be morally regrettable—constituting, perhaps, what Feinberg terms "non-grievance" or "free-floating" evils or "harmless immoralities"[47]—but they do *not* warrant holding risk takers culpable. And because such risks are permissible, there is neither a corresponding duty nor a reason to refrain from performing actions that beget these risks. After all, there can be no "absolute right not to be subject to any risk to which one has not consented, for this would seem to rule out virtually all action."[48]

Some have resisted this analysis, stressing instead that until a risk imposition creates some *de facto* harm—where the injury, its perpetrator, and the victim of the harm can be discerned and causal responsibility for the harm can be verified—it is misplaced to speak of assigning culpability.[49] Expressed differently, critics allege that there is no ground for holding actors culpable for actions that fall short of causing demonstrable material harm. Yet to suggest that risk impositions can never justify requiring a person to alter his behavior to strive to prevent harming others is to grant risk takers license to act in ways that will inevitably prove to harm some—provided they retroactively right these wrongs by compensating their victims. (This, of course, is to assume that compensation can right a wrong in the first place,[50] where an individual "is rendered neither better off nor worse off by the combination of suffering the rights violation and receiving the compensation for it."[51]) While the rights or interests of those who bear credible risks to be insulated from harm need to be balanced against the rights or interests of risk takers to engage in risky actions, even the most ardent proponents of freedom from interference admit that a principle of requisite compensation is inadequate to the task and that it is untenable to suggest that paying this compensation makes any risky action permissible.[52] This is especially so with potentially lethal risks (irreversible or irreparable harm), such as workplace exposure to asbestos or nuclear radiation, which may lead to life-threatening or life-altering illness like lung cancer or brain tumors.

In any event, the probable and substantive requisite of morally objectionable risks undermines the ability of conventional risk theory to account for uncertain threats of harm. First, it is dubious to treat all threats that do not allow for probabilistic assessments of likely outcomes as morally permissible—that uncertain threats of environmental harm lack the toxicity data necessary to draw conclusions about plausible outcomes of exposure and probability of harm upon exposure does not negate the potential for harm. Further, risks of harm presuppose clear causal connections, which permit, for example, the identification of risk takers and potential victims and verification of the risk takers' causal responsibility for creating the potential for harm. Yet given the complex causal chains characteristic of environmental harms, as discussed earlier, it is unlikely that with many environmental harms and risks of harm, it is possible to demonstrate causation to establish culpability as risk theory requires.

Now one might object and claim that we could assess risks statistically without ever having to establish clear causal connections. Suppose, for instance, that we observe that the rate of stomach cancer is twice as high among people who eat conventional meats that contain antibiotics and growth hormones than those who eat organic meats. With this statistical information, we could then conclude that to knowingly expose others to antibiotics and growth hormones is to violate our duty of due care—*even if* we never establish an actual causal connection between exposure and stomach cancer.

Beyond the fact that such inductive inferences may well be false (what Dewey terms "empirical coincidences"[53]), since we are assuming that no other factor could be causing the higher rate of stomach cancer we observe (which would make for a spurious correlation), there are only two ways that we could establish reliable statistics of the possibility for harm without studies involving people who are actually exposed to the substance—both of which are problematic. The first involves epidemiological studies of lab animals in controlled environments, from which scientists could extrapolate the likely effects to humans. The merits of extrapolation are contested—these controlled environments do not adequately represent the messy causal connections of exposure in the actual environment—and in this scenario there could not be a *clearer* causal connection, since all plausible variables are controlled for. The second is when a substance whose effects are uncorroborated shares key similarities to another substance whose effects and probability of causing harm *are* known—from which we can infer that similar pathways and degrees of exposure to the uncertain threat will yield similar harms. While this is helpful (as Figure 5.1 explicitly notes), this will only pertain to a subset of the thousands of uncertain environmental threats we face. More importantly, however, the importance of establishing more accurate causal connections has been central to industry's justification to delay regulation when available toxicity tests cannot confirm with a preponderance of evidence that exposure to the substance in question is the primary cause of the harm we observe (in lab animals or human beings). This is to say that critics of precaution, who insist that it is only impositions of probable risks of nontrivial harm that merit being restricted, and who advocate using quantitative risk assessments to discern thresholds of unreasonable risks—which require establishing clear causal connections—would likely resist this inductive method of assessing risk and delimiting our moral duties under uncertainty.

Moreover, as with cumulative environmental exposures, when one is exposed to numerous trivial risk impositions, each of which independently causes no "ill consequence,"[54] the aggregate effect *can*, in fact, create some actual harm.[55] And this casts doubt on the permissibility of risky but individually harmless actions that nevertheless contribute to some collective harm. Lastly, the only way we can make sense of uncertain threats in this view, the only way we can plausibly extend traditional risk theory to account for threats under conditions of uncertainty, is to conceive of uncertain threats as trivial risks.

Treating uncertain threats as trivial would mean that harm is highly improbable and/or that any resultant harm would be negligible[56] and, thus, that uncertain threats are morally permissible. Yet to equate uncertain threats to trivial risks, and to assert that uncertain threats are improbable and/or would constitute minor harms if they were to come to bear, is to assume knowledge to which we do not have access under conditions of outcome and probability uncertainty. It has been argued that uncertain threats of environmental harm pose a unique normative problem precisely because the potential for harm to others is indeterminate (and because these threats are pervasive). Thus, there is no epistemic ground for concluding that uncertain environmental threats pose negligible harm whose probability of occurring is nominal, and there is no moral ground for granting *ipso facto* the permissibility of endangering actions on the faulty epistemic basis that the threats they pose are trivial.

One may object that there also is no epistemic ground for claiming that uncertain environmental threats pose probable non-negligible harm, and so there is no moral justification for categorizing actions that engender these possibilities of harm as impermissible. And these antithetical arguments might seem to lead to insurmountable or paralyzing skepticism—of an analogous sort that characterizes the stalled debate between proponents and critics of the precautionary principle, as Chapter 2 explained. However, as the following discussion and Chapter 5.3 both detail, the objection is mistaken: for many uncertain threats of environmental harm, regardless of our inability to foresee potentially harmful outcomes or to calculate the probabilities that these outcomes will come to pass, there *is* compelling reason to suspect that some injury will come to those who are exposed.

4.3 Moral Luck and the Epistemic Limitation Excuse

It has been stressed that environmental public health threats created under conditions of uncertainty entail that the consequences are indeterminate, that the different possible ways in which people may be exposed to the substances are unclear, and that the probability that those who are exposed through one or more possible pathways may be injured upon exposure is unknown, due in part to their particular physiological dispositions to the substances to which they are exposed. These considerations may seem at first blush damning to P_7, which again states that prevailing outcome and probability uncertainty do not excuse culpability or justify the permissibility of uncertain threats. These considerations seem to create problems for this key premise of the argument for precaution because whether or not a person is predisposed or vulnerable to being harmed if exposed to an uncertain environmental threat, and whether one is likely to be exposed and what the injury would consist of if these consequences proved to be harmful, all seem to exceed the control of the actor who emits a potentially harmful substance under conditions of uncertainty. As such, it seems to be a matter of luck whether or not emitters who create uncertain threats are culpable, since it is a matter of luck whether some may be injured by their actions.[57] And in the absence of fault, one cannot be said to commit a wrongdoing: one is, as it were, blameless.

Arguments from moral luck, therefore, would suggest that given our epistemic limitations, given our inability to know whether an uncertain threat is likely to cause injury, culpability under uncertainty should be excused, for rational people, absent deficiencies in their cognitive faculties, cannot be expected to know better. This would *both* mean that creating uncertain threats is not morally objectionable (there is no justifiable normative reason for restricting or prohibiting actions that generate indeterminate threats) and that if others are, in fact, harmed (if an uncertain threat does prove injurious), the epistemic limitation excuse diminishes one's culpability for the ensuing harm.

Let us say, for example, that Mark rediscovers a resin that has been out of production for decades with which he can make durable plastic products at very low costs and that he decides to open a new manufacturing plant to produce plastic bottles and various cans for beverages and processed foods with this particular resin. Now suppose that this forgotten resin is one of the tens of thousands of grandfathered chemical substances under the Toxic Substances Control Act (TSCA) exempt from toxicity testing before its manufacture is permitted. And suppose that the toxicological profile of this resin, like that of countless other substances being manufactured in the United States, is incomplete and that Mark—in full compliance with the law—makes no effort to test the existing substance, whereby the possible adverse health effects of exposure to the resin remain uncorroborated. Arguments from moral luck should have us conclude that the fact that it is uncertain whether the resin in Mark's plastics may leach into the beverages and foods that others consume and cause them subsequent harm is, without qualification, sufficient to absolve Mark of any possible wrongdoing. Given Mark's reasonable epistemic limitations, even if we later learn that the resin imposes an unreasonable risk on the public (a high probability of substantive harm), and even if we later discover that exposure to these plastics caused irreparable harm to some consumers, Mark is not culpable for the uncertain threat, the unreasonable risk, or the actual harm that materializes. This is because, it is alleged, Mark could not have been expected to know that exposure to his resin would cause harm: certainly had he known, he would have acted differently, and so it would be unjust to blame him for any wrongdoing. As the following discussion bears out, however, as with conventional accounts of moral responsibility and risk theory, arguments from moral luck that strive to justify the permissibility of uncertain threats of environmental harm are also problematic.

It is important to note that this "ignorance of circumstance"[58]—unavoidable limits to what we can know and foresee about our actions and their outcomes[59]—is one of many excusing conditions that are conventionally said to mitigate culpability. This idea of diminished culpability is grounded in the prevalent belief that a person should not be held responsible for something she could not control.[60,61] Also, for ignorance to be excusable, it must be justifiable or reasonable, such that any normal, rational person would be unable to anticipate the outcomes of a course of action, given her knowledge of the situation. This qualification accounts for the limits to what objectively true knowledge we are privy to while preventing actors from skirting culpability by opportunistically claiming ignorance of, or intentionally remaining ignorant to, ascertainable facts about the consequences of their actions.

Dworkin explains that causing unintentional and unforeseeable harm to others ostensibly undermines one's responsibility, "since one is *always* liable [i.e., has the potential] to produce such harm whenever one acts, since there is no way of taking into account such harms."[62] Accordingly, whenever it is impossible to anticipate that one's action will cause others injury, Dworkin suggests that rather than hold the actor responsible, it would be "more reasonable to let such losses lie where they fall."[63] Reid analogously treats as axiomatic the claim that "no man can be under a moral obligation to do what it is impossible for him to do, or to forbear what is impossible for him to forbear."[64] In the context of reasonable ignorance, this implies that when it is not possible to ascertain or foresee the likely outcomes of an action, if an uncertain possibility of harm to others exists, then it cannot be expected that a person refrain from acting as he does and impose the uncertain threat on others.[65] In the absence of information necessary to render judgments about what actions are preferable or permissible, our capacity to exercise our freedom of the will—that is, our capacity to perform voluntary and deliberative actions—is frustrated. Instead, when we lack this information, our choices and actions, says Reid,

> must be made perfectly in the dark, without reason, motive, or end. They can neither be right nor wrong, wise nor foolish. Whatever the consequences may be, they cannot be imputed to the agent, who had not the capacity of foreseeing them, or of perceiving any reason for acting otherwise than he did.[66]

This parallels Nagel's notion of "resultant luck" and the idea that one cannot be blameworthy for actions from reasonable ignorance.[67] Plainly, resultant luck—one of four categories delineated by Nagel[68]—concerns the lack of control over "the way things turn out" (the lack of control over the consequences of one's actions).[69] Resultant luck aptly characterizes ignorance of circumstance, since a person cannot control outcomes that she is unable to foresee, the effects of which she is justifiably ignorant. For example, in his analysis of "innocent" versus "excused threats" and moral liability to defensive action, McMahan considers the case of the conscientious driver—a variation of Nagel's original example of the negligent driver. The conscientious driver is one who keeps her car in good repair and who drives cautiously and alertly at all times. Yet while driving on one occasion, the conscientious driver experiences a "freak event" that could not have been foreseen by anyone in her position and which—through no fault of her own—"causes her car to veer out of control in the direction of a pedestrian."[70] In Nagel's treatment of this case, it is a child who unexpectedly darts out into the street, compelling the driver to brake suddenly.[71] McMahan concludes that when considering the subjective justification that the conscientious driver has for her belief that driving her (well-maintained vehicle) will cause no harm to others, she is innocent and blameless for the harm that may come to the pedestrian toward whom her car now barrels (which, therefore, constrains the innocent pedestrian's ability to use lethal means to defend herself against the driver).[72] The driver is blameless because if harm were to befall the pedestrian, it would be a matter of sheer luck, as it is impossible for us to foresee these sorts of unexpected events—whether it is a mechanical failure, as with McMahan's example, or an independent, intervening action of another person, as with Nagel's thought experiment.[73] Thus, when considering the actions of two equally negligent drivers, Nagel maintains that because it is a matter of luck that the child runs into the street—whose wrongful death the driver's negligent vehicle maintenance facilitates (having failed, e.g., to ensure his brakes function properly[74])—it is equally a matter of luck that the other negligent driver who does *not* have to brake suddenly to avoid striking the child is only blameworthy for his negligence and not vehicular manslaughter. Both actors are equally responsible for failing to keep their cars in good repair and it is simply "bad luck" to which the child's injury seems attributable.[75]

While we can accept that certain causal factors are beyond our control that may warrant diminishing one's culpability or even fully exonerating a person for engaging in wrongdoing, ignorance of circumstance is *not* a legitimate excusing condition for exposing others to uncertain threats. Accepting that reasonable ignorance is excusable would mean that no uncertain environmental threat is morally problematic and that no requirement of due care under uncertainty is defensible—since emitters who release substances into the environment under conditions of uncertainty cannot reasonably be expected to know better or act differently than they do. They are, one might say, in McMahan's sense, like the conscientious driver: there is no way for emitters to objectively know that the uncertain potential for harm will prove to injure others. After all, in the absence of corroborating evidence to the contrary, there seems to be *as much* reason to believe that an uncertain environmental threat will be harmless as there is to believe that it will cause harm. And if emitters merit being absolved of culpability, then authoring uncertain threats of environmental harm is, in a word, permissible. It is mistaken, however, to treat reasonable ignorance as excusing culpability for uncertain environmental threats for at least the following four reasons.

(1) In perceiving uncertain threats as morally innocuous, arguments from moral luck essentially equate uncertainty to relative safety, treating uncertain threats as safe to human health. Yet it is erroneous to suggest that the absence of corroborating evidence of harm or unreasonable risk of harm equates to evidence of the benign nature of an uncertain threat. This is to beg the question against the very issue at hand. As Shrader-Frechette aptly notes in her authoritative analysis in *Taking Action, Saving Lives*, "from flawed or incomplete evidence—ignorance—no conclusion follows" about the relative safety or danger of exposure: "failure to have evidence does not prove anything, one way or the other."[76] If we reject, like Shrader-Frechette does, that the "absence of evidence" of harm equates to "evidence of absence" of harm, then until the potential for harm can be verified scientifically, we are obliged to suspend judgment about whether the consequences of exposure will be benign.

Advocates of the epistemic limitation excuse might deny that they draw this inference at all. They may insist that they suspend their judgment about whether or not uncertain threats are safe and conclude instead that it is because we cannot know whether the consequences will be harmful that assigning culpability would be unjustified. While semantically these are substantively different claims, the implication is the same. For proponents of excusable ignorance to argue that actors cannot be held culpable for actions whose outcomes are indeterminate is to imply that emitters cannot be expected to choose alternative courses of action that do not involve exposing others to uncertain threats. And to maintain that these actions are permissible is to give emitters unqualified license to release potentially harmful effluents into the environment. Yet prevailing uncertainty should prompt defenders of the epistemic limitation excuse—whose arguments are grounded in what we can or cannot know about the actual dangers to others—to suspend judgment about the permissibility or impermissibility of actions that beget uncertain threats, and thus to refrain from endorsing this license to emit. By not suspending judgment on the question of permissibility, proponents insinuate that these threats pose no legitimate safety concern to the public, for any judgment to the contrary would undercut the plausibility of their blanket denial that uncertain threats can ever justifiably be restricted and of their willingness to place the burden of the costs of any ensuing environmental harm squarely on the shoulders of the public.[77]

(2) Emitters cannot be excused for the uncertain threats they author because their ignorance is not reasonable. Even under conditions of outcome and probability uncertainty, we have access to at least two relevant facts, which we can reasonably expect emitters to know and which would make emitters culpable both for their ignorance and their actions from ignorance that put others in the way of potential harm: (a) we are aware of our environmental history, which is rife with examples of how the emission of substances into the environment has harmed public health and (b) we are aware of our ignorance—we know that we do not know the consequences of uncertain threats.[78]

Concerning (a), consider that despite the high-profile ban of DDT in 1972, the release of carcinogenic pesticides (like chlordane and dieldrin) and suspected carcinogenic pesticides (like atrazine, cyanazine, simazine, alachlor, and metolachlor) continues today. These substances are commonly found in the foods we consume and water we drink and in diverse public spaces and waterways.[79] It is estimated that such pesticides cause more than 13,000 deaths annually in the United States[80] (25 percent more than the yearly fatalities involving drunk drivers[81]), as well as various cancers and life-threatening or life-altering illnesses,[82] and their rates of consumption (and thus emission) are on the rise. As of 2011, the rate of consumption amounted to 5.1 billion pounds annually (or roughly 17 pounds per person per year).[83] And exposure to these "dietary pesticides"[84] constitutes *but one* example of myriad documented harms to public health in American environmental history.[85]

What we can and should glean from the prevalence of these sorts of environmental harms, as well as from specific cases like tetraethyl lead (a gasoline additive) in the 1920s, DDT (a pesticide) in the 1950s, and DES (a synthetic estrogen) in the 1970s is that because past exposure to substances whose effects were poorly understood and once deemed safe to public health have proven to be detrimental, future exposure to substances whose potential for harm is indeterminate is also likely to cause some actual harm. This is to say that irrespective of prevailing uncertainty about the severity and probability of harm of any particular threat, historical and contemporary trends substantiate the inference that because the release of substances into the environment has, in the past, commonly injured those who were exposed, we should expect that the release of substances in the present and future will eventually cause some material harm to some people.

And since it is reasonable to expect authors of uncertain threats of environmental harm to know that the release of chemical substances has, in the past, preceded injury to those who were exposed, they should be able to foresee *some*, if only vague, potential for harm to others when uncertainty prevails. Access to this morally relevant knowledge gives emitters *pro tanto* reason to exercise due care to mitigate the potential for harm to those who may bear the consequences of their endangering actions—undermining the plausibility of the epistemic limitation excuse. More strongly, as Section 4.3 subsequently details, this reason translates into a *pro tanto* duty to take due care with many uncertain environmental threats.

With regard to (b), it is unclear why arguments from moral luck neglect to consider the alternative upshot that rather than relax our moral obligations, knowledge of our own ignorance actually amplifies our duty not to harm others—galvanizing discrete duties under conditions of uncertainty. Again, excusable ignorance maintains that if I am incapable of knowing better, I have no reason and no obligation to act differently than I do, *even if* my action does ultimately bring undeserved harm to others. Yet there is more to the moral salience of ignorance. Knowledge of one's ignorance of circumstance may be sufficient reason to act differently; it may arguably require that one conscientiously and deliberately strive to minimize the possibility that her endangering actions may injure others. It may require, for example, that one deliberate about alternative courses of action that can still satisfy her ends, or further scrutinize the action to identify plausible outcomes, or reevaluate the ends that motivate her to perform the action in the first place if no feasible alternative action is possible.[86] And since this duty is triggered by one's lack of knowledge about how others may be affected, its disregard could not be excused on the grounds of ignorance. Reid, while sympathetic to the merit of excusing conditions, gestures toward this sort of auxiliary obligation.

Reid acknowledges that mitigating a person's culpability is sometimes justified: for instance, when one is judged to have been unable to resist a base impulse, that is, when one is judged to lack the capacity (at least in the moment of action) to act from "sober judgment." When some internal or external factor beyond a person's control determines one's action, Reid accepts that the wrongdoing should be attributed both to the agent and to the independent factor (here, the agent's brute impulse), such that one's blameworthiness diminishes "in proportion to" the efficacy or influence of this causal factor.[87] Nevertheless, Reid complicates the notion of reasonable ignorance, and the merit for treating it as an excusing condition, by suggesting that it is incumbent on the actor to try to overcome her ignorance, to try to ascertain the likely effects of her actions:

> Every man knows that it is in his power to deliberate or not to deliberate about any part of his conduct; to deliberate for a shorter, or a longer time, more carelessly, or more seriously [and] he may either honestly

> use the best means in his power to form an impartial judgment, or he may yield to his bias, and only seek arguments to justify what inclination leads him to do. In all these points, he determines, he wills, the right or the wrong. [. . .] *When the case is not clear*, when it is of importance, and when there is time for deliberation, we ought to deliberate with more or less care, in proportion to the importance of the action.[88]
>
> What we call a fault of ignorance, is always owing to the want of due deliberation. When we do not *take due pains to be rightly informed*, there is a fault, not indeed in acting according to the light we have, but *in not using the proper means to get the light*. For if we judge wrong after using the proper means of information, there is no fault in acting according to that wrong judgment; the error is invincible.[89]

Now Reid may overstate the implication that "due deliberation" fully absolves a person of her culpability for any harmful consequences her actions may cause, but he aptly illustrates how ignorance does not necessarily pardon the actor. The sentiments do more than merely restate the earlier mentioned requirement of reasonability: that ignorance cannot be intentional or calculated, or the result of passive indifference to available facts, but rather that it must be genuine. Reid's assertions call for a higher standard. Treating ignorance as a legitimate excusing condition requires more than determining that the actor was reasonably ignorant, that given our inherent epistemic limitations, he could not have known that his action may harm others. Rather, to excuse the actor's culpability, it is necessary to scrutinize how one alters his decision-making in response to his awareness of his ignorance—which is to say that ignorance of circumstance can only mitigate one's responsibility if one conscientiously strives to overcome his ignorance.[90]

Analogously, then, for an action that generates an uncertain threat of environmental harm to be morally permissible, and for the actor to merit having his culpability mitigated for the threat he authors and any harm his endangering action may prove to create, the actor must conscientiously take some preventative measures to mitigate the potential for harm to others.

(3) If we couple this line of reasoning with Dworkin's claim that one's subjectively justified belief in the adverse outcomes of her actions—versus corroborating evidence or knowledge of their actual effects—is reason enough to "[refrain] from acting,"[91] then we have *prima facie* sufficient reason to abstain from acting in ways that expose others to uncertain threats of environmental harm. If an actor could reasonably be expected to know that her emission of some substance whose effects are uncertain has some potential to cause others injury (which contemporary environmental history validates), and if this belief were a legitimate reason to refrain from performing the potentially harmful action as Dworkin posits, then if the actor nevertheless chooses to emit the substance into the environment, she is culpable and "must be able to account for [her] action."[92] (That is, of course, unless she took measures to investigate

the possibility of harm to others, which yielded reliable information that her emissions would not endanger others.)

This also aligns with McMahan's qualification that while the conscientious driver's act of driving is subjectively *permissible*—given the driver's epistemic limitation and, therefore, her inability to foresee the "freak event" that makes her lose control of her vehicle—the driver's act nevertheless is *not* subjectively *justified*. This is because the driver should know—*is expected to know*—that there is a small chance that innocent bystanders may be harmed as a result of her operating the car, and this knowledge undermines her "moral reasons for engaging in the activity."[93] That is, it precludes her moral justification for doing so. Furthermore, what renders her act of driving morally permissible, and what ultimately excuses her culpability if the marginal possibility for harm to bystanders proves to materialize in some actual injury, is precisely the conscientious manner in which she maintains and drives the car. McMahan suggests that it is the driver's conviction that her concerted efforts to keep the car in good repair and to drive cautiously will successfully prevent bystanders from being harmed that establishes the permissibility of her action. However, this permissibility presupposes that she *actually exercises this precaution* to mitigate the potential for harm—conscientious preventative measures on which any legitimate exculpatory plea, in turn, depends.

(4) Finally, believing that one's awareness of the possibility for harm gives one reason to refrain from performing the potentially harmful action, Otsuka maintains that if a person has the option to act otherwise and chooses not to, and if by some stroke of moral luck an unforeseeable causal factor intervenes such that the action proves to entail harm, then considerations of what is beyond the actor's control should be immaterial: the actor should be held culpable for the outcomes of his action.[94] More precisely, building on Dworkin's notion of "option luck"—which is a form of luck that one "exposes" herself to whenever one makes a "deliberate and calculated gamble" on the possible outcome of a potentially harmful action she performs[95]—Otsuka argues that when the actor "could have avoided being blameworthy altogether" by acting on an alternative available to her that entailed no such possibility for harm, then moral luck notwithstanding, the actor is *not* exempt from culpability for the unlucky harmful consequences her action begets.[96]

Suppose, then, that Mark, our manufacturer mentioned earlier, had available to him different resins with which he could have produced his plastic food and beverage packaging products: resins whose toxicity profiles were complete, whose health effects were therefore known, whose risks to public health were regulated by existing emission standards, and whose use would still allow him to make a profit (i.e., the alternatives were feasible). And suppose that Mark knew that these alternative resins were available to him, that he knew that any one of these options would have allowed him to avoid authoring an uncertain threat in the first place, and that he nevertheless ignored these alternatives. Finally, let us say that exposure to the resins in Mark's products, as with the first scenario, proves to cause some harm to consumers—but this harm occurs for reasons beyond Mark's control: for example, one of the automated machines that prepares the liquid resin mixture that will be molded into plastic containers malfunctions and disperses an unsafe quantity of the resin into the mixture, such that a batch of Mark's products contains an unsafe concentration of the substance. In Otsuka's account, even if we grant that Mark is not responsible for the malfunction and that the harm was a matter of unfortunate luck, Mark's ignorance and his stroke of bad luck are immaterial. Mark had the opportunity to avoid exposing others to potential harm and failed to take advantage of it: he should not benefit from his ignorance.

To further clarify the point, recall Nagel's example of the pair of negligent drivers, one of whom hits and kills a child who unforeseeably darts into the path of the poorly maintained car. According to Otsuka's "principle of avoidable blame," had this unlucky driver acted on any number of available (and presumably feasible) alternatives, he could have avoided blame for the ensuing harm.[97] The faulty driver could have opted to call a taxi, or to have a friend drive him, or he could have hopped a bus or ridden a bike instead of driving to his destination, or he could have stayed at home, or he could have thrown on his hazard lights and driven extremely slowly (ensuring that no impact would have been fatal), and so forth. Yet the driver disregarded such options and freely decided to gamble that his driving would harm no one. When this proves to be false and he strikes the child, in addition to being blameworthy for his negligence, Otsuka contends that the unlucky outcome is attributable *not* to moral luck but to the driver. And since the bad luck could have been avoided,[98] we should understand the luck and the culpability for the ensuing harm as voluntarily brought on by the actor himself—which is precisely why that although moral luck intervenes in these instances, diminishing the actor's culpability is not justified.

Now admittedly, Otsuka grounds this analysis in the actor's ability to "reasonably foresee" the effects of his wrongdoings. Conversely, one's culpability for a bad outcome *would* merit being attenuated when he cannot reasonably be able to anticipate the likely consequences of performing some action.[99] While this strongly resembles Nagel's notion of reasonable ignorance, which would excuse the harm as a matter of unavoidable resultant luck—an epistemic limitation that would ostensibly justify the actor "in choosing as he did, given the information available at the time of his choice," would thus absolve him of culpability.[100] Given this emphasis on "known risk[s],"[101] it would initially appear that Otsuka's analysis does not apply to uncertain threats of environmental harm, which preclude our ability to discern both the harmful effects and the likelihood that these effects will come to pass.

However, as (2) earlier argues (and as Chapter 4.3 initially suggested), even under conditions of uncertainty, emitters cannot claim to be ignorant of the possibility for harm: they do have adequate reason to believe that their emissions may injure others. Moreover, like Nagel, Otsuka also neglects to expand on what is reasonable to foresee, on what is reasonable to expect others to foresee. Examples commonly invoked of reckless driving, drunk driving, attempted murder, etc., may be helpful in clarifying difficult concepts or motivating complex conceptual problems, but such examples consist in (purposefully) overly simplified causal relationships, which provides a false impression that less clear or obvious or familiar outcomes cannot be foreseen. Stressing the historically harmful nature of the substances humans release into the environment, and underscoring McMahan's explicit suggestion that a person can *know* that an action she intends to perform entails even a small chance of harm to innocent people,[102] it *is* plausible that actors who intend to emit substances into the environment under conditions of uncertainty *can* foresee the possibility that their emissions may injure others—however ill-defined the actors' understanding is of what these injuries would be. After all, Dworkin makes plain that the key consideration is whether "we can say that the possibility of loss was part of [the decision the actor made]."[103] And if we grant that with this minimum morally relevant knowledge an emitter who disregards alternatives available to him and who voluntary chooses to gamble on the consequences of his emissions, effectively "exposes" himself to culpability for failing to exercise due care to mitigate the potential for harm, then he cannot claim that his ignorance of the actual outcomes excuses his blameworthiness.

4.4 Initial Objections

One might object that any requirement of due care under uncertainty imposes undue burdens on emitters. Since uncertain threats may prove to be harmless, it is unfair to expect emitters to bear the costs of working to mitigate the potential for harm—the costs, for example, of publicizing the existence of an uncertain threat and disclosing information pertaining to the possibility for harm, of investing in efforts to ascertain the health effects of exposure, of considering alternative courses of action that do not entail similar threats, etc. Indeed, because it is the public that benefits from the preventative measures, their cost should not be borne solely by authors of uncertain threats.

The argument for exercising due care, however, is sensitive to this worry. What exercising due care under uncertainty may consist of is explored at length in the following chapter, but it is important to offer three preliminary clarifications here. First, a feasible principle of due care under uncertainty, which requires authors of uncertain threats to take reasonable precautionary measures to avoid exposing others to possible harm, cannot be so stringent that if the threat fails to materialize into an actual harm, we would retrospectively find the measure unreasonable. We must keep in plain view that the aim here is to reconcile, as a matter of moral equality and reciprocity, the freedom of those who wish to exercise their autonomy and engage in endangering actions that entail the discharge of potentially harmful substances, with the freedom of those who are exposed to the potentially harmful effects of these actions to *not* have others gamble with their welfare and place them in potential harm's way. Consequently, for example, when due care is exercised and an endangering action does prove to be harmless, the reciprocity between moral equals may require that the beneficiaries of this due care, whose interests and welfare are safeguarded, compensate the actor for striving to diminish the potential for harm.[104]

Second, in this vein, any reasonable standard of due care—while grounded in a universal principle of respecting others as ends in themselves—must be sensitive to context. This is to say that what due care under uncertainty requires and how one's obligation to exercise due care is discharged will vary across contexts and actors. For instance, if a substance is being manufactured or emitted in large volumes, or if some vulnerable population may be disproportionately exposed to uncertain threats emitters create, or if feasible alternatives are available to emitters, or if authors of uncertain threats profit from their potentially harmful discharges, then the duty of due care may be stricter than if these factors were not present. Alternatively, for example, if the amount of the substance being manufactured or emitted is minimal, or if no vulnerable population bears a disproportionate threat of harm, or if emitters have no history of noncompliance (delinquency) with existing environmental regulations, then their duty to exercise due care may be attenuated. Our moral assessments of the permissibility or impermissibility of creating an uncertain threat of environmental harm—of the strength of one's obligation to exercise due care when exposing others to an uncertain threat would be impermissible, and of one's culpability for disregarding her duty of due care—must be able to accommodate diverse, context-dependent, and morally relevant factors. For the untenable alternative is that all uncertain threats are equally impermissible, which Section 4.3 explicitly denies.

Third, the one consistent (non–context-dependent) expectation when uncertainty prevails, the central pillar of the proposed standard of due care, is our obligation to take reasonable strides to investigate and discern the possible effects of our actions to others to mitigate the potential for harm. This would mean, for instance, that corporate emitters have an obligation to test for the toxicity of the substances they use in their production processes or discharge into the environment, and to forthrightly disclose this testing data to regulators, and to provide details to the public on the potential for harm in easily accessible and understandable ways for individuals to be able to better insulate themselves from potential harm.

Notably, these are among the broad aims of recent legislative revisions to the TSCA. The Lautenberg Chemical Safety for the 21st Century Act, ratified in June 2016, no longer requires that a credible risk or probable exposure be verified before the Environmental Protection Agency (EPA) can require companies to conduct toxicity tests, and expands the agency's capacity to require testing of both new and existing substances;[105] it affords the EPA discretion to designate substances as "high priority" whenever companies fail to provide adequate safety assessment data upon request (which would then require companies to conduct full-fledged risk assessments);[106] it prohibits new substances from being manufactured in the absence of safety assessments confirming that the substance "is not likely to present an unreasonable risk of injury";[107] it explicitly requires that vulnerable populations—including infants and children, workers, and the elderly—be identified and protected from exposure;[108] and it promotes greater public disclosure of information by substantively constraining the conditions under which companies can legitimately claim that health and safety information is confidential.[109] These developments to the regulation of substances whose health effects are uncertain or understudied, which closely overlap with the proposed standard of due care developed in Chapter 5, and the Lautenberg Act's emphasis on the need to better protect the public from potential harm of exposure, which closely overlaps with the foregoing defense of a duty of due care, should lend credence to the plausibility of the normative argument from equality.

Nevertheless, others might object that the subset of environmental threats whose effects and probability of causing harm are intractably uncertain (i.e., cannot be ascertained with current scientific practices or technologies) is relatively small. For example, Sunstein argues that "uncertainty will often move, over time, into the realm of risk, simply because knowledge grows over time."[110] And since the instances in which the argument for due care exists are the exception and not the norm, since genuinely uncertain environmental threats are rare, the moral force of this argument is undermined.

This counterargument, however, makes two problematic assumptions. First, exceptional (uncommon) cases of a moral problem should not inform our moral reasoning about more common instances of the problem and thus similarly should not shape our normative prescriptions for ordinary circumstances. Second, there is no analogous moral problem posed by the widespread incomplete knowledge of the probability and severity of injury for the myriad threats of environmental harm we face.

The first is shortsighted, admitting of a willingness to confine moral reasoning within the bounds of the conventional, the orthodox. Yet much can be gleaned from rare or extreme cases, uncommon manifestations of moral problems that are often invoked by philosophers to motivate a given problem, to substantiate a particular intuition, or to punctuate a proposed solution. One need only to consider, for example, Foot's runaway trolley thought experiment, or Thomson's colorful variation in which the only way to stop the trolley is by throwing an innocent fat man onto the tracks,[111] or Nozick's discussion of the "abject proletariat" who is alleged to choose freely despite having but two highly unpalatable alternatives (choosing to work for the exploitative capitalist or to starve).[112] To demonstrate that even in the most *prima facie* unlikely cases a normative argument holds is to reinforce the merit of one's conclusions—and this is precisely what justifying our obligations of due care under uncertainty is intended to accomplish. To show that prevailing uncertainty, which effectively obscures our ability to know whether our actions actually put others in danger, does *not* cloud our duty to prevent exposing others to potential harm, but serves to strengthen our obligations when we *do* have (at least partial) knowledge of the outcomes of our actions and/or the probability that some harm to others will come to pass. (Knowledge that, again, may be limited in many cases of uncertainty to the relevant information we can deduce or intuit from our observations and knowledge of prior probabilities.)

The second understates or misunderstands the problem that we lack understanding of the health effects of an overwhelming number of substances routinely and lawfully emitted into the environment. For instance, the TSCA's Toxic Release Inventory not only has permitted emitters to *self*-report their release of chemical substances, but it has limited the subset of chemicals whose emission must be reported to roughly 60 of the 80,000 substances in use—of which regulatory agencies have only tested 1 percent.[113] Similarly, basic toxicity profiles of 93 percent of the 3,000 high-production-volume (HPV) chemicals produced or imported in the United States are wholly absent or incomplete.[114] Consider further that of the 830 chemical companies that manufacture HPV chemicals[115] in the United States, 148 lack any Screening Information Data Set (SIDS) data—that is, test results of complex dose-response toxicity studies—for the chemical substances they manufacture, "459 companies sell products for which, on average, half or less of SIDS tests are available," and a meager "21 companies (or 3 percent of the 830 companies) have all SIDS tests available for their chemicals."[116] To grant that intractable uncertainty is rare—that it is possible to successfully test for and estimate the actual health effects of most environmental threats—diminishes neither the salience of the pervasive problem of unverified possibilities of harm nor the obligations we have to prevent putting others in the way of potential, unconsented-to harm. For so long as attainable scientific evidence eludes regulators and the public, as long as the actual effects of exposure remain uncorroborated, the implication is the same: emitters wrongfully gambling with the welfare of others, putting others in the way of potentially injurious emissions, and thus neglecting to afford them the respect that their equal moral standing requires.

One might also charge that there is no way to avoid acting in ways that place others in the way of potential harm: risk of harm in modern society is ubiquitous, and since it is an inescapable fact of our moral reality, one should not be liable to blame or punishment for failing to do that which he cannot do (that is, ought implies can). Yet preventing all possibilities of harm is not what is being suggested here, so our inability to eliminate all the various possibilities of harm to others that our actions may entail is not altogether material. Rather, what this chapter has argued is that we should *strive* to prevent exposing others to potential harm—reasonable measures we *do* have control over. For there is something disquieting about theories of responsibility and risk that tolerate one's knowingly exposing others to possible, albeit uncertain, harm *so long as* these threats are unquantifiable or never materialize into actual injuries. And there is something disquieting about tolerating pervasive environmental threats: giving license to emitters to expose the public to countless substances that may well bring harm to some and thus tolerating emitters gambling with the welfare and autonomy of moral agents who have their own interests and ambitions, which do not presumably include being placed in the way of possible harm.[117]

What this chapter has argued is that these gambles are blameworthy *even* if a threat proves to be harmless and that unless we are willing to accept the position that *no* uncertain threat of environmental harm warrants prohibition, conventional accounts of uncertain threats are untenable. Insisting that culpability is predicated both on one's causing some material harm or a probable risk of nontrivial harm, and also on the absence of mitigating factors that exceed one's control, like reasonable ignorance, arguments from traditional theories of responsibility and risk should have us dismiss as morally innocuous the pervasive potential for harm that uncertain environmental threats pose. Yet this chapter has denied that authors of uncertain threats of environmental harm are excusably ignorant and has underscored that obligations of mutual respect are not diminished by prevailing uncertainty: even (especially?) when the effects of our actions are indeterminate, taking seriously the equal moral standing of others and the demands of reciprocity requires that we regard others as ends in themselves and refrain from gambling with their welfare by putting them in potential harm's way. Uniquely, this means that the wrongfulness of creating undeserved and preventable uncertain threats of harm is *not* foremost that our actions endanger others—it is not the threat itself, since it may well prove to be harmless—but rather that our actions fail to respect those who we happen to endanger.

And this *prima facie* is especially true when a person who authors an uncertain environmental threat could have acted otherwise. Recall that Otsuka argues that if a person has a feasible alternative course of action available to her that entails no obvious possibility of harm but nevertheless chooses to perform the action that *does* carry some potential for harm, then if by luck some unforeseeable causal factor intervenes and the action does cause harm, it is irrelevant that this exogenous factor exceeded her control. Given that the actor could have avoided the "deliberate and calculated gamble" on the possible outcome of a potentially harmful action she performs, the actor is *not* exempt from culpability.[118] Analogously, if one has alternatives available to her but chooses to perform an action that exposes others to uncertain possibilities of harm and does so without exercising due care to try to mitigate the potential for harm, then even if no injury occurs, "one's voluntary choice to gamble"[119] with the interests and welfare of others makes her worthy of blame and sanction.

Similarly, consider that Scanlon suggests that a chief criterion for assigning blame should be the capacity of those accused of wrongdoing to have had the opportunity to avoid blame "by choosing reasonably"—which implies a range of alternatives that the actor could have reasonably been expected to choose from.[120] This parallels Watson's suggestion that to hold someone morally responsible depends on whether the person had a "reasonable opportunity" to avoid violating (i.e., to comply with) the moral demands for which he is blamed and sanctioned.[121] What we can glean from these ideas is that if actors who perform actions that put others in the way of possible harm have viable alternatives to act differently, in ways that do not entail uncertain threats, they may be obliged to do so. For example, while authors of uncertain threats may not be expected to bear unreasonable costs of exercising due care and mitigating the potential for injury, when they can implement the highest possible standards of environmental protection (e.g., using the best available control technologies) at low costs, they are obliged to do so. Chapter 5 explores such considerations in detail and delimits the components of a feasible standard of due care: a standard that centers on achieving and disclosing "better health information"[122]—that is, on striving to eliminate uncertainty and to improve public awareness of the threats of environmental harm we face.[123]

Notes

1. Much of the material in Section 4.3 is reprinted from Levente Szentkirályi, "Luck Has Nothing to Do with It: Prevailing Uncertainty and Responsibilities of Due Care," *Ethics, Policy, and Environment* (forthcoming). I am grateful to the editors at *Ethics, Policy, and Environment* for kindly granting permission to reprint this material.
2. For a revisionary account of blaming and sanctioning, see Thomas M. Scanlon, *Moral Dimensions: Permissibility, Meaning, and Blame* (Cambridge: Belknap Press, 2008): Chapter 4.
3. Supra note 4.
4. Joel Feinberg, *Doing and Deserving* (Princeton: Princeton University Press, 1970): 32–3, 222. Joel Feinberg, "Sua Culpa," in *Doing and Deserving* (Princeton: Princeton University Press, I970).
5. Gerald Postema, "Morality in the First Person Plural," *Law and Philosophy* 14 (1995): 35–64.
6. The relationship between moral liability and responsibility—with specific regard to uncertain threats of environmental harm—is detailed in Chapter 5, when the discussion turns to the implementation of the proposed standard of due care.
7. These considerations and how they can mitigate one's culpability are explained in Section 4.3, which explains how theories of moral luck try to account for the problem of uncertain threats.
8. Borrowed from Strawson, "Freedom and Resentment," 6–10; Bennett, "Accountability," 40; Watson, "Responsibility and the Limits of Evil," 259–60; and Wallace, *Responsibility and the Moral Sentiments*, Chapters 5–6.
9. Jeff McMahan, *Killing in War* (Oxford: Oxford University Press, 2009): 104–54, 159–73.
10. Feinberg, *Doing and Deserving*, 32–3.
11. Dworkin, "Intention, Foreseeability, and Responsibility," 342.
12. Ibid., 341–2.
13. Ibid.
14. Bernard Williams, *Ethics and the Limits of Philosophy* (Cambridge: Harvard University Press, 1985): 194.
15. Ibid.
16. Shrader-Frechette's *Taking Action, Saving Live*, 79–81.
17. Ibid., 80.
18. This consideration is borrowed from Nozick (*Anarchy, State, and Utopia*, 74) and his discussion on legitimate proscriptions of risk. See also Dworkin, "Intention, Foreseeability, and Responsibility," 343.
19. C. Arden Pope, III et al., "Health Effects of Particulate Air Pollution: Time for Reassessment?," *Environmental Health Perspectives* 103 (1995).
20. See, e.g., Dworkin, "Intention, Foreseeability, and Responsibility," 339–41.
21. Sierra Club, *Leaking Underground Storage Tanks: A Threat to Public Health and Environment* (San Francisco: Sierra Club, 2005); Sacoby Wilson et al., "Leaking

Underground Storage Tanks and Environmental Injustice," *Environmental Justice* 6 (2013).

22. Environmental Protection Agency (EPA), *Leaking Underground Storage Tanks* (Washington, DC: EPA, 1985); EPA, *Underground Storage Tanks Program Facts* (Washington, DC: EPA, 2016): https://epa.gov/sites/production/files/2016-06/documents/program-facts-5-10-16.pdf; see also Steven Cohen, *Understanding Environmental Policy* (New York: Columbia University Press): 62–75.
23. Dworkin, "Intention, Foreseeability, and Responsibility," 341.
24. Agency for Toxic Substances and Disease Registry, "Toxicological Profile for Asbestos" (Atlanta: U.S. Department of Health and Human Services, 2001): 6; Marilyn Browne et al., "Cancer Incidence and Asbestos in Drinking Water, Town of Woodstock, New York, 1980–1998," *Environmental Research* 98 (2005): 229; John Gamble, "Risk of Gastrointestinal Cancers from Inhalation and Ingestion of Asbestos," *Regulatory Toxicology and Pharmacology* 52 (2008): S149.
25. There may be other arguments that would not commit us to this conclusion. For example, a consequentialist could claim that we do not need to establish culpability to regulate uncertain threats of harm—it's not that an actor does something wrong by creating an uncertain threat and failing to exercise due care—but rather we can justify precautionary measures because a requirement of due care promotes most everyone's interest: uncertain threats of environmental harm constitute a collective problem that demands a solution. If this approach, then, could demonstrate empirically that the benefits of regulating uncertain threats is greater than the costs, which skeptics have denied, it would offer an alternative plausible justification of a requirement of due care.
26. See, e.g., Glen O. Robinson, "Risk, Causation, and Harm," in *Liability and Responsibility: Essays in Law and Morals*, Raymond Frey and Christopher Morris, eds. (Cambridge: Cambridge University Press, 1991): 320–1. In discussing the merits of "risk-based liability," Robinson equates "probabilistic injury" or the "probability of [expected] harm" to risk.
27. Joel Feinberg, *Harm to Others: The Moral Limits of the Criminal Law*, Vol. 1 (Oxford: Oxford University Press, 1984): 191.
28. See, for example, Ibid., 190–2.
29. Judith Jarvis Thomson, "Imposing Risks," in *To Breathe Freely: Risk, Consent, and Air*, Mary Gibson, ed. (Totowa: Rowman and Allenheld, 1985): 126, 131.
30. Undeserved implies innocence or having done nothing to merit this exposure to potential harm. Following Anscombe, the innocent engage in no "objectively unjust proceeding" and, thus, forfeit no right against being harmed (G.E.M. Anscombe, "War and Murder," in *The Collected Philosophical Papers of G.E.M. Anscombe*, Vol. 3 (Minneapolis: University of Minnesota Press, 1981): 51–61). Similarly, following Thomson, the innocent are "free of fault" (Judith Jarvis Thomson, "Self-Defense," *Philosophy and Public Affairs* 20 (1991): 284 fn. 1). Conversely, Thomson alleges ("Imposing Risks," 127) that when it is permissible to cause harm to another, it is *ceteris paribus* permissible to impose a risk of harm, but that it is unclear that whenever it is impermissible to cause another injury, it is also impermissible to impose a risk of harm. (While Thomson maintains in her final analysis ("Self Defense," 301–2) that neither fault nor agency is necessary to violate another's right to not be substantively harmed, this is a position she revises in *The Realm of Rights* (Cambridge: Harvard University Press, 1990)).
31. Robinson, "Risk, Causation, and Harm," 338–9.
32. *Summers v. Tice*, 33 Cal. 2d 80, 199 P. 2d 1 (1948).
33. *Sindell v. Abbott Laboratories*, 26 Cal. 3d 588, 607 P. 2d 924, cert. denied, 449 U.S. 912 (1980).
34. *Jackson v. Johns-Manville Sales Corp.*, 781 F.2d 394 (5th Cir. 1986).
35. Robinson, "Risk, Causation, and Harm," 339.
36. Ibid., 319.

37. Ibid., fn.5.
38. Ibid., 318.
39. It is unclear why Robinson's analysis would not extend beyond the indeterminacy of the probability that some harmful consequence—whose effects are known—may materialize, to the indeterminacy that marks uncertain threats of harm, both whose effects and probability remain unknown. Robinson's analysis may give us a *prima facie* justification for assigning moral responsibility for uncertain threats as with probabilistic risks.
40. Thomson, "Imposing Risks," 136; Feinberg, *Harm to Others*, 188–93, 216.
41. *Public Citizen Health Research Group v. Young*, 831 F.2d 1108 (D.C. Cir. 1987).
42. *Corrosion Proof Fittings v. Environmental Protection Agency*, 947 F.2d 1201 (5th Cir. 1991).
43. *Chlorine Chemical Council v. Environmental Protection Agency*, 206 F.3d 1286 (D.C. Cir. 2000).
44. *Chlorine Chemical Council v. EPA* (2000); Government Publishing Office, Toxic Substances Control Act, S.3149, 94th Congress Public Law 469 (October 11, 1976); and *EPA, Asbestos: Manufacture, Importation Processes, and Distribution in Commerce Prohibitions* (1989), and finally *Industrial Union Dept., AFL-CIO v. American Petroleum Institute* (1980), respectively.
45. See, e.g., Feinberg, *Harm to Others*, 190–1, 216.
46. See, e.g., Richard A. Epstein, *A Theory of Strict Liability* (San Francisco: Cato Institute, 1973): 25; Ernest J. Weinrib, "Toward a Moral Theory of Negligence Law," *Law and Philosophy* 2 (1983): 37; Richard W. Wright, "Causation in Tort Law," *California law Review* 73 (1985): 1741, 1821–6; Weinrib, "Causation and Wrongdoing," *Chicago-Kent Law Review* 63 (1987): 439–41; Stephen Perry, "Risk, Harm, Interests, and Rights," in *Risk: Philosophical Perspectives*, Tim Lewens, ed. (New York: Routledge, 2007): 190–210.
47. Joel Feinberg, *Harmless Wrongdoing: The Moral Limits of the Criminal Law*, Vol. 4 (Oxford: Oxford University Press, 1984): 7, 17–8, 321.
48. Hayenhjelm and Wolff, "The Moral Problem of Risk Impositions," e37; David McCarthy, "Rights, Explanation, and Risks," *Ethics* 107 (1997); Sven Hansson, "Ethical Criteria for Risk Acceptance," *Erkenntnis* 59 (2003).
49. See Epstein, *A Theory of Strict Liability*; Weinrib, "Toward a Moral Theory of Negligence Law" and "Causation and Wrongdoing;" and Perry, "Risk, Harm, Interests, and Rights."
50. On this controversial issue see, for example, Nozick, *Anarchy, State, and Utopia*, 54–87 and Richard J. Arneson, "The Shape of Lockean Rights: Fairness, Pareto, Moderation, and Consent," *Social Philosophy and Policy* 22 (2005): 261–6.
51. Arneson, "The Shape of Lockean Rights," 261 fn. 13.
52. Nozick, *Anarchy, State, and Utopia*, 74–83. While both this discussion of one's right against harm—direct, indirect, or risks thereof—and the standard of due care under uncertainty ultimately proposed in Section 4.2 assume a deontological approach, a similar conclusion would follow from a consequentialist position. For even if Samuel Scheffler ("The Role of Consent in the Legitimation of Risky Activity," in *To Breathe Freely: Risk, Consent, and Air*, Mary Gibson, ed. (Totowa: Rowman and Allenheld, 1985): 78) were correct that "the permissibility or impermissibility of imposing a particular risk . . . can be determined only by weighting the costs and benefits [understood more broadly than mere economic considerations] of the imposition against the costs and benefits of alternative courses of action," it is not implausible to expect that affording individuals license to engage in risky actions would *prima facie* entail greater costs than benefits.
53. John Dewey, *How We Think: A Restatement of the Relation of Reflective Thinking to the Educative Process* (Boston: D.C. Heath and Company, 1933).

54. Nozick, *Anarchy, State, and Utopia*, 74–83.
55. Feinberg, *Harm To Others*, 193–8, 217.
56. Sunstein, *Laws of Fear: Beyond the Precautionary Principle* (Cambridge: Cambridge University Press, 2005): 90, 173. Sunstein expressly equates trivial harms with (only) the improbability of their coming to pass, where improbable risks of substantive harm (say, death or contracting cancer) would be conceived of and treated the same as improbable risks of negligible harm. This understanding, however, overlooks the normative relevance of the severity of harm. Thomson, too, does not adequately distinguish trivial risks from trivial harms. It is unclear from her discussion, e.g., how trivial risks of severe harm should be appraised differently than nontrivial risks of trivial harm. For instance, at times she implies that it is morally impermissible to expose others to (*de facto* or objective) nontrivial risks of nontrivial or severe harm ("Imposing Risks," 131–2, 136). Yet elsewhere Thomson is explicit that it *is* permissible to expose others to (foreseeable) trivial risks of severe harm (ibid.: 134–5).
57. Consider Henning Jensen, "Morality and Luck," *Philosophy* 59 (1984): 326–7.
58. Nagel, "Moral Luck," in *Mortal Questions* (Cambridge: Cambridge University Press, 1979): 25. Nagel ostensibly draws on Aristotle (*Nicomachean Ethics*, J.A.K. Thomson, trans. (London: Penguin Books): 114–5 (Book III, 1110b31–1111a18)), who mentions ignorance "of the circumstances and objects of action"—ignorance of, for example, the blameworthy act and its effects (where the agent is unaware of what he is doing and/or the consequences of his action), the "object or medium" of the act, its aim, and so forth—details about which one's lack of awareness may render his action involuntary and, hence, may merit our pardon.
59. Ibid.; Norvin Richards, "Luck and Desert," *Mind* 95 (1986): 200.
60. Aristotle, for instance, argues that certain forms of compulsion—such as coercion, fear (as a kind of duress), or severely constrained alternatives to act otherwise—as with certain forms of ignorance, undermine the notion of acting voluntarily, of conscientiously choosing between good and evil. And since it is one's deliberate actions that define her moral character, Aristotle asserts that culpability for involuntarily acts may merit being excused, as they do not *prima facie* testify to one's genuine character (Aristotle, *Nicomachean Ethics*, 111–4 (Book III, 1109b30–1111a18), 116–7 (Book III, 1111b5–1112a17)). While scholars have explored several variations on these constraints, Feinberg (*Doing and Deserving*, 274) suggests that Aristotle should be understood as delineating *only* these two categories of factors that may undermine one's morally responsible agency.
61. For contemporary variations on these considerations, as well as discussions on the differences between excusing and exempting conditions and excuses and justifications, see Austin, "A Plea for Excuses," 2–3; Strawson, "Freedom and Resentment," 2–3, 8, 16; Bernard Williams, "Moral Luck," in *Moral Luck: Philosophical Papers 1973–1980* (Cambridge: Cambridge University Press, 1981 [1976]): 20–39; Bennett, "Accountability," 19; Dworkin, "Intention, Foreseeability, and Responsibility," 347, 351; Watson, "Responsibility and the Limits of Evil," 260; and McMahan, *Killing in War*, 104–54, 159–73.
62. Dworkin, "Intention, Foreseeability, and Responsibility," 351.
63. Ibid.," 347, 351.
64. Reid, *Essays On the Active Powers of the Human Mind*, 229, 259–60, 316.
65. Nagel's own sympathetic view of excusing conditions like ignorance aligns with Reid's conception of the liberty of moral agents, a liberty that implies "some degree of practical judgment or reason."
66. Reid, *Essays On the Active Powers of the Human Mind*, 260.
67. Ibid., 261; Nagel, "Moral Luck," 28. It also speaks to Williams's characterization of actions performed from ignorance as "involuntary" (Williams, "Moral Luck," 28).

68. The others include the following (Nagel, "Moral Luck," 26, 28–35). *Constitutive* luck pertains to biological, genetic, and environmental factors that we do not control, which shape who a person is: one's "inclinations, capacities, and temperament," or one's physical traits, psychological dispositions, upbringing, friendships, etc. *Causal* luck regards factors that influence one's volitions (the second-order desires one wills to be the desires on which she acts) and our subsequent deliberations and actions—factors that are "not subject to one's will" and thus contradict "genuine agency." *Circumstantial* luck concerns those factors that determine the broader context of our circumstances: the time in history in which we are born, the region of the world in which we live, and so forth. Nagel's own example is of ordinary citizens during World War II who did not have the opportunity to behave shamefully, as Nazi sympathizers did in Germany, or to act heroically, as did those German citizens who resisted the Nazi regime, in virtue of nothing more than the fact that these ordinary citizens did not live in Nazi Germany. It should be apparent that these different kinds of luck are not mutually exclusive. One's temperament or dispositions, e.g., shape one's volitions and decision-making and thus fall into the category of causal luck, but they are also constitutive of who a person is and thus also regard constitutive luck. Similarly, lacking control over "antecedent circumstances" is alleged to undermine our capacity to will our actions and thus is a form of causal luck, but antecedent circumstances help to produce the conditions under which we make choices and perform actions, and thus our lack of control is also a matter of circumstantial luck. Williams ("Moral Luck," 20–1, 25–7) also details various forms of luck, such as constitutive, extrinsic and intrinsic, epistemic, and shared luck.
69. Nagel, "Moral Luck," 28–9.
70. McMahan, *Killing in Self-Defense*, 165.
71. Nagel, "Moral Luck," 28–9.
72. More precisely, McMahan explains (165) that the conscientious driver's action is subjectively permissible, not subjectively justified, since her knowledge of the marginal risk of harm to innocent bystanders that operating a car entails undermines her "moral reasons for engaging in the activity" and precludes her justification for doing so.
73. Williams, "Moral Luck," 26; Bernard Williams, "Postscript," in *Moral Luck*, Daniel Statman, ed. (Albany: State University of New York Press, 1993): 251.
74. Nagel makes implicit that in the absence of this negligence, the driver would have been able to avoid striking the child by applying the properly functioning brakes. For concerns with Nagel's analysis, see Henning Jensen, "Morality and Luck," *Philosophy* 59 (1984).
75. Jensen ("Morality and Luck," 327–8) denies this claim and argues instead that while there may be justifiable reasons for treating one more harshly for the "bad outcome" his act entails, both negligent drivers are *equally* culpable for their faulty actions.
76. Shrader-Frechette, *Taking Action, Saving Lives*, 5.
77. Moreover, to fail to suspend judgment on the question of permissibility also implies that the interests and autonomy of emitters deserve priority at the expense of those who may be exposed to these emissions, since it is the public that stands to bear the costs of any ensuing environmental harm. In contrast, the proposed argument for due care under uncertainty tries to reconcile the interests and autonomy of emitters with those of the public—it aims, in other words, to give individuals in both groups *equal* priority (as a matter of their equal moral standing).
78. For a detailed discussion on the relevance of knowing or not knowing that we do not know to the assignment of culpability, see Alexander Guerrero, "Don't Know, Don't Kill: Moral Ignorance, Culpability, and Caution," *Philosophical Studies* 135 (2007): 59–97.

79. Ibid., 17, 20; see also Michael Alavanja, "Health Effects of Chronic Pesticide Exposure," *Annual Review of Public Health* 25 (2004): 156–8; John Wargo, *Our Children's Toxic Legacy*, 2nd ed. (New Haven: Yale University Press, 1998): x–xii, 262–3, 264–5, 274; Ken Sexton and Dale Hattis, "Assessing Cumulative Health Risks from Exposure to Environmental Mixtures," *Environmental Health Perspectives* 115 (2007): 825–6.
80. National Research Council, *Carcinogens and Anticarcinogens in the Human Diet* (Washington, DC: National Academy Press, 1996).
81. National Highway Traffic Safety Administration, "2014 Motor Vehicle Crashes" (March 2016): 3.
82. Richard Wiles et al., *Tap Water Blues* (Washington, DC: Environmental Working Group, 1994); National Research Council, *Carcinogens and Anticarcinogens in the Human Diet*; also supra note 131.
83. EPA, *Pesticide Industry Sales and Usage* (2011).
84. Shrader-Frechette, *Taking Action, Saving Lives*, 17.
85. Ibid., 12–3; 15–38.
86. Cf. Guerrero, "Don't Know, Don't Kill."
87. Reid, *Essays On the Active Powers of the Human Mind*, 72–3. See also 261–2.
88. Ibid., 81 (emphasis added).
89. Ibid., 81–2 (emphasis added).
90. This also accords with Rawls's claim (*A Theory of Justice*, 422–3) that while we cannot avoid limits to our knowledge, and while our actions may always have the potential to create some unforeseeable harm, acting from "deliberative rationality"—a cyclical process of moral learning where we scrutinize our previous actions and deliberate about how to improve on our choices in the future—can "ensure that our conduct is above reproach" (self-reproach or censure by others). Cf. Williams, "Moral Luck," 32–5.
91. Dworkin, "Intention, Foreseeability, and Responsibility," 347–8.
92. Ibid., 348. Cf. Forst, *The Right to Justification.*
93. McMahan, *Killing in Self-Defense*, 165 and fn. 197.
94. Otsuka, "Moral Luck: Optional, Not Brute," 381–2.
95. Ronald Dworkin, "What Is Equality? Part 2: Equality of Resources," *Philosophy and Public Affairs* 10 (1981): 293; Otsuka, "Moral Luck," 373, 377.
96. Otsuka, "Moral Luck," 375, 377, 379–80, 382–3.
97. Ibid., 379–80, 382; Michael Otsuka, "Incompatibilism and the Avoidability of Blame," *Ethics* 108 (1998): 688, 700.
98. This is the chief distinction between Dworkin's "option" versus "brute" luck, where brute luck concerns risky actions whose effects cannot be estimated, luck that is "unchosen and unavoidable" (Dworkin, "What Is Equality?," 293; Otsuka, "Moral Luck," 373).
99. Otsuka, "Moral Luck," 380.
100. Ibid., 373, 386 fn. 18.
101. Ibid., 386 fn. 18.
102. McMahan, *Killing in Self-Defense*, 165.
103. Dworkin, "What Is Equality?," 294.
104. Nozick, *Anarchy, State, and Utopia*, 78–84.
105. Government Publishing Office, Frank R. Lautenberg Chemical Safety for the 21st Century Act, H.R.2576, 114th Congress Public Law 182 (June 22, 2016): §4(a).
106. Ibid., §§6(b)(1)(C)(iii), 6(b)(3). It should be noted that this is the central tenet of the European Union's (EU's) 2006 Registration, Evaluation, Authorisation and Restriction of Chemicals (REACH) initiative (European Parliament and Council, Registration, Evaluation, Authorisation and Restriction of Chemicals, Regulation No. 1907/2006, Official Journal of the European Union, 396 (18 December 2006): 1–849), which requires that corporations that intend to sell chemical

substances within the EU first provide scientific evidence that their substances entail no adverse public health effects before they are given permission to enter the European market.

107. Ibid., §§5(a)(1)(B), 5(a)(3), 5(g).
108. Ibid., §§3(12), 5(e)(1)(A), 5(f)(1), 6(a), 6(b)(4)(A), and 6(b)(4)(F).
109. Ibid., §§14(c)(2)(G), 14(c)(3).
110. Sunstein, *Laws of Fear*, 61.
111. Philippa Foot, *The Problem of Abortion and the Doctrine of the Double Effect in Virtues and Vices* (Oxford: Basil Blackwell, 1978). This originally appeared in the *Oxford Review* (1967). See also Judith Jarvis Thomson, "Killing, Letting Die, and the Trolley Problem," *The Monist* 5 (1976): 204–17; Judith Jarvis Thomson, "The Trolley Problem," *Yale Law Journal* 94 (1985): 1395–415; Francis Kamm, "Harming Some to Save Others," *Philosophical Studies* 57 (1989): 227–60.
112. Nozick, *Anarchy, State, and Utopia*, 262–4.
113. Shrader-Frechette, *Taking Action, Saving Lives*, 70.
114. Office of Pollution Prevention and Toxics, Environmental Protection Agency, "HPV Chemical Hazard Data Availability Study" (April 1998); PSR, "U.S. Chemical Management."
115. Percival et al., *Environmental Regulation*, 213; Environmental Protection Agency, "Chemical Right to Know: High Production Volume Chemicals Frequently Asked Questions," EPA 745-F-09–002g Report (March 1999): HPV chemicals are those whose annual rate of domestic production and/or importation exceeds 1 million pounds.
116. Office of Pollution Prevention and Toxics, "High Production Volume Chemical Hazard Data Availability Study."
117. One might also object that the argument developed here is too weak, that there are too many qualifications and mitigating factors that afford industry too many opportunities to skirt their duties of due care. For instance, in *The Right to Justification*, Forst maintains that individuals have to answer for their actions: emitters, in this case, have to offer a justification for their emissions when the potentially harmful effects are unknown, and their failure to convincingly do so should prevent them from being able to perform the action that generates the emission.
118. Otsuka, "Moral Luck," 375, 377, 379–80, 382–3.
119. Ibid., 376.
120. Scanlon, *Moral Dimensions*, 183–4, 190. See also Mary O'Brien, *Making Better Environmental Decisions: An Alternative to Risk Assessment* (Cambridge: Massachusetts Institute of Technology Press, 2000).
121. Watson, "Two Faces of Responsibility," 235–7, 239. Also relevant here are: Joseph Raz, *The Morality of Freedom* (Oxford: Clarendon Press, 1986): 412–20; Michael Zimmerman, *An Essay on Moral Responsibility* (Totowa: Roman and Littlefield, 1988): Chapter 5; Wallace, *Responsibility and the Moral Sentiments*, 103–17; and Dana Nelkin, *Making Sense of Freedom and Responsibility* (Oxford: Oxford University Press, 2011): 31–50.
122. Shrader-Frechette, *Taking Action, Saving Lives*, 75.
123. Sunstein, *Laws of Fear*, 61, 113.

References

Agency for Toxic Substances and Disease Registry. "Toxicological Profile for Asbestos." Atlanta: Department of Health and Human Services, 2001.

Alavanja, Michael. "Health Effects of Chronic Pesticide Exposure: Cancer and Neurotoxicity." *Annual Review of Public Health* 25 (2004): 155–97.

Anscombe, G.E.M. "War and Murder." In *The Collected Philosophical Papers of G.E.M. Anscombe*, Vol. 3. Minneapolis: University of Minnesota Press, 1981.

Aristotle. *Nicomachean Ethics*, translated by J.A.K. Thomson. London: Penguin Books, 1976 [350 BCE].

Arneson, Richard. "The Shape of Lockean Rights: Fairness, Pareto, Moderation, and Consent." *Social Philosophy and Policy* 22 (2005): 255–85.

Austin, John L. "A Plea for Excuses: The Presidential Address." *Proceedings of the Aristotelian Society* 57 (1956): 1–30.

Bennett, Jonathan. "Accountability." In *Philosophical Subjects: Essays Presented to P.F. Strawson*, edited by Zak van Straaten. Oxford: Clarendon Press, 1980.

Browne, Marilyn, et al. "Cancer Incidence and Asbestos in Drinking Water, Town of Woodstock, New York, 1980–1998." *Environmental Research* 98 (2005): 224–32.

Chlorine Chemical Council v. Environmental Protection Agency, 206 F.3d 1286 (D.C. Circuit 2000).

Cohen, Steven. *Understanding Environmental Policy*. New York: Columbia University Press, 2006.

Corrosion Proof Fittings v. Environmental Protection Agency, 947 F.2d 1201 (5th Circuit 1991).

Dewey, John. *How We Think: A Restatement of the Relation of Reflective Thinking to the Educative Process*. Boston: D.C. Heath and Company, 1933.

Dworkin, Gerald. "Intention, Foreseeability, and Responsibility." In *Responsibility, Character, and the Emotions*, edited by Ferdinand Schoeman. Cambridge: Cambridge University Press, 1987.

Dworkin, Ronald. "What Is Equality? Part 2: Equality of Resources." *Philosophy and Public Affairs* 10 (1981): 283–345.

Environmental Protection Agency. *Leaking Underground Storage Tanks*. Washington: EPA, 1985.

———. "Chemical Right to Know: High Production Volume Chemicals Frequently Asked Questions." EPA 745-F-09–002g, March 1999.

———. *Pesticide Industry Sales and Usage: 2008–2012 Market Estimates*. Washington: EPA, 2011.

———. *Underground Storage Tanks Program Facts*. Washington: EPA, 2016. https://epa.gov/sites/production/files/2016-06/documents/program-facts-5-10-16.pdf.

EPA, Asbestos: Manufacture, Importation Processes, and Distribution in Commerce Prohibitions, 54 Fed. Reg. 29,640, 1989.

Epstein, Richard. *A Theory of Strict Liability*. San Francisco: Cato Institute, 1973.

European Parliament and Council. "Registration, Evaluation, Authorisation and Restriction of Chemicals." Regulation No. 1907/2006. *Official Journal of the European Union* 396 (December 18, 2006): 1–849.

Feinberg, Joel. *Doing and Deserving*. Princeton: Princeton University Press, 1970.

———. *Harm to Others: The Moral Limits of the Criminal Law*, Vol. 1. Oxford: Oxford University Press, 1984.

———. *Harmless Wrongdoing: The Moral Limits of the Criminal Law*, Vol. 4. Oxford: Oxford University Press, 1984.

Foot, Philippa. *The Problem of Abortion and the Doctrine of the Double Effect in Virtues and Vices*. Oxford: Basil Blackwell, 1978.

Forst, Rainer. *The Right to Justification*, translated by Jeffrey Flynn. New York: Columbia University Press, 2011.

Gamble, John. "Risk of Gastrointestinal Cancers from Inhalation and Ingestion of Asbestos." *Regulatory Toxicology and Pharmacology* 52 (2008): S124–53.

Government Publishing Office. "Toxic Substances Control Act, S.3149." *94th Congress Public Law 469*. October 11, 1976. https://congress.gov/bill/94th-congress/senate-bill/3149.

———. "Frank R. Lautenberg Chemical Safety for the 21st Century Act, H.R.2576." *114th Congress Public Law 182*, June 22, 2016. https://congress.gov/bill/114th-congress/house-bill/2576/text.

Guerrero, Alexander. "Don't Know, Don't Kill: Moral Ignorance, Culpability, and Caution." *Philosophical Studies* 135 (2007): 59–97.

Hansson, Sven. "Ethical Criteria for Risk Acceptance." *Erkenntnis* 59 (2003): 291–309.

Hayenhjelm, Madeleine and Jonathan Wolff. "The Moral Problem of Risk Impositions: A Survey of the Literature." *European Journal of Philosophy* 20 (2012): E26–51.

Industrial Union Dept., AFL-CIO v. American Petroleum Institute, 448 U.S. 607 (1980).

Jackson v. Johns-Manville Sales Corp., 781 F.2d 394 (5th Circuit 1986).

Jensen, Henning. "Morality and Luck." *Philosophy* 59 (1984): 323–30.

Kamm, Francis. "Harming Some to Save Others." *Philosophical Studies* 57 (1989): 227–60.

McCarthy, David. "Rights, Explanation, and Risks." *Ethics* 107 (1997): 205–25.

McMahan, Jeff. *Killing in War*. Oxford: Oxford University Press, 2009.

Nagel, Thomas. *Mortal Questions*. Cambridge: Cambridge University Press, 1979.

National Highway Traffic Safety Administration. "2014 Motor Vehicle Crashes." Report No. DOT HS 812 246. Washington: National Highway Traffic Safety Administration, March 2016. https://crashstats.nhtsa.dot.gov/Api/Public/ViewPublication/812246.

National Research Council. *Carcinogens and Anticarcinogens in the Human Diet*. Washington: National Academy Press, 1996.

Nelkin, Dana. *Making Sense of Freedom and Responsibility*. Oxford: Oxford University Press, 2011.

Nozick, Robert. *Anarchy, State, and Utopia*. New York: Basic Books, 1974.

O'Brien, Mary. *Making Better Environmental Decisions: An Alternative to Risk Assessment*. Cambridge: Massachusetts Institute of Technology Press, 2000.

Office of Pollution Prevention and Toxics. "High Production Volume Chemical Hazard Data Availability Study." Washington: EPA, 1998. Last updated August 2, 2010.

Otsuka, Michael. "Incompatibilism and the Avoidability of Blame." *Ethics* 108 (1998): 685–701.

———. "Moral Luck: Optional, Not Brute." *Philosophical Perspectives* 23 (2009): 373–88.

Percival, Robert, et al. *Environmental Regulation: Law, Science, and Policy*, 6th edition. New York: Aspen Publishers, 2009.

Perry, Stephen. "Risk, Harm, Interests, and Rights." In *Risk: Philosophical Perspectives*, edited by Tim Lewens. New York: Routledge, 2007.

Pope, C. Arden, et al. "Health Effects of Particulate Air Pollution: Time for Reassessment?" *Environmental Health Perspectives* 103 (1995): 472–80.

Postema, Gerald. "Morality in the First Person Plural." *Law and Philosophy* 14 (1995): 35–64.

Public Citizen Health Research Group v. Young, 831 F.2d 1108 (D.C. Circuit 1987).

Rawls, John. *A Theory of Justice*. Cambridge: Harvard University Press, 1971.

Raz, Joseph. *The Morality of Freedom*. Oxford: Oxford University Press, 1986.

Reid, Thomas. *Essays on the Active Powers of the Human Mind*. Cambridge: MIT Press, 1969 [1788].

Richards, Norvin. "Luck and Desert." *Mind* 95 (1986): 198–209.

Robinson, Glen. "Risk, Causation, and Harm." In *Liability and Responsibility: Essays in Law and Morals*, edited by Raymond Frey and Christopher Morris. Cambridge: Cambridge University Press, 1991.

Scanlon, Thomas M. *Moral Dimensions: Permissibility, Meaning, and Blame*. Cambridge: Belknap Press, 2008.

Scheffler, Samuel. "The Role of Consent in the Legitimation of Risky Activity." In *To Breathe Freely: Risk, Consent, and Air*, edited by Mary Gibson. Totowa: Rowman and Allenheld, 1985.

Sexton, Ken and Dale Hattis. "Assessing Cumulative Health Risks from Exposure to Environmental Mixtures: Three Fundamental Questions." *Environmental Health Perspectives* 115 (2007): 825–32.

Shrader-Frechette, Kristin. *Taking Action, Saving Lives: Our Duties to Protect Environmental and Public Health*. Oxford: Oxford University Press, 2007.

Sierra Club. *Leaking Underground Storage Tanks: A Threat to Public Health and Environment*. San Francisco: Sierra Club, 2005.

Sindell v. Abbott Laboratories, 26 Cal. 3d 588, 607 P. 2d 924, cert. denied, 449 U.S. 912 (1980).

Strawson, Peter. *Freedom and Resentment and Other Essays*. London: Methuen and Co., 1974 [1962].

Summers v. Tice, 33 Cal. 2d 80, 199 P. 2d 1 (1948).

Sunstein, Cass. *Laws of Fear: Beyond the Precautionary Principle*. Cambridge: Cambridge University Press, 2005.

Szentkirályi, Levente. "Luck Has Nothing to Do with It: Prevailing Uncertainty and Responsibilities of Due Care." *Ethics, Policy, and Environment* (forthcoming).

Thomson, Judith Jarvis. "Killing, Letting Die, and the Trolley Problem." *The Monist* 5 (1976): 204–17.

———. "Imposing Risks." In *To Breathe Freely: Risk, Consent, and Air*, edited by Mary Gibson. Totowa: Rowman and Allenheld, 1985.

———. "The Trolley Problem." *Yale Law Journal* 94 (1985): 1395–415.

———. *The Realm of Rights*. Cambridge: Harvard University Press, 1990.

———. "Self-Defense." *Philosophy and Public Affairs* 20 (1991): 283–310.

Wallace, R. Jay. *Responsibility and the Moral Sentiments*. Cambridge: Harvard University Press, 1996.

Wargo, John. *Our Children's Toxic Legacy: How Science and Law Fail to Protect Us from Pesticides*, 2nd edition. New Haven: Yale University Press, 1998.

Watson, Gary. "Responsibility and the Limits of Evil." In *Responsibility, Character, and the Emotions*, edited by Ferdinand Schoeman. Cambridge: Cambridge University Press, 1987.

———. "Two Faces of Responsibility." *Philosophical Topics* 24 (1996): 227–48.

Weinrib, Ernest. "Toward a Moral Theory of Negligence Law." *Law and Philosophy* 2 (1983): 37–62.

———. "Causation and Wrongdoing." *Chicago-Kent Law Review* 63 (1987): 407–50.

Wiles, Richard, et al. *Tap Water Blues*. Washington: Environmental Working Group, 1994.

Williams, Bernard. *Moral Luck: Philosophical Papers 1973–1980*. Cambridge: Cambridge University Press, 1981.

———. *Ethics and the Limits of Philosophy*. Cambridge: Harvard University Press, 1985.

———. "Postscript." In *Moral Luck*, edited by Daniel Statman. Albany: State University of New York Press, 1993.
Wilson, Sacoby, et al. "Leaking Underground Storage Tanks and Environmental Injustice." *Environmental Justice* 6 (2013): 175–82.
Wright, Richard. "Causation in Tort Law." *California law Review* 73 (1985): 1735–828.
Zimmerman, Michael. *An Essay on Moral Responsibility*. Totowa: Roman and Littlefield, 1988.

5 Obligations of Due Care Under Uncertainty

The previous chapters have bridged arguments in environmental policy over the merits of precautionary risk regulation with debates in normative ethics over the moral permissibility of performing actions that expose others to uncorroborated possibilities of harm. Chapter 2 explained that contemporary defenses of precautionary risk regulation are vulnerable to criticism because their justificatory appeals to epistemic limitations do not provide a strong foundation for exercising precaution because they employ a narrow conception of what uncertainty means and because they overstate their position—maintaining that a precautionary approach is appropriate with most, if not all, cases of environmental health risks. In addition to distinguishing traditional "risk impositions" (whose potential for harm is measurable and probabilistic) from what this book terms "uncertain threats" (whose potential for harm is unquantifiable and, thus, indeterminate), Chapter 2 also explored attempts by proponents of precaution to respond to the battery of objections critics raise about the implausibility of health-based precautionary risk regulations and illustrated that these arguments cannot adequately defend preventative safeguards of public health. The chapter closed with a brief sketch of a normative, rights-based formulation of the precautionary principle, which was purported to withstand these common objections of critics.

Demonstrating how the litany of charges leveled against precautionary measures can be averted was tabled until this chapter to allow us to first explore the viability of this normative argument for precaution, which was subsequently developed and defended in Chapters 3 and 4. This third chapter explained that we have a duty of due care under uncertainty to strive to prevent exposing others to the potentially harmful consequences of our actions—that outcome and probability uncertainty do not give us license to act in ways that may prove injurious to others. This is to say that as a matter of moral equality and the deontological principle of treating others as ends in themselves, individuals have a corresponding right not to have others gamble with their welfare. Yet as this chapter underscores in practical terms, Chapter 4.4 emphasized that it is the same moral equality and the demands of reciprocity between moral equals that require that restrictions on endangering actions that beget uncertain threats be reasonable. When we are unable to know whether the consequences of one's actions will be harmful or harmless, when we lack the justification to either prohibit or permit actions that entail potential harm to others, it is necessary to reconcile the right of actors to perform actions that may adversely affect others with the right of those who stand to bear the consequences of these actions not to be put in possible harm's way. The aim, in other words, is to establish a reasonable compromise between these parties: a mutually acceptable approach to managing environmental threats under uncertainty, which serves to diminish the potential for harm to public health without prohibiting emitters from exercising their autonomy and pursuing ambitions that involve the release of effluents into the environment so long as outcome and probability uncertainty prevail.

Having shown that contemporary normative arguments from moral responsibility, moral luck, and the ethics of risk offer questionable explanations of the permissibility of uncertain threats, and having defended the claim that emitters can be obliged to exercise due care under conditions of uncertainty, this chapter shifts the discussion to how this obligation may be discharged. And in concert with this book's broader aim of defending the precautionary principle as a normatively justified and pragmatically tenable policy alternative to environmental risk management under conditions of uncertainty, the primary standard of due care that is relevant here regards the duties of industry. What the exercise of due care may entail for particular individuals and the government also merits discussion, but will not be featured here.[1] The substance of this context-dependent industrial standard of due care—that is, how authors of uncertain threats can satisfy their duties toward others, or how emitters can respect the correlative rights of others to be safeguarded against potential harm—initially turns on identifying what it is we already know about the possibility for harm that an effluent may entail. Accordingly, Sections 5.1 to 5.3 propose a practical framework by which we may determine the precautionary measures that industry is obliged to take by exploring three broad scenarios in which the degree of uncertainty varies: one in which the actual risk to public health can be deduced, another in which the actual risk to public health can be tested and corroborated, and a third in which the actual risk to public health cannot be empirically verified with existing technologies—or where the toxicity data we *can* collect are still insufficient to eliminate outcome uncertainty. (Recall that if outcome uncertainty can be eliminated such that we can confirm the consequences of exposure, then we are no longer in the realm of uncertainty, but rather in the domain of risk: whose measurable and probabilistic possibilities of harm come under the purview of the quantitative, risk assessment–based regulatory regime.) As the following discussion explains, and as Figure 5.1 illustrates, each scenario is defined by a different degree of uncertainty, which will entail different means by which industry can discharge its duties of due care—a flexibility and sensitivity to context that are further explained in Section 5.4, which explores various morally relevant contextual factors that can either diminish or amplify an emitter's obligation to exercise due care before releasing a potentially harmful substance into the environment. Finally, Section 5.5 explores several possible problems with the proposed industrial standard of due care—returning to the series of objections to the precautionary principle initially introduced in Chapter 2 and arguing that the rights-based account can respond to these charges.

5.1 When Risk can be Deduced

In the first scenario, the actual risk of exposure to human health is unknown, but the substance in question shares similarities to pollutants whose effects *have* been scientifically verified and from which the effects of the former may reasonably be inferred. In this way, the uncertainty that obscures the threat to which others are exposed diminishes. Thus, barring future evidence to the contrary, these uncertain threats can tentatively be treated as comparable to traditional risk impositions, where the adverse outcomes of exposure can be foreseen and what remains unknown is only the probability that exposure will cause harm, which can be estimated. And if such risks are judged to be unreasonable—judged, that is, to entail probable and nontrivial harm—then they are subject both to conventional accounts of moral responsibility and the ethics of risk (see Chapter 4), and also to existing environmental regulations.

Consider, for example, that in *Reserve Mining Company v. EPA* (1975), the U.S. Court of Appeals issued an injunction against the emission of taconite tailings on the basis of the apparent likeness to asbestos fibers. In 1972, the Department of Justice, in conjunction with the states of Minnesota, Wisconsin, and Michigan and various environmental organizations, sued Reserve Mining for the company's discharge of taconite tailings (low-grade iron pellets) into Lake Superior.[2] At the time, Reserve Mining was releasing 67,000 tons of taconite tailings each day, or 47 tons per minute, which raised serious concerns for communities like Duluth, Minnesota, which depended on Lake Superior for its public drinking water. Even though the actual health effects or threat of harm from exposure remained inconclusive, the district court ruled that air and water discharges were "substantially endanger[ing] the surrounding population."[3] Although taconite tailings contain asbestiform fibers, which are similar to asbestos fibers known to cause diseases with prolonged *inhalation*, Reserve Mining claimed that its discharges into water and any subsequent *ingestion* of these fibers in drinking water "posed no legally cognizable risk to public health."[4] The court therefore insisted that an epidemiological (skin tissue) study of Duluth residents be conducted, along with a gastrointestinal study of animals exposed to taconite, as well as a gastrointestinal study of workers occupationally exposed to asbestos dust, in order to ascertain the possible health effects of ingesting asbestiform fibers.

These subsequent studies yielded mixed results. Yet the federal Court of Appeals concluded that exposure to asbestiform in drinking water was "comparable" to occupational exposure to asbestos dust at levels that were known to cause gastrointestinal cancer. The court acknowledged that the probability of harm from ingestion and inhalation of taconite tailings is inconclusive (there is no conclusive evidence of any actual harm), that all that can be concluded is that exposure to taconite tailings creates *some* possibility of harm and that concern for public health is *prima facie* reasonable. Given this uncertain but potential threat to the public, the court felt justified in issuing an injunction against Reserve Mining, requiring the company to cease the discharge of tailings as a preventative measure to protect public health from a substance that may reasonably "be considered a carcinogen."[5] It is worth noting that this injunction was justified on the grounds that evidence of potential, albeit indeterminate, harm—here, the likeness between asbestiform and asbestos fibers can also be understood as "endangering" the public and, thus, can be "legally cognizable."[6] Also of note is that following this decision, Congress saw fit "to shift the burden of proof to polluters to prove the safety of their discharges" once it was established that the discharges posed a "reasonable risk of being a threat to public health."[7] It is this notion of increasing the stringency of mandatory testing by industry to strive to determine the potentially harmful effects of the substances that corporations release into the environment that is central to the standard of due care that is proposed here.

As such, as Figure 5.1 illustrates, when it is possible to infer the measurable and probabilistic risk of harm that an uncertain environmental threat poses, existing environmental regulations and emission standards apply—compliance with which substitutes for the requirement of exercising due care. We may presume that complying with existing environmental protections satisfies one's moral obligation to strive to prevent exposing others to potential harm (since this is the objective of risk regulations) and relieves one of his culpability for the threat he creates.

5.2 When Risk can be Scientifically Verified

In the second scenario, the actual risk of exposure to human health could feasibly be scientifically tested and verified, but it has not yet been and, thus, it remains uncertain. A substantial number of threats of environmental harm fit this description. Recall from Chapter 2.3 that most of the more than 60,000 chemical substances grandfathered under the Toxic Substances Control Act (TSCA) and exempt from any mandatory testing of their relative safety to public health have gone untested or remain understudied—even though the Environmental Protection Agency (EPA) suggests that "basic toxicity assessments" or Screening Information Data Sets (SIDS) for at least the high production volume chemicals on this exemption list *can* be ascertained with existing technologies.[8] (With many of these chemicals falling out of production for various reasons since TSCA's enactment, some maintain that the number of chemicals currently being manufactured, processed, or imported for commerce in the United States is closer to 10,000.[9] However, this figure is highly speculative, since the EPA has no central, comprehensive, and accurate list of the chemical substances in current production, including those pre-1976 substances that were exempt from mandatory testing under TSCA: the Agency for Toxic Substances and Disease Registry, the Toxic Release Inventory Program, the TSCA Hotline, and the office on Chemical Data Reporting have not only failed to confirm which grandfathered chemical substances are still being produced and at which volumes, but they have also failed to confirm what toxicity data exist or are lacking for these pre-existing substances.)

Consider further that the costs of running the tests "necessary for a minimum understanding of a chemical's toxicity,"[10] and therefore a minimum understanding of its actual dangers to public health, would cost roughly $200,000 per chemical substance[11]—which is but a small fraction of the profits that many corporations make on the manufacture, distribution, and use of these substances (see Section 5.5 below).

That emitters are unaware of the possible harm to public health because they have not tested for the health effects of exposure clearly does not relieve them of their culpability for the uncertain threats they author. The uncertainty in these cases arises and persists precisely because emitters neglect to take reasonable measures to ascertain the likelihood of harm—reinforcing the need for some standard of due care that requires emitters to take reasonable measures to avoid gambling with the welfare of others by putting them in the way of untested possibilities of harm. As such, when it is possible to corroborate the actual risks to human health, once toxicity tests are conducted and it is determined whether or not exposure is likely to cause harm, the environmental threat moves from the realm of uncertainty into the domain of risk and under the purview of formal risk assessment and existing environmental regulations and emission standards.

As the center branch of Figure 5.1 details, what is required of industry in these circumstances is to test in earnest the health effects of their products and the effluents they release into the environment: for the equal moral standing of those who may be adversely affected and the reciprocity that defines their moral relationships with emitters demand that industry refrain from gambling with the welfare of others. The first step in treating those who stand to bear the harms that one's uncertain threats may cause is to discern the outcome of exposure to substances one discharges into the environment and the likelihood that exposure will beget this harm. However, respecting the moral standing of others also obliges emitters to disclose the findings of their toxicity tests to regulatory agencies and the general public—not only to subject their emissions to existing environmental protections but also to afford those who may be exposed to these emissions the information necessary to help insulate themselves from potential harm. This duty may be carried further to require not just toxicity tests but "transparent, independent and reproducible health studies" that may allow us to achieve a fuller understanding of the potential for harm.[12] (This conception of the duty of due care is strongly motivated by the European Union's [EU's] 2006 REACH initiative,[13] which prohibits corporations that aim to produce or sell chemical substances within the EU from entering the European market until they first provide scientific evidence corroborating the absence of adverse health effects of exposure to these substances. Though in

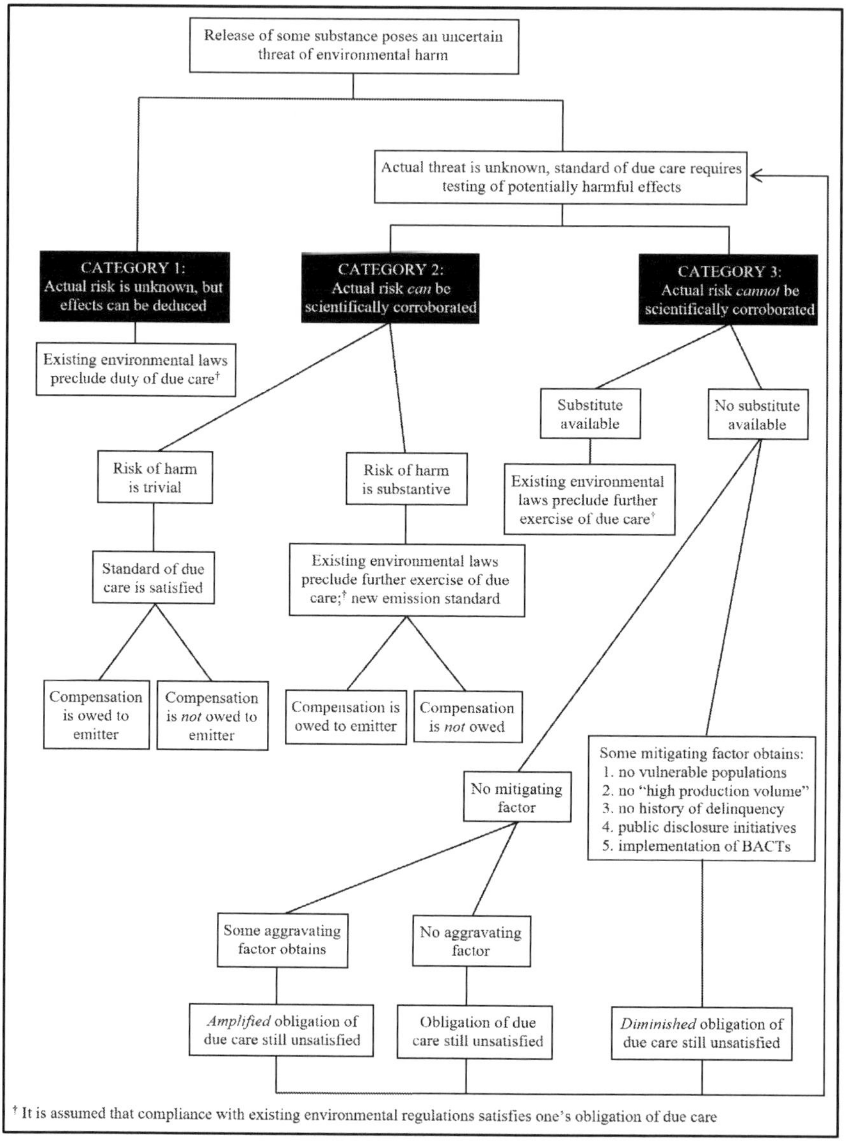

Figure 5.1 Discharging the Industrial Standard of Due Care

an effort to take seriously the interests of industry and reconcile them with the broader public interests, the expectations of industry proposed here are more relaxed than REACH.)

And when this mandatory testing reveals a trivial risk of harm such that the estimated probability of experiencing injury upon exposure is low and/or the foreseeable injury from exposure is minor (findings that would be subject to and dependent on external audits by an independent regulatory agency), the emitter will have satisfied his obligations of due care. Alternatively, if this testing verifies a nontrivial risk of harm, where the likelihood of injury is high or the foreseeable harm from exposure is severe, then the environmental risk and any actual injuries resulting from exposure fall under the scope of existing environmental laws. It may well be that regulatory agencies will have to establish new emission standards for these particular substances, which may impose further legal and moral constraints on the emitter with regard to his future emissions of such substances, but the emitter will have satisfied his obligation to exercise due care. As noted earlier with the first scenario, it is presumed that compliance with existing environmental laws satisfies one's duty to avoid exposing others to possibilities of harm and relieves one of his culpability for the threat he authors.

It should be added that when industry exercises due care under uncertainty, if it is verified that industry's emissions are harmless, it may be appropriate to consider compensating corporations. It is the same reciprocity among moral equals that obliges those who wish to perform actions that entail uncertain threats to others to bear some burden in safeguarding against potential harms, which should also oblige those whose autonomy and welfare are protected in this way to bear some burden when the exercise of due care proves unnecessary (i.e., when an uncertain threat of harm proves to be harmless). As Nozick suggests, however, in his discussion on the plausibility of compensating people "for having certain risky activities prohibited to them,"[14] this is a controversial suggestion—if only because we generally presume that if one has a right against being exposed to threats of harm, no compensation is owed. Having this right implies that one is entitled to its enforcement, such that forbidding endangering actions does no wrong to, or constitutes no infringement on the liberties of, the would-be risk taker—thereby requiring no compensation. This consideration reiterates the notion that rights entail correlative duties, whose satisfaction does not entitle one to compensation. Although these issues will not be resolved here, the merit of such compensation is explored later, when the discussion turns to the objection that any moral standard of due care under uncertainty is likely to be unduly burdensome on industry.

One might object here and insist that rather than disproportionately burden industry with the costs of exercising precaution, a more equitable solution would involve distributing the costs of preventative safeguards among everyone through some taxation scheme and to allocate these funds to industry to test the health safety of their products and the substances they manufacture and emit into the environment, or to allocate these public funds directly to regulatory agencies like the EPA, Food and Drug Administration (FDA), Centers for Disease Control (CDC), Occupational Safety and Health Administration (OSHA) to enable the agencies themselves to conduct the toxicity tests. After all, we all have a stake in preventing pollution, which is to say that we all stand to benefit from precautionary risk regulations.

Some common pool fund might be part of the solution. However, it seems more plausible to retroactively compensate emitters should their uncertain threats prove to be harmless—where industry's efforts to strive to safeguard the public from harm prove unnecessary and, thus, where industry needlessly absorbs costs in exercising precaution—as opposed to having the public front the costs of having industry satisfy its moral duties. This is because the public fund alternative would mean that the public is not only expected to bear the costs of any eventual harm that uncertain threats may entail but also to subsidize efforts to corroborate the presence or absence of actual risks to public health—all the while industry profits handsomely. An alternative that would only begin to place burdens on industry (in the form of emission standards) when actual risks to human health are corroborated hardly seems equitable—especially if we acknowledge the common practice among corporations to undermine efforts of public health scientists and regulatory agencies to confirm the presence of credible health risks: deliberately falsifying or withholding scientific data that would verify adverse health effects of exposure, funding studies to contradict and discredit the findings of public health scientists, misleading the public with embellished or false public relations campaigns about actual dangers to human health, and intimidating whistleblowers and advocacy groups.[15] As Section 5.5 below notes, the costs of toxicity testing are quite modest in relation to the profits that related industries record, and because emitters profit from the uncertain threats while the public stands to absorb the costs of any ensuing harm, it seems more reasonable—and to more closely align with the notions of reciprocity and the duty to exercise due care—to expect industry to shoulder more of the costs of mandatory toxicity testing.

5.3 When Risk Remains Unverifiable

Finally, in the third scenario, the actual health effects of exposure are unknown, and this uncertainty cannot currently be eliminated even with diligent empirical testing using extant technologies and scientific standards—or, conversely, the toxicity data we *can* gather are insufficient to corroborate the severity and/or likelihood that exposure will entail harm. It is precisely those actions that beget uncorroborated threats of this sort that motivate the unique challenge of uncertain threats to conventional theories of moral responsibility. Accordingly, beyond striving to eliminate the uncertainty that persists from the absence of testing, as defined by the duty of due care in the second scenario, the standard of due care delineated here requires industry to take additional measures to try to mitigate the potential for harm. More specifically, in addition to initial toxicity testing, which is the first and principal component of the due care required of industry, when the health effects of some substance are tested in earnest and remain inconclusive, as the right branch of Figure 5.1 indicates, the next requirement of corporations is to find what substances could feasibly be substituted in their various business practices, whose effects we *do* know or whose probability of causing harm we *can* estimate. Whenever such substitutes are available, existing environmental laws serve to regulate their release, and so long as emitters utilize these substitutes and comply with these laws, their obligation to exercise due care is once again satisfied. (Some might argue that with regard to the creation of new substances, when the health risk of exposure remains unverifiable, a duty of due care might require that industry refrain from introducing the new substance in the first place.[16])

Admittedly, some substitutions may counterproductively impose known risks of harm on others. This concern is illustrated, for example, in *Public Citizen v. Young* (1987), where the U.S. Court of Appeals invalidated the FDA's relaxation of the zero-risk standard for known carcinogens established under the Delaney Clause of the 1958 Food Additives Amendment—clarifying that Congress had "permitted no *de minimis* exception" in the 1958 amendments.[17] The court *did* acknowledge, however, the FDA's conclusion that the cancer-causing risks of the two additives that had been exempted, Orange #17 and Red #19, were "so trivial as to be effectively no risk."[18] Moreover, in underscoring the misguidedness and irresponsibility of the "failure to employ a *de minimis* doctrine" with environmental risk regulations, the court stressed that the Delaney Clause and its zero-risk standard may well increase overall risk to public health by motivating industry to substitute higher-risk noncarcinogenic toxins for low-risk carcinogens, stating that it is "a clear loss for safety" when "makers of drugs and cosmetics . . . are barred from [substituting] a carcinogenic dye carrying a one-in-20-million lifetime risk [for] a non-carcinogenic, but toxic, dye carrying, say, a one-in-10-million lifetime risk."[19]

It certainly would defeat the purpose of a principle of due care if it were to be counterproductive in this way, creating the very sort of environmental harm it aims to prevent. However, the problem with this objection is that under conditions of uncertainty, we cannot determine the danger of an uncertain threat relative to a substitute whose health effects are known. To suggest that when available substitutes entail known credible risks of harm we are obliged to permit (as a matter of precaution?) the uncertain threat is to equate uncertainty with relative safety. It is, in other words, to treat uncertain threats as safer or less risky than the substitutes. Yet as the previous chapters have argued, it is mistaken to regard uncertain threats as safe or as constituting trivial risks of harm. In the absence of adequate scientific evidence corroborating the actual dangers or lack of measurable risk to public health—that is, until the uncertainty is eliminated—there is no way to verify whether the uncertain threat will entail a greater or lesser likelihood of harm than the substitutes available to emitters.

Further, as detailed in the broadly Kantian justification for exercising due care under uncertainty in the previous chapter, it is not the presence of an uncertain threat of harm itself that can make an endangering action morally objectionable, for the consequences to others may well prove to be harmless. Rather, it is what the creation of the unconsented-to and preventable threat implies about the moral relationship between the author of the threat and those he may expose to potential harm—namely, the disregard of the equal moral standing and capacity of self-authorship of others. This is to say that conditions of uncertainty diminish or suspend the relevance of consequence to our assessments of the wrongfulness of putting others in the way of uncertain harm. In the context of possible substitutes, since it is not possible to ascertain the potential danger of exposing others to a substance with unknown health effects relative to exposure to a substitute substance whose health effects are known, respecting others as ends in themselves would involve adopting an available substitute so long as the known risk of harm is reasonable—as defined by existing accounts of moral responsibility and risk theory, which would apply in the absence of uncertainty.

In contrast, the absence of a suitable substitute and persisting uncertainty does not give license to emitters to impose uncorroborated, albeit potential, threats of harm on others. If we take seriously the equal moral standing of others and the subsequent obligations we have to respect their capacity for self-authorship, we are obliged to refrain from gambling with their welfare to serve our own ends. Thus, a standard of due care must be stringent enough that satisfying its conditions effectively demonstrates one's due regard for others as moral ends. This means that a viable standard of due care must be strict enough to ensure that strides are actually taken to mitigate the potential for harm to others. Consequently, when uncertainty prevails and no substitute is to be had, further efforts must be made to ascertain the actual risk of harm the endangering action poses. This aligns with the EPA's suggestion that further SIDS tests are required in circumstances when basic toxicity testing "will not provide sufficient understanding to adequately assess the hazards and risks presented by some chemicals."[20]

Nevertheless, our standard of due care cannot be so demanding that if the uncertain threat of harm never does materialize into an actual injury (or unreasonable risk of harm), we would retrospectively find the measure unreasonably burdensome. Again, the aim here is to reconcile the competing rights—as a matter of moral equality and reciprocity—of emitters to exercise their autonomy and engage in those practices that entail the discharge of potentially harmful substances, with the rights of those who may be exposed to these substances to *not* be placed in the way of possible harm. In this vein, several factors may attenuate the further obligation of due care industry has to continue testing for the health effects of the potentially harmful substances to which they expose the public. Some of the considerations that may warrant mitigating a corporation's outstanding duty of due care include those noted in Figure 5.1. In contrast, when examining whether any of these mitigating factors apply, should we discover egregious examples or a history of corporate social irresponsibility, these factors can aggravate or amplify a corporate emitter's outstanding duty of due care.

Consider, for instance (as Chapter 6 explores in detail), that in the late 1920s, corporations like General Motors, Standard Oil of New Jersey, and Ethyl Gas

Corporation—three key companies in the oil and automotive industries with both vested interests in the production of leaded gasoline and proprietary rights to the evidence that would have revealed the adverse health effects of exposure to tetraethyl lead (TEL) from vehicle exhaust—began to mount a campaign against scientific studies aiming to confirm the effects of TEL exposure, as well as policy initiatives aiming to implement mandatory emission standards for leaded gasoline. Several tactics these companies used to ensure the expanded production of leaded gasoline were deceitful—including but not limited to purposefully misleading public relations campaigns that stressed the economic benefits but ignored the suspected health risks of the additive, funding government-led research and manipulating the reports to understate the risks to public health, undercutting any possibility of establishing a preponderance of evidence of the actual dangers of TEL exposure by funding industry-friendly research of independent scholars to reject the findings of public health studies and inject doubt into the discussion (thereby thwarting the justification for mandatory emission standards), and making false and inflammatory public statements about the occupational safety at TEL processing plants that blamed workers themselves for their exposure-related injuries and deaths. These considerations are morally relevant and should factor into our assessments of what burdens of due care are reasonable to impose on emitters, especially when considering that the example of exposure to tetraethyl lead involved highly vulnerable populations like infants, children, and industrial workers. This sort of history of socially irresponsible behavior—which contradicts the fundamental principle of exercising precaution under uncertainty for the sake of showing others due regard as ends in themselves—may justify amplifying emitters' outstanding duties of due care. They may lend credence, for instance, to sanctioning the emitter by prohibiting any use of the substance in question despite the prevailing uncertainty.

5.4 Context-Dependent Mitigating Factors

The previous discussion provided an initial sketch of how context matters in determining what the exercise of due care may consist of and how this duty may be discharged by corporate emitters. With regard to those uncertain environmental threats whose potential harm to public health cannot be corroborated with existing detection capabilities (scenario 3), it was suggested that testing is still a necessary component of the duty of due care—otherwise, the absence of testing would have the *de facto* effect of branding these effluents and the uncertain threats they beget as safe. Nevertheless, since initial testing will merely confirm that health effects cannot currently be corroborated, this prevailing uncertainty should motivate emitters to employ feasible substitutes when available, whether this means incorporating an alternative substance into a corporation's business practices or choosing an alternative course of action altogether that does not entail the uncertain public health threat. When no substitutes are available or feasible, it was suggested that the next step in our assessment of what the duty of due care consists of is to examine whether any morally relevant mitigating factor applies, which might reduce (or conversely amplify) an emitter's obligation to strive to diminish the potential for harm. Five such mitigating factors are discussed in this section.

First, there is no vulnerable population that bears a disproportionate threat of harm. This is to say that the uncertain threat a corporation creates does not target, or even unintentionally affect, any particularly vulnerable populations, such as infants and children, the elderly, pregnant women, racial and ethnic minorities, the poor, and so forth. If, for instance, a company like Vestergaard[21] were to aim to use a substance in its manufacture of water filtration straws to be sold in developing countries—where it is estimated that more than 2 million people die each year due to diarrhea and other water-related diseases resulting from the consumption of contaminated water[22]—the company's residual duty (or unsatisfied obligation) to exercise due care may not be deserving of attenuation.

Second, the substance in question is not a "high production volume" chemical, which means that less than 1 million pounds of the material is either manufactured in or imported to the United States each year.[23] It can reasonably be assumed that the greater the amount of substances used in consumer goods or discharged into the environment that pose uncertain threats to public health, the greater the possibility for actual harm becomes—for these high rates of production and consumption make the public's exposure to the substances more likely. Accordingly, smaller industries that emit fewer substances whose effects are uncertain face a more relaxed residual duty to exercise *further* due care.

Third, there is no history of delinquency or negligence with a corporation's compliance with existing environmental regulations. We might, all things considered, accept that legally responsible industries are deserving of some leniency, since it may be that strict compliance with environmental standards regarding the discharge of pollutants known to be harmful demonstrates an actor's commitment to protecting public health and welfare. And this outward commitment may merit the assumption that the industry is also acting in good faith with the use and release of substances whose potentially harmful effects are empirically uncorroborated.

Fourth, beyond disclosing information to regulatory agencies and the public pertaining to uncertain possibilities of harm, the corporation proactively engages in informational campaigns to raise public awareness of the uncertain threats they author—providing individuals who may be exposed to these threats information in highly visible ways that can easily be consumed. One example of this sort of initiative might consist of a labeling scheme for products containing, services involving, or workplaces using substances whose effects remain scientifically unverified. As an analogy, consider that California state law, in accordance with Proposition 65,[24] requires (among other disclosures) that all products manufactured or distributed in California that contain, as well as all workplaces in California that employ, substances that the Office of Environmental Health Hazard Assessment (OEHHA) estimates to produce a 1/100,000 chance of causing cancer "over a 70-year lifetime" to be labeled with a "clear and reasonable warning."[25] A few examples of mandatory warnings are provided in Figure 5.2.[26]

More to the point on uncertain threats, producers and distributors of various dairy products have adopted new labeling schemes to inform consumers of the absence of synthetic growth hormones and antibiotics in their products. Starting in the spring of 2015, for example, as Figure 5.3 illustrates, Breyers ice cream temporarily altered its tamper band by including the following statement:

> No Artificial Growth Hormones. The FDA states that no significant difference has been shown between dairy derived from rBST-treated and non-rBST-treated cows. We use only milk and cream from cows not treated with artificial growth hormones. Suppliers of other ingredients such as cookies, candies, and sauces may not be able to make this pledge.

This redesigned tamper band preceded Breyers' introduction of its new product packaging, which has since included some version of the labels illustrated in Figure 5.4, which similarly inform consumers that Breyers ice cream products are free of synthetic growth hormones.

Companies like Whole Foods, Kroger, Horizon, and Tillamook have also, for some time, included on their packaging various statements to the effect that their products are "Made with Milk from Cows Not Treated with rBGH." Recombinant bovine growth hormones (rBGH) are commonly used as catalysts

WARNING: This product contains a chemical known to the State of California to cause cancer.

WARNING: This product contains a chemical known to the State of California to cause birth defects or other reproductive harm.

WARNING

Detectable amounts of chemicals known to the State of California to cause cancer, birth defects or other reproductive harm may be found in and around this facility.

Figure 5.2 California Proposition 65 Warning Content

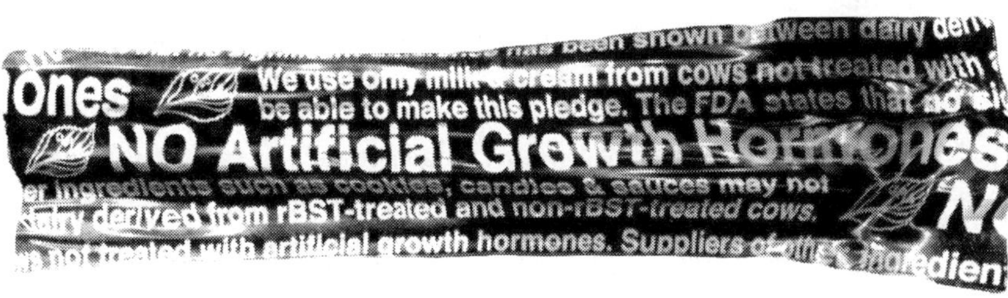

Figure 5.3 Breyers' Growth Hormone–Free Label for Tamper Band (2015)

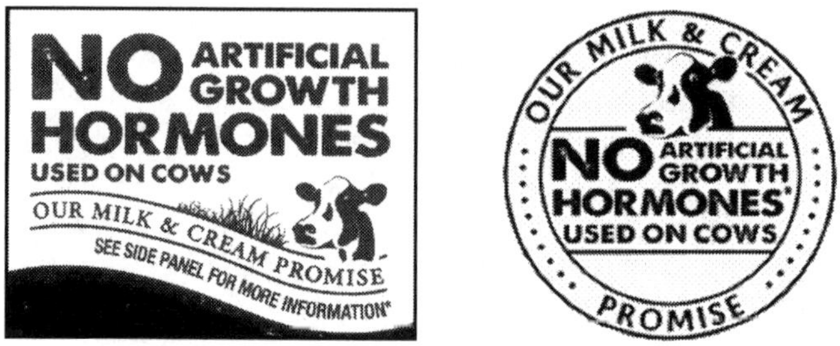
NO ARTIFICIAL GROWTH HORMONES
USED ON COWS
OUR MILK & CREAM PROMISE
SEE SIDE PANEL FOR MORE INFORMATION*
OUR MILK & CREAM
NO ARTIFICIAL GROWTH HORMONES*
USED ON COWS
PROMISE

Figure 5.4 Breyers' Growth Hormone–Free Product Labels (2016)[27]

for lactating dairy cattle to produce greater volumes of milk, and traces of rBGH residues have been found in all possible dairy products produced with milk from rBGH-treated cattle—whose consumption entails uncertain human health effects.[28] And since cattle given rBGH are more prone to develop infections of their udders, they are also given higher levels of antibiotics than non–rBGH-treated cattle—the ingestion of which is suspected to pose further long-term health risks to consumers.[29] And despite the FDA's firm denial of the potential adverse health effects of consuming rBGH-treated dairy and its insistence that there is no salient difference between milk from treated and untreated cows,[30] many corporations have proactively chosen to disclose details of the contents of their products to allow consumers to make more informed decisions about the products they purchase and, thus, about the possible environmental threats to which they expose themselves. The same can be said for other existing initiatives, such as the diverse variations of "BPA-free" product labels that companies like Nalgene and Philips AVENT have implemented, or "All Natural" or "100% Natural" labeling schemes per the FDA's definition of "natural,"[31] or—as Figure 5.5 depicts—the U.S. Department of Agriculture's Certified Organic label and the Non-GMO Project's compliance label for foods produced free of genetically engineered components. In this same spirit, dedicated uncertainty labels and notices could be implemented to inform the public of the uncorroborated potential for harm that a corporation's products, services, or workplace environments entail. A few prototype designs follow in Figure 5.6.

We may at once feel some fear for uncorroborated possibilities of harm, as well as indignation toward legislators, regulators, and industry for their respective failures to require and invest in basic toxicity tests of the substances the public is routinely exposed to, and thus for irresponsibly tolerating and perpetuating uncertainty. However, the intention of a new uncertainty warning is neither to instill fear by implying that uncertain threats are dangerous, nor to indict stakeholders in the private and public sectors for their lack of due care. Rather, the impartial aims of the proposed public disclosure

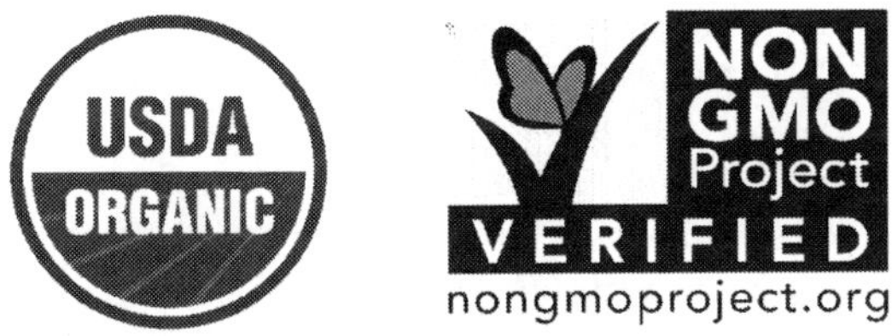

Figure 5.5 Examples of Existing Consumer Protection Labels[32]

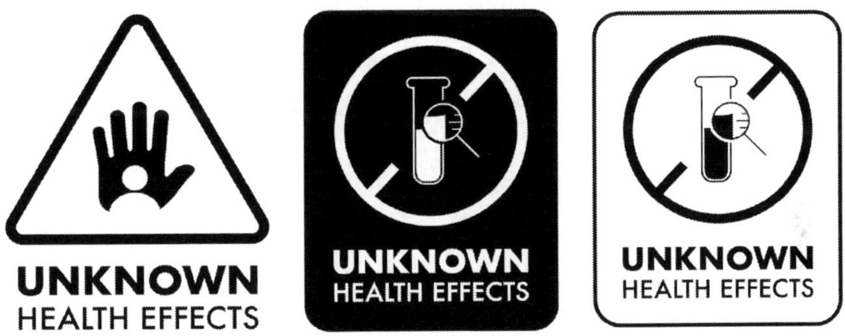

Figure 5.6 Proposed Uncertain Threat Warnings (© Szentkirályi 2019)

initiative—which hopefully will follow the publication of this book—are to underscore the prevalence of uncertain threats, to motivate the elimination of scientific uncertainty, and to promote greater transparency and the public's right to know[33] so that individuals may better insulate themselves from potential injury (the corollary of which may well be greater pressure for industry to be socially responsible and greater accountability among regulatory agencies and policy-makers).

In any event, such efforts to forewarn consumers, employees, and the broader public of potential, albeit uncertain, threats of environmental harm enable individuals to make more informed choices about the threats they knowingly and willingly accept. And by enhancing one's capacity for autonomous decision-making in this way, public disclosure initiatives may attenuate the residual obligations industries have to exercise due care under conditions of uncertainty.

Finally, if "best available control technologies" (BACTs), "maximum achievable control technologies" (MACTs), or even the less demanding "best available technology economically achievable" (BAT), were implemented to further mitigate the potential for harm that a corporation's emissions may entail, the emitter's residual obligation to exercise further due care may also merit being attenuated—in large measure because of the significant burden that the costly implementation of these control technologies involves. While BACT and MACT standards have pertained specifically to the emission of effluents into the ambient air, similar standards could be applied more generally to the release of substances whose effects are scientifically uncertain.

Whenever one or more of these possible mitigating factors is present, the responsibility corporations have to continue testing for the health effects of the potentially harmful substances they emit into the environment diminishes. In the absence of these mitigating factors, the outstanding or residual duties corporations have to verify the effects of the uncertain threats they author remain unaltered, and testing must begin anew. And again, if our assessment of whether a corporation merits a diminished duty of due care reveals egregious instances or a history of socially irresponsible corporate behavior—what we might call aggravating factors, then it may be appropriate to amplify the corporation's residual obligation to strive to mitigate the potential for harm. The general aim here is to shift the burden of proof to industry to strive in earnest to demonstrate the absence of unreasonable risks to public health. As some regulators have stressed, with regard at least to those substances being emitted in large quantities,

> It is time to fill the gap in information. . . . U.S. companies need to do much more testing and generate basic toxicity assessments in a form that is publicly available and usable by consumers, community groups, chemical users, and workers. Industry has committed to increase testing, but their progress has been slow; meanwhile companies continue to reap significant profits from the production and sale of these HPV chemicals.[34]

However, this compulsory exercise of due care should *not* entail forbidding corporations from engaging in those practices that beget uncertain threats until they can prove the relative safety of their potentially harmful actions, for the results of this testing may prove to be inconclusive and uncertainty may still persist. Moreover, the point is not for industry to retest again and again what current technologies and scientific standards cannot currently determine. Thus, when the initial phase of testing fails to reveal the actual risk of exposure and when due care requires that further testing be conducted, we may conclude something like the following.

Some reasonable standard amount of time (one year, perhaps) between compulsory tests will be necessary to allow for technological and scientific advancements that could be implemented in future phases of testing. Also, even if the potential for harm has not been successfully corroborated, eventually this cycle of testing and retesting must cease: eventually industry has to be relieved of any further obligations of due care. After a reasonable number of attempts and years (perhaps a decade), during which time corporations *are* permitted to release the potentially harmful substance into the environment, then despite the possibility that the uncertain threat may ultimately prove to be harmful, restrictions on the manufacture, distribution, consumption, and emission of these substances should be suspended—unless or until future evidence confirms that a credible (measurable and probabilistic) risk of harm to public health exists. The moral reciprocity between authors of uncertain threats and the public that benefits from precautionary safeguards would justify shifting the burden of proof onto the public and regulatory agencies. This assumes, of course, that corporations forthrightly disclose all data on the health safety studies they conduct to regulators and the public, and that if corporations are found to falsify data or to manufacture doubt to discredit findings that corroborate the actual risks a particular substance poses to human health, these corporations would be sanctioned and prohibited from any use of the substance in question. (And perhaps these derelict corporations could be issued fines that would then be used to invest in research and development in toxicological studies to improve our testing capabilities.)

This certainly is not an exhaustive list of mitigating (and aggravating) factors that should inform our assessments of what due care under outcome and probability uncertainty should consist of. However, the point of these considerations is to underscore again the salience of context and to reiterate that any feasible standard of due care must be able to accommodate variation in a host of morally relevant factors. This book's normative defense of the exercise of precaution is grounded in the deontological principle that as moral equals we ought to treat each other with due regard and that this equality demands—as a matter of the reciprocity that defines our moral relationships with each other—that we refrain from gambling with the welfare of others and from projecting our perceptions of acceptable risk onto our fellows. However, the application of this universal principle cannot be uniform if it is to account for the variable and highly complicated causal contexts of environmental harms (see Chapter 2.1), or if it is to withstand the numerous practical, policy-oriented objections against the precautionary approach to regulating environmental risk—objections to which we now turn.

5.5 Rejoinders to Standard Objections to Precaution

Recall that Chapter 2 explained why contemporary defenses of precautionary environmental risk regulation are flawed and introduced the rights-based conception of the precautionary principle. Chapter 3 then developed the normative justification of this right against being exposed to uncertain possibilities of harm—which was grounded in our obligations of mutual respect and the idea that treating others as moral equals, as ends in themselves, obliges us to strive to prevent putting them in the way of potential harm. Building on this defense of precaution, Chapter 4 showed how contemporary arguments from moral responsibility, moral luck, and the ethics of risk do not adequately demonstrate (either explicitly or by implication) the permissibility of uncertain environmental threats. Finally, Sections 5.1 to 5.4 in this chapter have given substance to a reasonable standard of due care by which authors of uncertain threats can satisfy their duties toward others (that is, by which emitters can respect the correlative rights of others to be safeguarded against potential harm). What remains, then, is to show how the proposed rights-based account is capable of avoiding the common objections against the precautionary principle that were introduced in Chapter 2.2. Returning to this litany of charges and demonstrating the proposed normative defense of exercising precaution can adequately respond to these worries not only illustrates the viability of this reformulated understanding of the precautionary principle but also promises to revive the stalled debate over the merits of precaution.

Recall from Chapter 2 that the charges commonly leveled against the precautionary approach to environmental risk regulation include the following: (1) The precautionary principle tolerates unfounded restrictions on actions that beget merely speculative risks. The idea here is that until a preponderance of evidence confirms empirically that an actual risk to public health exists, we lack the justification to regulate the possible risk: we cannot make sense of imposing restrictions on industry when their emissions, products, and workplaces may prove to be harmless. In this way, the precautionary principle has no epistemic basis to justify its regulatory decisions. (2) Precautionary policies are commonly subjective and highly political.[35] This objection parallels the worry in (1) that proponents of precaution lack justificatory grounding for their regulatory decisions in the absence of corroborating empirical evidence. Accordingly, the notion that precautionary regulations are subjective and political implies their proponents ground the legitimacy of preventative measures in intuitive, fallible, and inconsistent "lay" perceptions of risk that are vulnerable to being influenced (co-opted) by political agendas, as opposed to grounding regulatory decisions in objective scientific evidence and reasoning. (3) The precautionary principle effectively "paralyzes" all policy making.[36] The charge here is that all actions carry some inherent risk to others and that all policy prescriptions have the potential to cause some (unintended and/or unforeseeable) harm to others. And since the precautionary principle aims to mitigate this risk, it commits us to prohibiting all risky action, which amounts to prohibiting *all* action—including, counterintuitively, the implementation of (potentially harmful) precautionary measures themselves.

(4) Preventative measures may create more risk than they ameliorate and are thus incoherent. The general concern here is that precautionary regulations are counterproductive: as a matter of principle, to mitigate possible risks of harm, proponents of precaution would opt to prohibit the use of substances whose effects are suspected to cause harm, *even if* the probability of injury coming to pass is estimated to be low, and even if the indirect consequences of exercising precaution would themselves be harmful. The example of how the precautionary ban of dichlorodiphenyltrichloroethane (DDT) in developing nations prompted a rise in malaria-related illnesses and deaths, as well as the claim that precautionary bans of genetically modified foods would lead to higher

rates of illness and death from malnutrition and starvation in the world's poorest countries, illustrate this worry. (5) Precautionary regulations "selectively" acknowledge certain costs of nonregulation while imprudently ignoring others. This is an extension of objection (4) and suggests that the exercise of precaution consists of a perverse and irrational risk–benefit calculus, which justifies eliminating speculative risks at the expense of broader social policies and values or the benefits of nonregulation—the forfeiture of which entails costs that never enter into the equation. For instance, that genetically modified crops can require less irrigation and fewer fertilizers, which are benefits of accepting the health risks that consumption of genetically modified organisms (GMOs) may entail, is disregarded by precautionary calls for the ban of genetically modified (GM) foods.

(6) The principle fails to be "action guiding"; it is rather vacuous.[37] This criticism has to do with the notion that calls for precaution are vague, that precautionary prescriptions are superficial—neglecting to explain or justify what specifically the exercise of precaution would consist of. Perhaps precaution entails informing the public about the presence of an environmental threat (as with the labeling schemes noted earlier), or working to diminish the potential health effects of exposure (perhaps by providing individuals better access to healthcare), or eliminating the causes of potential public health threats (as blanket prohibitions intend to do). A commitment to the precautionary principle does not straightforwardly translate into any substantive regulatory decision. (7) Rigid precautionary standards fail to balance the benefits with the costs of regulation and, hence, unfairly burden industry.[38] Since proponents, as a matter of principle, err on the side of caution whenever the potential harm to public health is unclear, they are willing to tolerate the potentially high costs of their regulatory decisions—in large measure because they are prepared to direct those costs to industry. For instance, a commonly alleged implication of the precautionary principle is that industry must bear the burden of proof and demonstrate that exposure to a particular substance poses no actual risk to human health (that exposure is safe) before the manufacture of the substance is permitted. (8) The precautionary principle stifles technological innovation.[39] Since a commitment to the precautionary principle tolerates high costs to industry and entails a general aversion to risk, precaution disincentivizes industry's investment in research and development and the introduction of new innovations, because these novel advancements (whose benefits and drawbacks may take years to fully understand) would be subject to severe restriction or prohibition on the precautionary account. Each of these criticisms is addressed in turn.

The first two objections claim that the precautionary principle condones regulating speculative risks and that its policy recommendations are suspiciously nonobjective—which, in both cases, amounts to suggesting that the precautionary principle ignores the science of environmental risk and grounds its preventative measures in some form of "intuitive toxicology."[40] First, it would be misguided for any proponent of the principle to suggest that the precautionary approach is appropriate for all, or for even most, threats of environmental harm. As was already stated, a plausible defense of precautionary risk management must acknowledge that the precautionary principle should only supplement science-based, quantitative risk assessment: it is not a substitute for this alternative approach. After all, many potential environmental harms *are* probabilistic. That is, they constitute traditional risk impositions, where we know the outcomes associated with exposure to a particular substance and we know enough about its toxicity to conduct risk assessments and quantify the actual dangers to the public. And risk assessments *can* effectively account for many environmental harms and risks. Sunstein notes, for example, that mitigating the release of, exposure to, and harm from asbestos and lead are among the noteworthy success stories of risk cost–benefit analysis.[41] Therefore, more specifically, the purview of the precautionary approach should be limited to those cases in which *both* outcome and probability uncertainty are present—that is, when we lack the information necessary to conduct formal risk assessments and when any such assessment will consequently fail to yield justifiable policy recommendations to safeguard the public from potential harm.

As such, key to the proposed rights-based account—which espouses the limited scope or applicability of the precautionary principle—is embracing the need for scientifically grounded regulations, which in turn entails rejecting the merit of subjective risk perceptions when we are faced with environmental risks of harm. In contrast, when responding to uncertain threats of environmental harm, the inferences we could draw from formal risk assessments about the nature of the threat and the actual possibility for harm are unfounded (unverifiable) and thus are as speculative as the precautionary approach is alleged to be by its critics. In other words, under dual conditions of outcome and probability uncertainty, the threat to public health is inescapably speculative given our epistemic limitations.

That said, in the rights-based account, erring on the side of caution to prevent an uncertain threat from materializing in some harm to public health is neither speculative nor subjective in the way critics envision. For rights-based precautionary measures are not based on what we know or think we know about the threat of harm, but rather they are grounded in a deontological conception of what it is we owe each other as moral equals. The nature and our knowledge of the threats to which we may expose others are salient contextual factors that will alter the stringency of our obligation of due care and how we may discharge this obligation. Yet our duty to exercise precaution under uncertainty is present, regardless of whether the threats of harm our actions beget are imminent and nontrivial and scientifically verified, or speculative and subjective.

What of the third objection, then, that the precautionary principle is "incoherent" and "paralyzes" all policy making, since its justificatory force (of prevailing uncertainty) undermines *all* policy alternatives, *including* any precautionary risk regulation? Again, critics allege that since *any* policy decision has the potential to cause some harm, and since exercising precaution requires that possibilities of harm be prevented, the precautionary approach *ipso facto* can justify no policy option. Some proponents of precautionary risk regulation have dismissed this charge as a caricature of what the exercise of precaution entails. Deville and Harding, for instance, insist that preventative policies naturally vary in their stringency and that full bans of activities, technologies, or risk regulations that expose the public to uncertain possibilities of harm are simply the most restrictive alternatives. But this need not mean that a commitment to the precautionary principle amounts to endorsing the most restrictive response to uncertain environmental threats. Less restrictive measures to mitigate the potential for harm under conditions of uncertainty might include requiring further research on the effects of exposure or requiring suitable substitutes or control technologies.[42] Moreover, there are those like Shrader-Frechette who argue that policy making is not paralyzed by a willingness to err on the side of caution under conditions of uncertainty,[43] but rather it is paralyzed by proponents of formal risk assessment who exploit "uncertainties about various mechanisms of harm" and call for ever-greater risk analysis.[44] By underscoring the inconclusiveness of our knowledge of public health threats, it is alleged that opponents of precaution commonly insist on the need for a preponderance of evidence to delay regulation.[45]

However, if we take the objection seriously, in the rights-based interpretation, its salience is no longer obvious. For the rights-based account of precaution effectively shifts the discussion from trying to minimize or eliminate threats that remain uncertain to adjudicating competing rights claims—namely, reconciling the rights of some to engage in potentially harmful activities, whose outcomes may in fact prove to be benign, with the rights of others not to be placed in the way of possible harm.

The question, then, is not whether the precautionary principle can overcome the apparent contradiction of proposing preventative policy prescriptions that are themselves vulnerable to the uncertainty that they aim to manage. Rather, the question becomes whether we can justify preventative measures that constrain an emitter's right to perform actions that expose the public to potential, albeit uncertain, threats of environmental harm. And the answer to this question, while it is challenging and dependent on various contextual factors, suffers no contradiction. It turns *not* on what we can or cannot know about the potential for harm and the residual threat of harm that constraining an emitter's autonomy may entail, but rather on our conception of what moral equality and reciprocity demand of us—which entails, at base, that emitters make a reasonable effort to avoid exposing others to potential harm. And as is stressed again below, it is possible to reconcile the competing rights claims of emitters with the claims of those who are exposed to the uncertain threats emitters create in such a way that does not presume that precautionary measures are implausibly stringent.

With regard to the analogous fourth criticism, which suggests that precautionary policies may well create greater threats of harm than they ameliorate and, thus, that they are irrational, proponents have underscored that the precautionary principle entails no such obtuse conclusion. If the exercise of precaution were expected to create a serious potential for harm, this would be compelling reason *not* to preventatively regulate the uncertain environmental threat.[46] If a precautionary ban of GM crops, for instance, would threaten to beget widespread malnutrition or starvation, this possibility for harm may well undermine the proponent's justification for exercising precaution. Yet this sort of conventional response quickly stalls the debate once again, for its focus remains on what we can know about the threat of environmental harm and how this knowledge or lack of knowledge justifies regulating or not regulating the threat. The rights-based interpretation of the precautionary principle, however, tables the usual epistemic justification for taking precaution. Accordingly, while rights-based precautionary efforts *could*, in principle—given prevailing uncertainties—entail greater potential harm than the uncertain threat it attempts to prevent, the *de facto* success or failure of mitigating the possibility for harm is largely immaterial here. What justifies rights-based precaution is the intention and effort to respect the equal moral standing and the fundamental rights of others not to be harmed or put in potential harm's way. Invariably there will be occasions where we will fail to prevent undeserved harm, and there is nothing preventing us from retaining a further standard of fault liability, which could ensure that if one's actions prove to harm others despite her exercise of due care, she can still be held liable for the injury.[47]

As for the sixth objection noted earlier, that the precautionary principle fails to provide any substantive policy guidance, that it is vacuous or fails to be action guiding, there are numerous plausible criteria for discharging one's moral obligation to exercise due care—criteria that can provide a foundation for substantive policy objectives. Again, perhaps one way in which an emitter may satisfy his duty to exercise due care under uncertainty is to inform those whom he exposes to his emissions of the indeterminate possibility for harm. For industry, this may take the form of a labeling scheme on products containing substances whose potential for harm is scientifically unverified. Like existing organic, non-GM, hazardous materials, choking hazard, or fair trade labels, such an initiative would provide those who are exposed to uncertain threats salient information to avoid possible injury. Another way to satisfy one's duty of due care would be to proactively strive to prevent exposing traditionally vulnerable populations to uncertain threats (including infants and children, the elderly, pregnant women, racial and ethnic minority groups, the poor, etc.). Alternatively, industry might work to discharge the standard of due care under uncertainty by implementing BACTs in their various production processes, or by substituting substances in their business practices whose potential for harm remains scientifically uncorroborated with those whose effects of exposure have been verified[48] (i.e., whenever such substitutes exist).[49]

At base, however, any feasible standard of due care would require corporations to try to discern the actual risk of harm their emissions pose to others. This would entail shifting the burden of proof to require that industrial emitters demonstrate the absence of unreasonable harms to public health by testing in earnest the potential dangers to public health before they are permitted to release substances into the environment. However, this criterion does *not* equate to the usual claim that emitters must prove the relative safety of their potentially harmful actions, since the results of this mandatory testing may still prove inconclusive and (outcome and probability) uncertainty may still persist. What is important to note is that any defensible standard of due care must be flexible or context dependent. For not all uncertain threats of environmental harm are the same: the nature of the emitted substance will vary, as will the reasons for the emission; the costs and benefits of the emission; the population that is exposed; the vulnerability or physiological predisposition to being injured of those who are exposed; the timing, duration, intensity, and frequency of exposure; the availability of alternative courses of action or substitute technologies; and so forth. Consequently, what the exercise of precaution (or due care) entails will also be context dependent. Thus, while other criteria for discharging the obligation to exercise precaution under uncertainty may be found to be more appropriate, the examples provided earlier illustrate that the foregoing objection to the precautionary principle is unfounded.

Alternatively, objections (5) and (7) claim that precautionary policy prescriptions are overly demanding and are unduly costly to emitters. Some might insist that from mandatory toxicity testing, to implementing suitable substitutes, to adopting BACTs, and so forth, the burdens on industry are extensive—which is to say that the benefits of mitigating the uncertain potential for harm are outweighed by the costs of these preventative measures. Indeed, as the EPA has acknowledged, basic toxicity testing for any given chemical substance would amount to approximately $200,000.[50] At this rate, even conducting toxicity testing for only the roughly 3,000 high production volume chemicals being manufactured in and/or imported into the United States would likely exceed $600 million. Similarly, the costs of the research and development required for a company to find suitable substitute substances—whose toxicity data *have* been collected and whose risk of harm to the public *can* be estimated—which could be suitable for a given product or service, as well as the costs of altering its manufacturing and service processes to accommodate these substitutes, could be exorbitant. The same could be said of retrofitting existing machinery or incorporating newer, improved available technologies ("add-on control systems")[51] to satisfy more stringent BACT or MACT regulations.

With the express aim of adjudicating—as a matter of moral equality and reciprocity—the competing interests and rights claims of those who wish to engage in potentially harmful actions to exercise their moral autonomy, with the interests and rights of those who are exposed to the potentially harmful effects of these actions to *not* have others gamble with their welfare, this objection seems misplaced. In other words, this rights-based formulation of the precautionary principle is uniquely capable of taking seriously the right of emitters to engage in potentially harmful activities under uncertainty. Indeed, it is the same reciprocity between moral equals that obliges emitters to exercise due care that also protects emitters from undue burdens on their autonomy. In fact, as was suggested earlier, when due care is exercised and one's potentially harmful action retroactively proves to cause no actual harm, the reciprocity between moral equals may require that the beneficiaries of due care compensate the actor for a portion of the costs entailed by her efforts to mitigate the uncertain potential for harm. What is more, the series of context-dependent mitigating factors is specifically intended to underscore that any plausible standard of due care under uncertainty must be stringent enough to ensure that efforts are actually taken to mitigate the potential for environmental harm, but it must nevertheless be flexible enough that if the threat never does materialize into an actual harm, we would not retrospectively find the measure unreasonable. As some have aptly noted, exercising precaution (taking due care to prevent exposing others to possible injury) "is *not* tantamount to systematic renunciation, prohibition, stalling, and stonewalling."[52]

For these reasons, it might in fact be argued that the proposed standard of due care can actually be hyper-accepting of environmental threats of harm. Since the appeal to rights of moral equals that grounds preventative measures of due care simultaneously grounds the right of individuals to engage in potentially harmful behavior, flipping this justification for taking care on its head would mean that as a matter of right and moral equality, we are obliged to accept widespread environmental threats as opposed to championing substantive precautionary safeguards. Moreover, the proposed standard of due care under uncertainty, as noted earlier, does *not* require that emitters prove that the uncertain threats they create will not endanger public health and welfare. Again, more modestly, if an emitter satisfies her duty of due care, then even if the threat to others remains inconclusive, this proposed account would permit the emitter to perform the potentially harmful action. And this, too, may draw criticism for being too lax.[53]

Nevertheless, to assuage some concerns about unfair burdens to industry, we might note that BAT, BACT, and MACT regulations all take explicit account of the cost-effectiveness or economic feasibility of new control technologies[54] and that the list of mitigating factors briefly explored here is neither mandatory nor inclusive: companies would be free to seek more cost-effective alternatives to further attenuate their moral obligation of due care, or to decide to do nothing beyond testing the toxicity of the substances they emit.

Less sympathetically, however, it should be underscored that the costs of basic toxicity testing are nominal relative to the profits the chemical industry customarily enjoys. Suppose we focus, again, only on the few thousand high production volume chemical substances being manufactured and sold in the United States—whose rates of production and consumption make our exposure to these substances more likely and which thus should amplify our concerns about the indeterminacy of these particular threats to public health. The estimated figure of $600 million to test and collect the toxicity data for these 3,000 high production volume substances may seem like an undue imposition on the chemical industry when taken out of context. However, consider that Dow Chemical, which is but one of the leading chemical manufacturing companies in the United States, in the fourth quarter of 2015 alone recorded $11.5 billion in sales and $2.4 billion in earnings (or net income) and "returned $2.7 billion to shareholders through paid dividends and share repurchases."[55] Should Dow alone bear the burden of conducting the aforementioned toxicity tests, this would amount to 25 percent of its fourth-quarter earnings, or 6.3 percent of its net income in 2015.[56] And yet there is no reason to presume that the financial burden of collecting toxicity data on those substances whose potentially harmful effects and probability of causing harm remain uncertain could not be fairly distributed among the myriad American chemical companies. Dow Chemical, Exxon Mobil, DuPont, PPG Industries, Chevron Phillips, Praxair, and Huntsman Corp. are among the leading firms of more than "830 companies making HPV chemicals in the U.S."[57] In this proper context, the objection of unfairness is simply absurd: the imposition of costs of toxicity testing is not just feasible, but it is so negligible that it is difficult to comprehend how, after 40 years since the enactment of the TSCA, mandatory testing is just now being implemented under the 2016 Lautenberg Act and its fundamental corrections to the TSCA provisions.

In any event, among the virtues of this rights-based precautionary principle is that it is *not* "exclusive," yet it *is* "determinative"[58]—which is to say that it neither considers only environmental threats in prescribing policy alternatives, nor is it a vacuous policy tool (as explained earlier). The rights-based precautionary principle can heed relevant factors other than the presence of environmental risk: taking into consideration, for example, the interests and rights of the polluters to engage in their risky activities, the competing interests and rights of others not to be exposed to potential harms, whether polluters exercise due care in striving to prevent harm to others, and so forth.[59] In this way, while the rights-based account is still exclusionary—precluding, for example, the salience of the various costs and benefits of risk regulation—it is not as narrow or rigid as other formulations of the principle.

Finally, recall the criticism that the precautionary principle stifles technological innovation. Claims that the economic costs imposed on industry to comply with stricter precautionary environmental standards directly undermine innovation and progress or claims that precautionary policies are inherently hostile to technology because they sometimes entail banning technologies that may have some benefit (like pesticides and GMOs) are highly contentious, if only for the selective examples that are invoked to make the point. It seems equally plausible to claim that the upshot of requiring industries to conduct tests on the possible dangers of the pollutants they aim to emit into the environment—the first condition of the liability standard of this proposed rights-based account—would, in fact, be greater technological innovation. Consider, for instance, that a company that extensively tests some chemical it wishes to use in some manufacturing process might discover how to effectively abate the environmental impacts of the pollutant. In so doing the company would have incentives to patent and manufacture new control technologies that it could profit from when they are adopted as BACTs by regulatory agencies.[60]

This discussion may seem to leave much unsettled. Some might argue, for instance, that a deontological standard of due care cannot be reconciled with the purported context-dependent nature of environmental threats. Others may insist that the account developed here only gestures at what exercising due care would require in any given circumstance, and it offers no substantive explanation of *how* we adjudicate between the competing interests and rights of emitters and the interests and rights of those who are exposed to the uncertain threats of harm emitters author. Further still, some might charge that this deontological defense of precaution fails to explain how a rights-based precautionary approach toward environmental risk regulation can be reconciled with or can effectively augment a consequentialist system of risk management that is firmly rooted in formal risk assessment and utilitarian cost–benefit balancing.

Some of these concerns are addressed in the following chapter of the book, which explores the environmental health hazard that the manufacture and emission of TEL involved for more than five decades to further demonstrate the plausibility and necessity of the foregoing, context-sensitive industrial standard of due care. As a gasoline additive that prevented engine knocking and improved automotive efficiency and prolonged the life of internal combustion engines, TEL began to be mass-produced in the early 1920s. At the time, little was known about the subclinical (low-dose) effects of exposure to lead, as well as the immediate or long-term health effects of exposure to leaded gasoline exhaust in the ambient air. The broader foreseeable dangers to public health, and earlier warnings by public health scientists, seemed to be validated when the mass production of TEL and the subsequent increased workplace exposure revealed several high-profile instances of severe illness and death from acute lead poisoning. The numerous deaths and hundreds of cases of severe lead poisoning at the Standard Oil of New Jersey research labs and refinery in Elizabeth, New Jersey; at the DuPont manufacturing plant in Deepwater, New Jersey; and at the General Motors research facility in Dayton, Ohio, provoked public outcry and cast doubt on the benefit of the additive. Yet, these opportunistic companies, which had strong vested interests in preventing the implementation of mandatory emission standards for TEL and leaded gasoline, capitalized on and helped to perpetuate the uncertainty of the dangers to the public to ensure the continued production of leaded gasoline for more than 50 years. Chapter 6 demonstrates that the disregard with which these corporations put others in the way of possible injury testifies to the need to hold emitters accountable, despite prevailing uncertainty, by imposing on them reasonable measures to try to prevent this harm.

Nevertheless, before the discussion turns to this case study, a few words in closing regarding the previous concerns are in order. As noted earlier at the end of Section 5.4, it is a virtue of the proposed argument for precaution (and an improvement on previous defenses of the precautionary principle) that it is sensitive to context, and there is nothing outwardly contradictory with espousing a deontological (universal) principle of due care that we all should, in all contexts, strive to mitigate the potential for undeserved and preventable harm that our actions may have on others, while concomitantly maintaining that how this obligation is satisfied shall vary across contexts and actors. Indeed, many environmental harms and risks are marked by incredibly complex causal chains. Different forms and degrees of uncertainty often obscure our understanding of the dangers to human health. New chemical substances are consistently introduced into industrial and commercial manufacturing processes, which broaden and amplify the (cumulative and interactive) environmental threats we face. Toxicological studies and detection capabilities are constantly evolving, which shapes our subsequent understanding of the health effects of long-term, low-dose exposure and safe thresholds of risk. The morally relevant efforts that emitters may take to proactively mitigate the potential for harm under uncertainty are variable. And the acknowledgement that not all uncertain environmental threats are the same means that different individuals may infer or intuit different reasons for believing or disbelieving in the potential for harm, which tentatively may help to establish when (mere) reasons to exercise due care translate into duties to do so. These considerations all lend credence to the central assumption that any tenable argument for taking responsibility for our uncertain environmental threats must be contextual.

With regard to the second worry that this book's normative defense of precaution neglects to adequately explain what exercising due care would require in any given circumstance, each of the five sections in this chapter have made plain that the fundamental tenet of the proposed standard of due care is making toxicity testing mandatory in an effort to determine the potentially harmful effects of uncertain threats, so as to eliminate the various uncertainties that prevent their regulation under existing environmental laws. As stated previously, by eliminating uncertainty, uncertain threats become traditional, probabilistic risk impositions, whose danger to public health can generally be mitigated with the alternative quantitative, risk assessment–based regulatory regime and existing environmental protections. At base, then, the exercise of due care will require that we strive to determine the uncorroborated effects of our actions. Beyond this central tenet, given the necessary flexibility of a feasible standard of due care, what the exercise of precaution will consist of very much depends on the particular circumstance. The lengthy discussion of Figure 5.1 and how one might discharge her duty of due care under uncertainty, as well as the discussion in Section 5.4 on various morally relevant mitigating factors that should inform our assessments of what due care may require in particular circumstances, have tried to address this very concern.

Let us turn, then, to the charge that the proposed normative defense of precaution fails to provide a substantive explanation of *how* we can reconcile the competing interests and rights of those who wish to exercise their autonomy and perform actions that entail uncorroborated threats of harm to others with the interests and rights of those who stand to bear the outcomes of these actions *not* to have others gamble with their welfare and place them in potential harm's way. As Sections 5.3 and 5.5, as well as Chapter 4.4, have suggested, this account of precaution strives to construct the framework for arriving at mutually acceptable regulatory decisions under conditions of uncertainty. The intention is to prevent affording emitters license to perform actions that may cause preventable harm to others, while neglecting to impose unreasonable restrictions on these moral agents for the sake of insulating others from uncorroborated risks that may in the end cause no harm. With conventional normative arguments from moral responsibility, moral luck, and the ethics of risk all understating or dismissing—explicitly or by implication—the problem of uncertainty, and hence offering insufficient guidance on this subject, in developing a cursory framework for mutually acceptable and normatively justified regulatory decisions, the purpose here has been to defend a guiding principle for taking due care—a principle we might more modestly understand as a helpful heuristic to inform our responses to uncorroborated environmental health threats. Expressed differently, developing a thorough explanation of how the proposed standard of due care can be implemented to reconcile the competing interests and rights of parties involved (beyond what has already been said) would make for an ambitious subsequent project—integrating a more detailed discussion of environmental laws and relevant regulatory decisions that speak to this question, markedly expanding the discussion on cost–benefit balancing, engaging considerations of moral liability and relevant tort law; integrating substantive discussions on corporate social responsibility, corporate citizenship, and greenwashing; and developing similar standards of due care for individuals and governments.

Finally, in response to the objection that the proposed deontological defense of precaution fails to explain how a rights-based approach to environmental risk regulation can be squared with or augment a consequentialist system of risk management that is grounded in formal risk assessment and cost–benefit balancing, the answer has already largely been provided. This book's intention is not to develop a comprehensive moral theory of mutual respect and due care. Rather, much more modestly, the aim has been to defend a general framework for responding to environmental risk when we lack the information necessary for quantitative risk assessments (QRA) and cost–benefit analyses (CBA) to provide any policy guidance. QRA and CBA are nonstarters under conditions of uncertainty. Unless we are prepared to accept all uncorroborated environmental threats as safe or reasonable or permissible, we require an alternative approach to resolve the unique moral problem that uncertainty begets. Further, environmental risk management is not foremost motivated by statistical death and cancer rates, scientific dose-responses and tolerance thresholds, and the impersonal calculus of weighing the economic costs with the benefits of regulatory decisions. While regulatory decisions often turn on these considerations because we care about aggregate harms and the distribution of risk, we trust in science and realist conceptions of truth, and we value efficient or cost-effective policies. Nevertheless, environmental risk regulations aim, at base, to protect citizens from preventable and foreseeable harm: it is a fundamental commitment to human welfare and environmental justice that grounds the institution of environmental protection, and it is these values that operate in the background of our seemingly cold or distant statistical, scientific, and economic calculations. This is to say that there is nothing contradictory in suggesting that we can espouse values that stem from discrete and ostensibly competing comprehensive moral theories.

Notes

1. An individual standard of due care, e.g., might require that actors take reasonable measures to (1) become more knowledgeable of the complexity of environmental harms and the ways in which their individual emissions (namely via consumption and waste) could adversely affect others, (2) determine what substances the products they purchase contain and to utilize information that is publicly disclosed to try to discern the potential for harm of exposure to these substances or of the product's entering the waste stream, (3) use alternative products whenever possible that do not contain substances whose effects are unverified, (4) take advantage of public services that allow for the safe disposal of household waste (e.g., to avoid throwing fluorescent bulbs or spent paint or batteries into the garbage but rather to recycle them), and (5) review the companies whose products they purchase or invest in to determine (a) the rate at which they emit and (b) their compliance with existing environmental regulations.
2. *United States v. Reserve Mining Company* (1974); *Reserve Mining Company v. EPA* (1975).
3. Robert V. Percival et al., *Environmental Regulation: Law, Science, and Policy*, 6th ed. (New York: Aspen Publishers): 184.
4. Ibid.
5. Ibid., 189.
6. Ibid.
7. Ibid., 191.
8. Office of Pollution Prevention and Toxics, *High Production Volume Chemical Hazard Data Availability Study* (Washington, DC: EPA, 1998, last updated: August 2, 2010): 2, 34–5.
9. Steve DeVito, *Senior Scientist and Advisor*, Environmental Protection Agency, personal correspondence, February 15, 2017.
10. These include acute, chronic, and developmental and reproductive toxicity; mutagenicity; ecotoxicity; and environmental fate (ibid.).
11. Office of Pollution Prevention and Toxics, Environmental Protection Agency, "HPV Chemical Hazard Data Availability Study," 10, 34–5.
12. Joël Spiroux de Vendômois et al. "Debate on GMOs Health Risks after Statistical Findings in Regulatory Tests," *International Journal of Biological Sciences* 6 (2010): 597.
13. European Parliament and Council, "Registration, Evaluation, Authorisation and Restriction of Chemicals, Regulation No. 1907/2006," *Official Journal of the European Union*, 396 (December 18, 2006): 1–849.
14. Nozick, *Anarchy, State, and Utopia*, 83; see 78–84.
15. See §§1–2 in Chapter 6, as well as Kristin Shrader-Frechette, *Taking Action, Saving Lives: Our Duties to Protect Environmental and Public Health* (Oxford: Oxford University Press, 2007): Chapters 1–3.
16. My thanks to Joel Tickner for this suggestion.
17. Percival et al., *Environmental Regulation*, 285.
18. Ibid., 283.
19. Ibid., 284–5.
20. Office of Pollution Prevention and Toxics, "HPV Chemical Hazard Data Availability Study," 11, 34–5.

21. LifeStaw by Vestergaard: www.vestergaard.com/our-products/lifestraw.
22. World Health Organization, "Water Sanitation Hygiene: Water-Related Diseases," drawn from WHO, *Global Water Supply and Sanitation Assessment* (Geneva: WHO, 2000): http://who.int/water_sanitation_health/diseases-risks/diseases/diarrhoea/en/.
23. Percival et al., *Environmental Regulation*, 213: HPV chemicals are those whose annual rate of domestic production and/or importation exceeds 1 million pounds.
24. Formally known as the Safe Drinking Water and Toxic Enforcement Act of 1986 (or Chapter 6.6 of Division 20: Miscellaneous Health and Safety Provisions of the California Health and Safety Code).
25. Percival et al., *Environmental Regulation*, 148; see also California Environmental Protection Agency (CalEPA), Office of Environmental Health Hazard Assessment (OEHHA), "Proposition 65 in Plain Language," https://oehha.ca.gov/proposition-65/general-info/proposition-65-plain-language, last updated February 1, 2013; CalEPA, OEHHA, *California Code of Regulations*, Title 27, Article 6: Clear and Reasonable Warnings (amended on November 20, 2017).
26. These are drawn from the California Health and Safety Code, Sections 25249.6 and 25249.11.
27. My sincere thanks to Unilever for permission to reprint these labels and tamper band.
28. Food and Drug Administration, "Interim Guidance on the Voluntary Labeling of Milk and Milk Products from Cows That Have Not Been Treated with Recombinant Bovine Somatotropin," *Federal Register* 59 (February 10, 1994): https://gpo.gov/fdsys/pkg/FR-1994-02-10/html/94-3214.htm; Program on Breast Cancer and Environmental Risk Factors, Cornell University, "Consumer Concerns about Hormones in Food," June 2000: http://envirocancer.cornell.edu/factsheet/diet/fs37.hormones.cfm, last updated May 2, 2003; Food and Drug Administration, U.S. Department of Health and Human Services, "Report on the FDA's Review of the Safety of Recombinant Bovine Somatotropin," April 23, 2009: http://fda.gov/AnimalVeterinary/SafetyHealth/ProductSafetyInformation/ucm130321.htm, last updated July 28, 2014.
29. Program on Breast Cancer and Environmental Risk Factors, Cornell University, "Consumer Concerns about Hormones in Food;" American Cancer Society, "Learn about Cancer: Recombinant Bovine Growth Hormone," http://cancer.org/cancer/cancercauses/othercarcinogens/athome/recombinant-bovine-growth-hormone, last updated September 10, 2014.
30. Food and Drug Administration, "Interim Guidance on the Voluntary Labeling of Milk and Milk Products From Cows That Have Not Been Treated with Recombinant Bovine Somatotropin;" Program on Breast Cancer and Environmental Risk Factors, "Consumer Concerns about Hormones in Food;" Food and Drug Administration, "Report on the FDA's Review of the Safety of Recombinant Bovine Somatotropin."
31. Food and Drug Administration, "Use of the Term Natural on Food Labeling," www.fda.gov/food/food-labeling-nutrition/use-term-natural-food-labeling, last updated October 22, 2018.
32. My sincere thanks to the USDA Agricultural Marketing Service and its National Organic Program, as well as the Non-GMO Project for permission to reprint these labels.
33. Shrader-Frechette, *Taking Action, Saving Lives*, 122.
34. Office of Pollution Prevention and Toxics, "HPV Chemical Hazard Data Availability Study," 2.
35. Miller and Conko, "The Perils of Precaution," 26, 29, 36. Sunstein, *Risk and Reason*; Sunstein, *Laws of Fear*.
36. Edward Soule, "Assessing the Precautionary Principle," *Public Affairs Quarterly* 14 (2000); Sunstein, *Risk and Reason*; Sunstein, *Laws of Fear*; Martin Peterson,

"The Precautionary Principle Is Incoherent," *Risk Analysis* 26 (2006); Per Sandin, "Commonsense Precaution and Varieties of the Precautionary Principle," in *Risk: Philosophical Perspectives*, Tim Lewens, ed. (New York: Routledge, 2007).

37. Daniel Bodansky, "Scientific Uncertainty and the Precautionary Principle," *Environment* 33 (1991); Per Sandin, "Dimensions of the Precautionary Principle," *Human and Ecological Risk Assessment* 5 (1999); Soule, "Assessing the Precautionary Principle;" Harris and Holm, "Extending Human Lifespan and the Precautionary Paradox;" Per Sandin, "Commonsense Precaution and Varieties of the Precautionary Principle," in *Risk: Philosophical Perspectives*, Tim Lewens, ed. (New York: Routledge, 2007).
38. Miller and Conko, "The Perils of Precaution;" Whiteside, *Precautionary Politics*, 39, 42.
39. Cross, "Paradoxical Perils of the Precautionary Principle;" Miller and Conko, "Genetically Modified Fear and the International Regulation of Biotechnology;" Morris, "Defining the Precautionary Principle;" Goklany, *The Precautionary Principle*; Stone, "Is There a Precautionary Principle?;" John Graham, "The Role of Precaution in Risk Assessment and Management: An American's View," Remarks Prepared for "The US, Europe, Precaution and Risk Management: A Comparative Case Study Analysis of the Management of Risk in a Complex World" (January 11–12, 2002): http://whitehouse.gov/omb/inforeg/eu_speech.html.
40. Sunstein, *Risk and Reason*, 35; Sunstein, *Laws of Fear*, 83.
41. Sunstein, *Risk and Reason*, 27.
42. Adrian Deville and Ronnie Harding, *Applying the Precautionary Principle* (Annandale: Federation Press, 1997): 25–42.
43. Sunstein, *Laws of Fear*, 4–5, 26; see also Soule, "Assessing the Precautionary Principle;" Peterson, "The Precautionary Principle Is Incoherent;" Sandin, "Commonsense Precaution and Varieties of the Precautionary Principle," 101. Sunstein, e.g., argues that even precautionary regulations—efforts to prevent the actualization of some potential harm—run the risk of imposing (new) harms on those it aims to safeguard. And in some cases, it is alleged (Wildavsky, *But Is It True?*; Goklany, *The Precautionary Principle*) that precautionary regulations counterproductively beget greater (risk of) harms than which it strives to prevent.
44. Shrader-Frechette, *Taking Action, Saving Lives*, 109.
45. Ibid.
46. Deville and Harding, *Applying the Precautionary Principle*, 44.
47. How a proactive or forward-looking obligation of due care relates to a retroactive or backward-looking notion of moral culpability is explored in detail in Chapter 2.1.
48. Among the possible objections to these criteria that comprehensive defense of this rights-based conception of the precautionary principle would have to address is the concern that these substitutions may well entail greater risk impositions—as clarified, e.g., in *Public Citizen v. Young* (1987): "As a result, makers of drugs and cosmetics who are barred from using a carcinogenic dye carrying a one-in-20-million lifetime risk may use instead a noncarcinogenic, but toxic, dye carrying, say, a one-in-10-million lifetime risk. The substitution appears to be a clear loss for safety."
49. While the focus here is on the risky actions of industry, a similar standard of due diligence could extend to the actions of and interactions between particular individuals.
50. Office of Pollution Prevention and Toxics, "HPV Chemical Hazard Data Availability Study."
51. Environmental Protection Agency, "EPA Air Pollution Control Cost Manual, 6th Edition," EPA/452/B-02–001 (January 2002): www3.epa.gov/ttncatc1/dir1/c_allchs.pdf, 8.
52. Whiteside, *Precautionary Politics*, 55 (emphasis added).

53. Indeed, in this vein, one may well reject the very suggestion that emitters enjoy the same moral standing as particular individuals or the broader public, and thus one may reject the idea that industry has a right to perform actions that put the public in potential harm's way. More to the point, it seems dubious that industry has a right to emit potentially harmful substances in the first place. After all, corporations are not moral agents, the legal classification of personhood notwithstanding. My thanks to Carolyn Raffensperger for this suggestion, and as a cursory response here (more certainly deserves to be said), there is nothing inherently problematic with viewing corporations as we do groups or peoples—attributing to them, for instance, collective interests and observing those interests manifest in collective actions. Thus, like other communities of individuals, it seems *prima facie* plausible to grant corporations moral rights that parallel traditional group rights, as well assign to them corresponding moral duties. In any event, since corporations are, at base, aggregates of individuals, we may at least view the actions of a corporation as manifestations of the actions of key decision makers in the company, who *are* moral agents and who have the right to exercise their autonomy. Accordingly, it is these particular decision makers who we would then also hold culpable for a corporation's failure to exercise due care.
54. Environmental Protection Agency, "EPA Air Pollution Control Cost Manual," 3; Massachusetts Department of Environmental Protection, "Best Available Control Technology (BACT) Guidance," (June 2011): http://mass.gov/eea/docs/dep/air/approvals/bactguid.pdf, 4–5.
55. Dow Chemical Company, "Dow Reports Fourth Quarter and Full-Year Results" (February 2, 2016): http:// dow.com/en-us/investor-relations/financial-reporting/earnings/q4-2015.
56. Ibid.
57. Office of Pollution Prevention and Toxics, *High Production Volume Chemical Hazard Data Availability Study*; Alexander Tullo, "Top 50 U.S. Chemical Producers," *Chemical and Engineering News* 92 (2014): 16–8.
58. Gardiner, "A Core Precautionary Principle," 47, 53.
59. Though this proposed rights-based precautionary principle is not "inclusive," as Gardiner alleges his account is. He underscores that his *Rawlsian Core Precautionary Principle* in no way restricts "the kinds of considerations [that are] relevant to outcome assessment" and the justification of precautionary risk regulation.
60. Other objections that this book, as a future book project, will need to respond to may include the following: (1) "mandatory labels suggest a danger that might not exist" (Sunstein, *Laws of Fear*, 128: note that Sunstein is critical of this idea); (2) an obligation to exercise due care under uncertainty may well be self-defeating; (3) the proposed industrial standard is arbitrary; (4) by incorporating various mitigating factors that attenuate one's culpability, the standard is too lax (qua Rainer Forst, *The Right to Justification*, Jeffrey Flynn, trans. (New York: Columbia University Press, 2011); (5) the standard, which requires testing for the unknowable, is implausible; (6) the proposed standard does not explain how particular individuals (or private citizens) and government entities can satisfy their own obligations of due care under uncertainty; and (7) uncertain threats of harm may have *some* moral import, but do not warrant limits on autonomy in order to prevent them (qua Feinberg's analysis of "non-grievance" evils (Joel Feinberg, *Harmless Wrongdoing: The Moral Limits of the Criminal Law*, Vol. 4 (Oxford: Oxford University Press, 1984): 7, 17–8, 321).

References

American Cancer Society. "Learn About Cancer: Recombinant Bovine Growth Hormone." Last updated September 10, 2014. http://cancer.org/cancer/cancercauses/othercarcinogens/athome/recombinant-bovine-growth-hormone.

Bodansky, Daniel. "Scientific Uncertainty and the Precautionary Principle." *Environment* 33 (1991): 4–44.

California Environmental Protection Agency, Office of Environmental Health Hazard Assessment. "Proposition 65 in Plain Language." Last updated February 1, 2013. https://oehha.ca.gov/proposition-65/general-info/proposition-65-plain-language.

———. *California Code of Regulations*, Title 27, Article 6: Clear and Reasonable Warnings. Last updated November 20, 2017.

Cross, Frank. "Paradoxical Perils of the Precautionary Principle." *Washington and Lee Law Review* 53 (1996): 851–925.

de Vendômois, Joël Spiroux, et al. "Debate on GMOs Health Risks after Statistical Findings in Regulatory Tests." *International Journal of Biological Sciences* 6 (2010): 590–8.

Deville, Adrian and Ronnie Harding. *Applying the Precautionary Principle*. Annandale: Federation Press, 1997.

Dow Chemical Company. "EPA Air Pollution Control Cost Manual." 6th edition. EPA/452/B-02-001, January 2002. www3.epa.gov/ttncatc1/dir1/c_allchs.pdf.

———. "Dow Reports Fourth Quarter and Full-Year Results." February 2, 2016. http://dow.com/en-us/investor-relations/financial-reporting/earnings/q4-2015.

European Parliament and Council. "Registration, Evaluation, Authorisation and Restriction of Chemicals." Regulation No. 1907/2006. *Official Journal of the European Union* 396 (December 18, 2006): 1–849.

Feinberg, Joel. *Harmless Wrongdoing: The Moral Limits of the Criminal Law*, Vol. 4. Oxford: Oxford University Press, 1984.

Food and Drug Administration. "Interim Guidance on the Voluntary Labeling of Milk and Milk Products from Cows That Have Not Been Treated with Recombinant Bovine Somatotropin." *Federal Register* 59 (February 10, 1994). https://gpo.gov/fdsys/pkg/FR-1994-02-10/html/94-3214.htm.

———. "Report on the FDA's Review of the Safety of Recombinant Bovine Somatotropin." April 2009. Last updated July 28, 2014. http://fda.gov/AnimalVeterinary/SafetyHealth/ProductSafetyInformation/ucm130321.htm.

———. "Use of the Term Natural on Food Labeling." Last updated October 22, 2018. https://fda.gov/food/food-labeling-nutrition/use-term-natural-food-labeling.

Forst, Rainer. *The Right to Justification*, translated by Jeffrey Flynn. New York: Columbia University Press, 2011.

Gardiner, Stephen. "A Core Precautionary Principle." *Journal of Political Philosophy* 14 (2006): 33–60.

Goklany, Indur. *The Precautionary Principle: A Critical Appraisal of Environmental Risk Assessment*. Washington: Cato Institute, 2001.

Graham, John. "The Role of Precaution in Risk Assessment and Management: An American's View." Remarks prepared for "The U.S., Europe, Precaution and Risk Management: A Comparative Case Study Analysis of the Management of Risk in a Complex World." January 11–12, 2002. http://whitehouse.gov/omb/inforeg/eu_speech.html.

Harris, John and Søren Holm. "Extending Human Lifespan and the Precautionary Paradox." *Journal of Medicine and Philosophy* 27 (2002): 355–68.

LifeStaw by Vestergaard. www.vestergaard.com/our-products/lifestraw.

Massachusetts Department of Environmental Protection. "Best Available Control Technology Guidance." June 2011. http://mass.gov/eea/docs/dep/air/approvals/bactguid.pdf.

Miller, Henry and Gregory Conko. "Genetically Modified Fear and the International Regulation of Biotechnology." In *Rethinking Risk and the Precautionary Principle*, edited by Julian Morris. Oxford: Butterworth-Heinemann, 2000.

———. "The Perils of Precaution: Why Regulators' 'Precautionary Principle' Is Doing More Harm Than Good." *Policy Review* 107 (2001): 25–39.

Morris, Julian. "Defining the Precautionary Principle." In *Rethinking Risk and the Precautionary Principle*, edited by Julian Morris. Oxford: Butterworth-Heinemann, 2000.

Nozick, Robert. *Anarchy, State, and Utopia*. New York: Basic Books, 1974.

Office of Pollution Prevention and Toxics. "High Production Volume Chemical Hazard Data Availability Study." Washington: EPA, 1998. Last updated August 2, 2010.

Percival, Robert, et al. *Environmental Regulation: Law, Science, and Policy*, 6th edition. New York: Aspen Publishers, 2009.

Peterson, Martin. "The Precautionary Principle Is Incoherent." *Risk Analysis* 26 (2006): 595–601.

Program on Breast Cancer and Environmental Risk Factors, Cornell University. "Consumer Concerns about Hormones in Food." June 2000. Last updated May 2, 2003. http://envirocancer.cornell.edu/factsheet/diet/fs37.hormones.cfm.

Public Citizen Health Research Group v. Young, 831 F.2d 1108 (D.C. Circuit 1987).

Reserve Mining Company v. EPA, 514 F. 2d 492 (8th Circuit 1975).

Sandin, Per. "Dimensions of the Precautionary Principle." *Human and Ecological Risk Assessment* 5 (1999): 889–907.

———. "Commonsense Precaution and Varieties of the Precautionary Principle." In *Risk: Philosophical Perspectives*, edited by Tim Lewens. New York: Routledge, 2007.

Shrader-Frechette, Kristin. *Taking Action, Saving Lives: Our Duties to Protect Environmental and Public Health*. Oxford: Oxford University Press, 2007.

Soule, Edward. "Assessing the Precautionary Principle." *Public Affairs Quarterly* 14 (2000): 309–28.

Stone, Christopher. "Is There a Precautionary Principle?" *Environmental Law Reporter* 31 (2001): 10790–9.

Sunstein, Cass. *Risk and Reason: Safety, Law, and the Environment*. Cambridge: Cambridge University Press, 2002.

———. *Laws of Fear: Beyond the Precautionary Principle*. Cambridge: Cambridge University Press, 2005.

Tullo, Alexander. "Top 50 U.S. Chemical Producers." *Chemical and Engineering News* 92 (2014).

United States v. Reserve Mining Company, 380 F. Supp. 11 (D. Minnesota 1974).

Whiteside, Kerry. *Precautionary Politics: Principle and Practice in Confronting Environmental Risk*. Cambridge: MIT Press, 2006.

World Health Organization. "Water Sanitation Hygiene: Water-Related Diseases." In *Global Water Supply and Sanitation Assessment*. Prepared by World Health Organization. Geneva: WHO, 2000. http://who.int/water_sanitation_health/diseases-risks/diseases/diarrhoea/en/.

6 Feasibility of a Precautionary Standard of Due Care

Prevailing uncertainty about the health effects of environmental exposure prevents us from being able to discern actual risks to public health that many chemical substances pose. Since this uncertainty means that we cannot ascertain the potentially harmful consequences of exposure or the probability that exposure will cause harm, the plausibility of regulatory decisions based on quantitative risk assessments is undermined, as risk analysis presupposes the availability of this knowledge. The same can be said of conventional theories of moral responsibility and normative arguments in moral luck and the ethics of risk—which narrowly conceive of uncertainty as probability uncertainty and assume that whenever the probability of harm cannot be estimated, the risky action in question is morally innocuous. However, as the previous chapters have established, an alternative, precautionary approach to risk management is necessary to regulate the subset of effluents that entail uncertain threats of environmental harm. And by developing a deontological foundation for a precautionary standard of due care under uncertainty that is grounded in principles of moral equality and reciprocity—as opposed to appealing to our epistemic limitations and the indeterminate potential for harm to justify the need to exercise precaution—Chapters 4 and 5 also defended precautionary risk regulation against common objections to restricting the emission of substances in the absence of evidence corroborating a probable risk of nontrivial harm.

As Chapter 5 stressed, however, precautionary measures to protect the public from uncertain threats of environmental harm must be reasonable: while a precautionary standard of due care must be stringent enough to mitigate exposure to potential environmental harms, it must be flexible enough that if the threat ultimately proves to be harmless, we would not retrospectively judge that the restrictions on emitters were unfair (unduly burdensome). The sliding scale of uncertainty and the qualification that with some uncertain threats emitters may only have a *reason* to exercise due care as opposed to an *obligation* to do so (Chapter 3), as well as the various context-sensitive criteria and possible mitigating factors that not only influence how emitters may discharge their duty of due care but also further shape the strength of their obligation to take reasonable preventative measures (Chapter 5), all work to establish the plausibility and feasibility of implementing a standard of due care under uncertainty.

To underscore the feasibility of this normatively motivated policy proposal, this chapter explores a high-profile and precedent-setting example of an uncertain public health threat involving tetraethyl lead (TEL), which highlights the adverse consequences of the absence of a compulsory standard of due care.

It should be clarified at the outset, however, that this case study is largely intended to motivate answers to fundamentally normative questions, so its purpose deviates from conventional process-tracing case study analysis. While the chief objective of conventional qualitative research is to explain the tapestry of causal relationships that shape a given phenomenon we observe in the world, this chapter aims primarily to highlight the normative and policy implications of these causal relationships. More specifically, the case involving TEL is intended to illustrate the context-dependent nature of problems of environmental risk, the different ways that corporations may respond to the potential harm that their emissions create, and the different ways emitters may satisfy their moral obligation to exercise due care—which should inform the normative and policy standards to which we hold them.

6.1 Tetraethyl Lead: A Brief History

Our American environmental history is peppered with examples of corporations deliberately falsifying or withholding scientific data that verify risks to human health, misleading the public with embellished or utterly false public relations campaigns about the actual health threats their business practices create, manufacturing and emitting substances without ever testing their potentially harmful health effects, delaying the implementation of policies that could prevent harm to public health, intimidating whistle-blowers and advocacy groups, and using their political clout to influence business-friendly environmental policies.[1] "[I]nvestigations of the regulatory database of a wide range of consumer products and industrial chemicals," says Epstein,

> have revealed a pattern of constraints, including gross negligence, manipulation, distortion, suppression and destruction of data, which are so frequent as to preclude their dismissal as exceptional aberrations. [. . .] Such constrained data have served as the basis for the past and continuing successful strategies of some segments of the industry, which have minimized or denied risk to workers and the public-at-large, and have maximized product or process efficacy and the apparent preoccupations with short-term economic growth to the detriment of considerations of long-term adverse public health and environmental impacts, [and] have resulted in a burgeoning toll of cancer and other preventable diseases.[2]

The case of TEL in the early 20th century is no exception. And given the gravity of harm that lead exposure entails, the lengths to which the chemical and automotive industries went to understate the effects of exposure, and the success of these efforts, which allowed the manufacture and emission of TEL to continue unabated for five decades, this case effectively illustrates the sort of corporate irresponsibility and lack of regulatory oversight we should wish to avoid.

TEL was introduced as a gasoline additive to prevent engine knocking, to improve automotive efficiency, and to promote the life of internal combustion engines.[3] By the early 1920s, as the substance started to be mass-produced, the observable effects of extreme lead exposure (that is, of lead poisoning) had been well documented for more than two centuries. Various observable symptoms of occupational lead exposure had been catalogued as early as 1713, when Ramazzini studied the attributes of potters who worked with lead and found that they consistently became "paralytic, splenetic [irritable], lethargic, cachectic [fatigued and emaciated], and toothless."[4] In 1767, Sir George Baker proved that an epidemic that had been known as "Devonshire colic" (later termed "lead colic") was caused by lead poisoning from the consumption of cider that had been produced with and contaminated by lead-based apple crushers.[5] Confirming Ramazzini's earlier finding, Paul (1860)[6] and Oliver (1911)[7] demonstrated that reproductive problems and higher infant mortality rates were associated with employment in lead industries: female workers were found to experience disproportionately high numbers of abortions and stillbirths, and both women and men were found to be significantly more likely to be sterile than those who did not experience occupational exposure to lead.[8] (In fact, throughout the 19th and early 20th centuries, "lead compounds were widely used to induce illegal abortions."[9]) Similarly, associative muscular and arthritic pain was documented as early as 1854,[10] lead blindness as early as 1908,[11] and kidney failure as early as 1929.[12]

While our knowledge of the dangers of acute exposure and "lead toxicity"[13] was firmly rooted and improving during the early 1900s, it was not until the 1960s that public health scientists and regulators began to explore and better understand the immediate and long-term adverse health effects of low-level exposure to lead. Standard existing clinical examinations focused on outward behavior and demonstrable early symptoms of lead poisoning (or "insensitive toxicity indicators"), such as the ability to straighten or extend one's fingers ("extensor strength of the hand"), joint pain, or the blueish discoloration of one's gums ("lead line" or the "Burton line").[14] Alternative methods to diagnose lead exposure consisted of highly limited and inaccurate "biochemical" testing, such as measuring the level of hemoglobin in one's blood:[15] for a low concentration of hemoglobin (the vital protein that carries oxygen through the bloodstream) is a mark of anemia, and anemia was a known indicator of lead poisoning as early as 1831.[16] Yet, similarly, such tests could only establish whether or not a person already suffered lead poisoning.

Advances in the medical sciences allowed for more sophisticated and reliable epidemiological, blood lead level, psychological, and neurophysiological testing, which could confirm the "subclinical" or low-level effects of lead exposure, which do not present "distinctive symptoms."[17] These newfound "dose-response" exposure measurements could determine the adverse health effects of a given substance at particular levels and durations of exposure, through different media (e.g., air, soil, dust, water, and food) and through different pathways of exposure (e.g., inhalation, ingestion, absorption) of the substance in question. What these improved tests revealed is that lead exposure was incredibly prevalent and that even at low levels it has harmful and irreversible neurological effects, such as impaired brain development, hyperactivity, and mental retardation.[18] With a broader and more nuanced understanding of the adverse consequences to public health, scientists not only began settling on stricter definitions of lead poisoning—lowering the qualifying blood lead level from 40 to 10 μg/dL between 1970 and 1990[19]—but with the repeated discovery that "levels previously thought to be safe posed significant risks to health," scientists and regulators gradually realized that lead affords no safe level of exposure.[20]

While scientific advancements and our more comprehensive understanding of the effects of lead exposure catalyzed various precautionary policies and regulations to better protect public health (some of which are discussed below), these achievements were delayed for decades because of the automotive and oil industries' efforts—both scientifically and politically, nationally and globally—to bury the truth of the prevalence and gravity of lead exposure so as to prevent restrictions on the continued manufacture and emission of leaded gasoline. Contrary to public interest and trust, these efforts facilitated countless preventable and undeserved injuries to physiologically and socially vulnerable groups like children, the poor, minority communities, and industrial workers—decades of corporate irresponsibility, harm, and negligence that this book's proposed precautionary standard of due care is intended to prevent.

6.2 "Intentional Externalizing" and the Orchestrated Failure to Protect Public Health

Patented in 1922 by General Motors (GM), despite neglecting to first test the potential occupational health hazards or adverse health effects on the general public of exposure to lead in the ambient air,[21] TEL was quickly moved into production, and "ethyl" gasoline was first put on the market in February 1923, for GM executives believed that the technological and economic benefits of TEL could not be understated.[22] Motivated by the unique opportunity to corner the motor fuel market and reap enormous profits, GM trumpeted the ability of its newfound anti-knocking agent to increase engine efficiency and to prolong the life of an automobile, which would allow consumers and the country to conserve money and fuel—during a postwar era when demand for cars and petroleum was booming and concerns over oil shortages were looming.[23] These circumstances would give GM and other opportunistic companies that became involved in the production and sale of TEL (namely, Standard Oil of New Jersey [now ExxonMobil] and DuPont) the political cover necessary to justify and excuse their actions to regulators and the public if occupational or environmental exposure proved to be harmful. After all, it would befit the unbridled benefits of this "apparent gift of God" (as Standard Oil infamously proclaimed), which was the alleged "key to the industrial future of the nation," if the development of TEL, like much historical progress, "required some sacrifice."[24] In this vein, central to GM's public relations and sales campaigns, the company "portray[ed] its interests and those of the public as synonymous, as if they had merged into one common interest," suggesting that its business practices were driven by what was good for the American people.[25] However, the duplicity of GM and Standard Oil—who merged their TEL patents in August 1924 and partnered to establish the Ethyl Gasoline Corporation to market the lead additive[26]—and the companies' indifference to the interests of the American public were soon realized.

For example, after five industrial workers died at Standard Oil's TEL research labs and refinery in Elizabeth, New Jersey, in October 1924, as well as dozens more hospitalized for "severe palsies, tremors, hallucinations, and other serious neurological symptoms of organic lead poisoning"[27]—events whose scrutiny also revealed similar deaths and hundreds of cases of severe lead poisoning at the DuPont plant in Deepwater, New Jersey, and GM's research facility in Dayton, Ohio,[28]—the companies ardently disavowed responsibility, stating publicly that the preventable deaths and illnesses were due to the carelessness of employees. GM Chemical Company vice president, Thomas Midgley (who had discovered TEL) was quick to indict workers for recklessly putting themselves in harm's way by knowingly mishandling the substance: failing, for example, to heed "warnings and provisions for their protection" and ignoring "dangers of constant absorption of the fluid by their hands and arms."[29] Brashly suggesting that strict punishments be implemented to deter such carelessness, Midgley explicitly proposed that whenever employees begin to display "signs of exhilaration" (i.e., demonstrable symptoms of lead poisoning) or spill TEL on themselves, they should immediately be fired and that this negative incentive would prevent future tragedies.[30] In parallel fashion, Standard Oil insisted that "every precaution was taken" to ensure workplace safety.[31] Yet as some have noted, preventative measures of the time, including "exhaust ventilation, wettening dusty processes, and personal protective equipment" (like rubber gloves and boots), while intuitive, were not scientifically tested or verified to safeguard workers against occupational exposure; further, many workers were found to be neither aware of the dangers they faced nor informed about how to protect themselves to the extent that limited conventional means would allow.[32]

These high-profile events cemented broader concerns that "lead exhausted from autos using leaded gasoline would accumulate in ambient settings and present a public health hazard"[33]—concerns that begun taking root with the publication of the first comprehensive study of the occupational and environmental safety of TEL. This was not because the study had confirmed adverse health effects of TEL exposure, but rather because the study had been strongly influenced by corporate interests, which both torpedoed the reliability of the study and eroded the public's trust in the oil and automotive industries' intentions and the reassurances they had publicly given about the relative safety of TEL. While the U.S. Bureau of Mines, an independent third party, had conducted the investigation in its own facilities and prepared the report, the study had been commissioned by the GM Research Corporation. As the auto and oil industries had strong vested interests in the continued and expanded production of TEL and leaded gasoline,[34] this partnership created a clear conflict of interest,[35] which was perhaps most evident by the numerous restrictions that GM and DuPont imposed on the contractual arrangement. For example, as part of its "blackout of information" stipulation, GM insisted that neither the report nor correspondences regarding the study should make mention of "lead," but rather should refer to TEL by its nonscientific trade name: "ethyl." While the justification had to do with worries over "leaks to the newspapers" that might mislead and confuse the public, it was clear that the companies simply wanted to prevent the release of information that could prejudice public attitudes toward "ethyl" gasoline and "arouse" public anxiety.[36]

Similarly motivated, GM and its subsidiary, Ethyl Gasoline Corporation, also required the bureau to refrain from communicating any information about the research to the press and to submit all research materials and manuscripts "for comment, criticism, and approval" before they would be released for publication.[37] These controversial provisions, which enabled corporations with strong vested interests to shape what findings the study would reveal and how the bureau's report would frame these findings, all but ensured a favorable, foregone conclusion that TEL and leaded gasoline posed no public health threat.[38] Testifying to the dubious nature of this report, several months before the research was made public, GM announced to the American Medical Association that the analysis would confirm "that there is no danger of acquiring lead poisoning through even prolonged exposure to exhaust gases of cars using Ethyl Gas."[39]

These revelations amplified the public's scrutiny of GM, Standard Oil, Ethyl Gas Corp., DuPont, and the alleged safety of TEL and prompted Surgeon General of the U.S. Public Health Service (PHS), Hugh Cummings, to convene industry leaders and public health scientists to explore mutually acceptable solutions to the public health concerns that the manufacture and emission of leaded gasoline entailed.[40] Corporate representatives exploited this forum by proposing that industry voluntarily self-regulate TEL and leaded gasoline, such that if subsequent independent studies could prove "an actual danger to the public," the companies would immediately halt production altogether[41]—knowing full well the meaningless commitment this proposal entailed.[42] What public health officials and scientists party to the conference failed to appreciate at the time was that by opportunistically skirting a responsibility to verify the *absence* of harm to public health, and consequently by shifting the burden of proof to regulators and public health scientists to corroborate the *presence* of a credible public health threat, industry would only need to demonstrate that the matter remains unresolved to justify its continued manufacture and sale of TEL and leaded gasoline.[43] So long as this issue was to be decided "solely on the basis of facts,"[44] as emphasized by Robert Kehoe, Ethyl Corporation's medical director, the lack of a preponderance of evidence would warrant delaying regulation.[45] After all, "In a world of imperfect knowledge, especially if the industry controlled most of the information, it would always be easy to find uncertainty in any study."[46] (And as GM et al. underscored their willingness to cooperate, the precedent this group set with voluntary self-regulation further undercut the justification for implementing mandatory standards to regulate the release of TEL under conditions of uncertainty.[47])

Accordingly, what followed the conference were decades-long calculated initiatives by General Motors and others to generate outcome, probability, causal, and scientific[48] uncertainty about the actual health risks of TEL through industry-led studies and to discredit the research of public health scientists that ostensibly confirmed the harmful effects of exposure.[49] It was common practice, for instance, for industry to hire as consultants or to commission the research of academic scholars and public health scientists, whose consulting work and research, which was legitimized by their university and affiliations and prominent statuses, served to validate industry's position that TEL posed no public health threat. Robert Kehoe, for instance, a premier scholar of physiology and industrial medicine, whose work influenced the "development of industrial hygiene and public health," became a "key" consultant for the lead industry and was eventually hired as the medical director of Ethyl Gasoline Corporation. With his laboratory and research funded by these corporate interests, Kehoe was a vocal proponent of the expansion of TEL production, he helped to forestall mandatory lead emission standards from being implemented (e.g., by proposing a system of voluntary self-regulation that shifted the burden to the public to prove that TEL was harmful), and his "private-interest" scientific research[50] became part of a broader effort to "embellish the industry's particular views" and to discredit other scholars' antithetical findings that exposure to leaded gasoline emissions were deleterious to human health.[51]

A paradigmatic example of this sort of industry-sponsored research can be found in Ramirez-Cervantes et al. (1978), who denied the merits of lowering the "action level" for occupational lead exposure and suggested instead that the existing 80 μg/dl blood lead level was an acceptable threshold to ensure workplace safety.[52] (Conversely, subsequent studies have shown that blood lead levels as low as 10 to 15 μg/dl are sufficient to cause irreversible health problems.) The study of Ramirez-Cervantes et al., whose aim was to cast doubt on the adverse health effects of non-demonstrable, low-level exposure to lead, was subsequently rejected as highly flawed, incomplete, and thus misleading.[53]

Richard Doll, noted Oxford University professor and scholar, regarded epidemiologist, and once consultant for GM (as well as other firms), has also been harshly criticized for his conflicts of interest—testifying, for example, on GM's behalf "that exposure to lead from leaded gasoline was not harmful to children" and "misleading the public about potential cancer causes."[54] One of the more controversial historical examples involved respected industrial hygienist, Emery Hayhurst, who was working as a consultant for Ethyl Corp.

while concurrently advising the PHS and the Workers Health Bureau. Hayhurst not only supplied "advocates of tetraethyl lead with information regarding the tactics to be used by their opponents" but also published materials testifying to the "complete safety" of TEL after the suspect Bureau of Mines report was released with the intention of creating the misleading "impression that public health professionals had determined that leaded gasoline posed no threat to the public's health."[55]

As consumer advocate, Ralph Nader, unveiled in *Unsafe at Any Speed*,[56] for decades automakers also proactively worked to stall environmental policies and emissions standards that would have significantly restricted the production, sale, and emission of TEL and leaded gasoline. One such strategy was to discourage competition and technological innovation that would have permitted an opportunistic company to introduce a cleaner vehicle: in the mid-1950s, for instance, automakers like GM collaboratively agreed with one another to "jointly license any pollution control technologies they might develop" and to refrain from making "any public announcement of breakthroughs in emission control technologies without prior approval of all other signatories"—the intention of which was to deter advances in emission control technologies to prevent the implementation of new mandatory emission control standards.[57] Similarly, while automakers had developed new control technologies (like the catalytic converter), whose introduction could have extensively reduced the public's exposure to the dangers of leaded exhaust fumes, these technologies were intentionally withheld from the public and the market until the 1970s.[58]

This is plainly evident by the marked reduction in blood lead levels that was associated with the eventual phase-out of TEL in gasoline (which began in 1976), as Figures 6.1 and 6.2 depict. And since 1980, as many have noted, the mandate against leaded gasoline in the United States has succeeded in more than halving the pre-1976 average blood lead level of both adults and children.[59]

Efforts to "shift the costs to the public," what some have referred to "intentional externalizing,"[60] were also manifest in the auto and oil industries' rejection of the Environmental Protection Agency's (EPA's) standing under the 1970 Clean Air Act to regulate gasoline additives. Spearheaded by Ethyl Gasoline Corporation, PPG Industries, DuPont, NALCO Chemical Company, and National Petroleum Refiners Association (all of which were producers of TEL), the suit against the EPA charged that the agency had exceeded its authority in presuming to regulate the additive—for the EPA had failed to demonstrate "beyond reasonable doubt the levels of airborne lead in ambient air at which health effects in persons would be caused."[61] The EPA argued that it was authorized to regulate gasoline additives if their emissions "will endanger the public health or welfare," and though studies on the effects of lead emissions from gasoline exhausts were inconclusive (that is, no cases of lead poisoning by gasoline emissions could be proven), the EPA insisted that lead in gasoline constituted a "substantial risk of harm."[62] In response to the EPA's mandated reduction of lead in gasoline, Ethyl Corp. "sought judicial review"

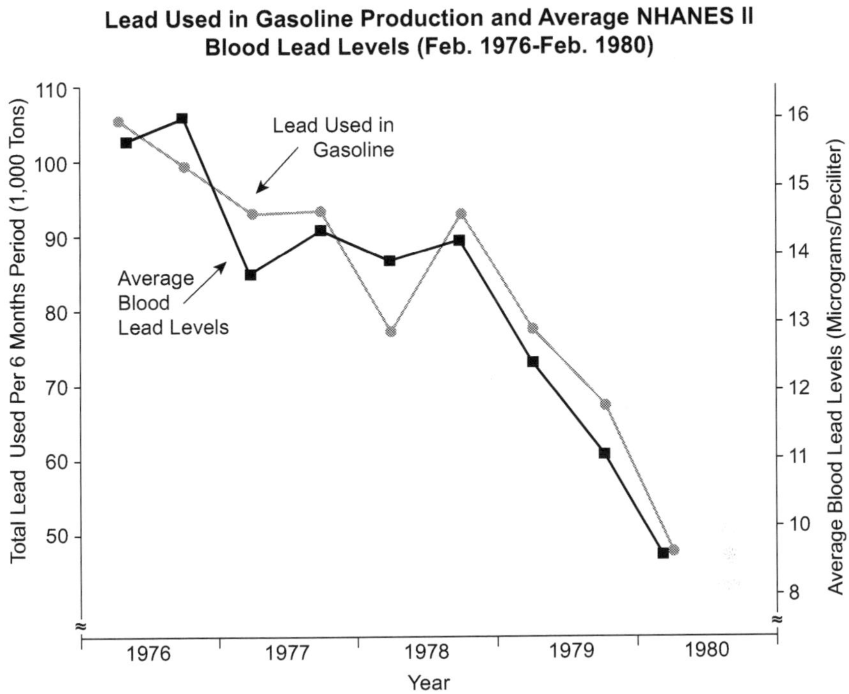

Figure 6.1 Correlation Between Lead Phase-Out and Reduced Environmental Exposure[63]

of the agency's capacity to extend its regulatory reach in this way from tailpipe emissions to gasoline content. In this landmark 1974 Supreme Court case,[64] the court ruled that before any preventative action could be warranted, some form of proof of the adverse effects to public health of exposure to TEL would have to be provided by regulatory agencies. Yet companies like Ethyl Corp. and DuPont enjoyed proprietary rights to the scientific data that could corroborate the health effects of TEL, and these corporations had deliberately chosen to withhold this information from regulators and the public and, as noted earlier, worked to shroud the independent findings of public health scientists in uncertainty.[65]

Nevertheless, when the court reheard *Ethyl Corp. v. EPA* in 1976, it reversed its earlier ruling. Conventionally, justifying the regulation of environmental risks has required demonstrating that an effluent "endangers" public health or welfare, which means that regulators are able to show empirically that beyond some baseline threshold, exposure to the substance creates adverse human health effects. The court argued, however, that to endanger public health can mean merely to "threaten" it—at least as it pertains to lead exposure, the detrimental effects of which were generally known and widely suspected at the

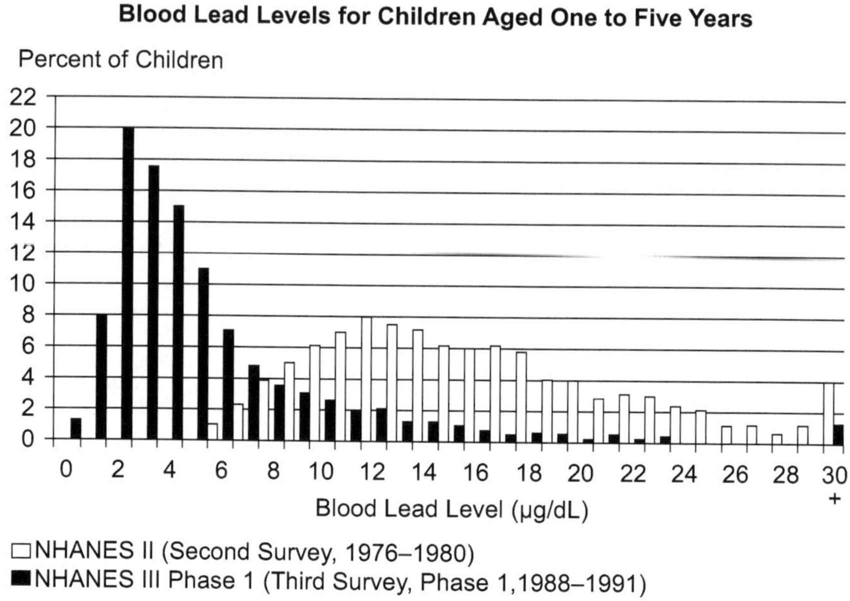

Figure 6.2 Reduced Environmental Exposure in Children During Leaded Gasoline Phase-Out[66]

time. That is, the endangerment condition could be satisfied (an "endangerment finding" could be supported) in the absence of an empirically verifiable threshold beyond which harm occurs. Accordingly, the court suggested that no actual harm must be proven to justify precautionary regulatory action aimed at preventing the perceived threat of exposure to leaded gasoline emissions.[67] More specifically, the court amended its position and ruled that "while no specific blood lead level could be identified as the threshold for danger," there nevertheless was compelling reason to believe that the lead additive did pose "a significant risk to public health."[68]

6.3 Motivating the Need for a Standard of Due Care

The experience with TEL and the oil and automotive industries illustrates precisely the sort of situation we should want to avoid, and it offers a decisive example of when the absence of a preponderance of evidence of the actual dangers to human health should be irrelevant to our regulatory decisions. Yet beyond the compelling reasons there were to believe that the uncertain threat leaded gasoline entailed would likely cause harm[69] (reasons that were grounded, at base, in clinical evidence of the demonstrable effects of lead poisoning), there are several defining features of this case involving

TEL that validate the plausibility of adopting a standard of due care under uncertainty.

First, TEL was a "high production volume" chemical.[70] At the height of its production in the early 1970s, roughly 300,000 tons (or 660 million pounds) of the additive were being manufactured annually.[71] This, by some estimates, amounted to the production of 5.3 trillion gallons of leaded gasoline or 125 billion barrels in the United States between 1926 and 1985: an average of 5.7 million barrels each day during this period.[72] (That is, between the time production of TEL resumed in 1926—following the brief period the PHS investigated the health effects of TEL exposure after the rash of deaths and hospitalizations from occupational lead poisoning caused public alarm—and the EPA-directed, near-total phase-out of TEL in gasoline was completed.) Coupled with the steady increase in the number of registered vehicles in the United States during the 60 years TEL was in mass production (from 22.2 million vehicles in 1926 to 171.7 million in 1985[73]), these figures speak to the pervasiveness of the public's exposure to airborne lead emissions.[74] In fact, with these levels of production and consumption, in concert with the finding that TEL emissions accounted for more than 90 percent of environmental lead pollution in the United States prior to its eventual phase-out, geochemists studying the atmospheric concentration of lead in ice core samples in Greenland dated a three-fold increase in the concentration of lead in the ice to TEL's introduction.[75]

Second, particularly vulnerable populations, including industrial workers, pregnant women, and children, were disproportionately exposed to the threat of harm. As noted earlier, industrial workers commonly were unaware of the dangers they faced in handling the lead additive, they were not informed about how to take preventative measures to increase their workplace safety, and they were not provided protective gear to mitigate occupational exposure. Similarly, as numerous studies have since confirmed, children's immature and developing physiological and neurological systems make them highly susceptible to being harmed once exposed to lead (even during gestation).[76] Infants who experienced low-level exposure to lead while in the womb have been found to be more likely to be born prematurely and underweight.[77] Also, toddlers and young children are likely to encounter more sources of lead and to experience more intense levels of exposure—in large measure because they absorb and ingest lead dust from vehicle exhaust emissions that settles on the ground and mixes with the dirt with which kids play.[78] This is consistent with the finding that children's "normal hand-to-mouth activities may introduce many non-food items into their gastrointestinal tract," and a National Research Council study on lead absorption in the gastrointestinal tract that found that pregnant women and children absorb nearly five times the amount of lead than average adults.[79] And since lead deposits in soil and dust do not "dissipate, biodegrade, or decay," they pose constant threats to the health of children, especially when considering that as late as 1988 (three years after the near-total ban of TEL in motor fuel took effect), "4.5

million metric tons of lead used in gasoline remain[ed] in dust and soil."[80] Further disquieting is the fact that since lead bioaccumulates (concentrates over time) in the body, given the different sources and pathways of exposure, "[m]ultiple, low-level inputs of lead can result in significant aggregate exposure."[81]

Given the prevalence of enduring lead deposits from vehicle exhaust, it may be of little surprise that nearly 1 million children under five years old "have blood lead levels able to cause irreversible cognitive, behavioral, internal-organ, blood-forming, and growth damage."[82] Some have called pediatric lead poisoning in the United States "an epidemic" (i.e., prior to the 1980s before stricter protections were implemented), with roughly 250,000 recorded occurrences of lead poisoning in children each year—due in no small measure to the emission of airborne lead from leaded gasoline exhaust.[83] Amplifying these concerns is the fact that poorer and minority children living in urban areas (with heavy traffic and, thus, higher volumes of airborne lead emissions[84]) are especially vulnerable to developing dangerous blood lead levels.[85] In fact, public health scientists have found that 8 percent of children living in poverty have blood lead levels that constitute lead poisoning, whereas on average only 1 percent of children living above the poverty line experience lead poisoning. And whereas roughly 2 percent of white children are generally found to exhibit lead poisoning, an average of 11 percent of black children suffer the effects of extreme exposure.[86]

Third, feasible substitutes and alternatives were available to the oil and automotive industries. For instance, several years prior to the discovery of TEL, the GM research division found that adding ethyl alcohol (or grain alcohol) to gasoline "could produce a suitable motor fuel" that protected against damaging engine "knock." While GM and Standard Oil of New Jersey had explicitly appealed to the conservation of petroleum to justify their marketing of TEL, the contradictory rationale for tabling this alternative blended fuel was that "the addition of ethanol to gasoline would have reduced vehicle's use of gasoline by 20–30 percent, thus making cars less dependable on petroleum products."[87] In contrast, since only a small volume of TEL was necessary to mix with each gallon of petroleum, it would not alter gasoline consumption and the oil industry's profit margin.[88] Alternatively, developing a viable, more efficient, albeit smaller, engine that could run on higher-quality gasoline without succumbing to engine "knock," which European and Japanese manufacturers opted for, was dismissed by American automakers. With the endorsement of Ethyl Corp., though contrary to the recommendation of some of its own researchers, it was decided that the solution was to improve the viability of lower-grade fuel.[89] The introduction of either alternative, while less profitable to GM et al., would have averted the public health threat that TEL ultimately created.

In a similar vein, as part of its "planned and coordinated strategy," industry also worked to "stifle the development and use" of better emission control technologies that could have mitigated the potential for harm to public health.

For example, technology for the "lead-intolerant" catalytic converter had been available for decades preceding its mandate in 1975, and its concealment has been criticized by some for transferring the costs of the health and environmental externalities of leaded gasoline production onto an unsuspecting public—and violating public trust and its right to know.[90] (This behavior also characterized the oil and automotive industries' later efforts to reduce National Ambient Air Quality [NAAQ] standards, to eliminate Corporate Average Fuel Economy [CAFE] standards, to deny the existence and causes of anthropogenic climate change, and to forestall policies to mitigate the effects of global warming.[91])

Fourth, as noted earlier, the corporations that had strong vested interests in the continued and expanded production of TEL proactively worked to understate the suspected adverse health effects of exposure to airborne lead emissions—and the industries' various public disclosure initiatives purposefully withheld important information about the potential for harm, both to preserve its consumer base and to generate uncertainty about the actual health risks TEL posed in order to undercut possible justifications for mandatory regulations. Ethyl Gasoline Corporation's advertisements, for instance, commonly omitted the word "lead," referring to leaded gasoline instead as "ethyl gas,"[92] so as to prevent drawing attention to the fact that the central compound in its product included a substance that was "known at the time to be poisonous" (at least with extreme exposure) and possibly alienating a fearful public.[93] Moreover, these publications, as Figure 6.3 illustrates, only highlighted the advantages of TEL (such as increasing fuel efficiency and engine power, prolonging engine life, and preventing costly engine repairs) and neglected to note the potential for adverse health effects. This misinformation and deceit through omission is evident in the advertisement's highly selective "facts" list—which *does* make mention of TEL, but only details the various ways the additive enhances engine performance—and its blatantly false statement that "The price of Ethyl Gasoline is simply the price of good gasoline, plus the few extra pennies the Ethyl ingredient costs."[94] In fact, the price for many individuals proved to entail chronic health issues, diverse developmental problems, and death.[95]

Finally, as the previous discussion has demonstrated, the case of TEL and leaded gasoline reveals a sordid history of delinquency and negligence among key oil and automotive companies and their executives. Recklessly flaunting their disregard of the interests and welfare of the public, and appealing to the very uncertainty that their industry-led studies generated and which they proactively promulgated, GM, Standard Oil, Ethyl Corp., and DuPont worked for decades to delay the regulation of lead emissions by insisting that regulators and public health officials must first produce a preponderance of evidence that confirms an unreasonable risk to public health. By withholding evidence of the effects of low-level exposure, shifting the burden of proof, manufacturing doubt, dismissing viable alternatives, and lobbying for laxer regulations, industry actors failed to take any reasonable measures to safeguard its workers, consumers, and the public from preventable harm.

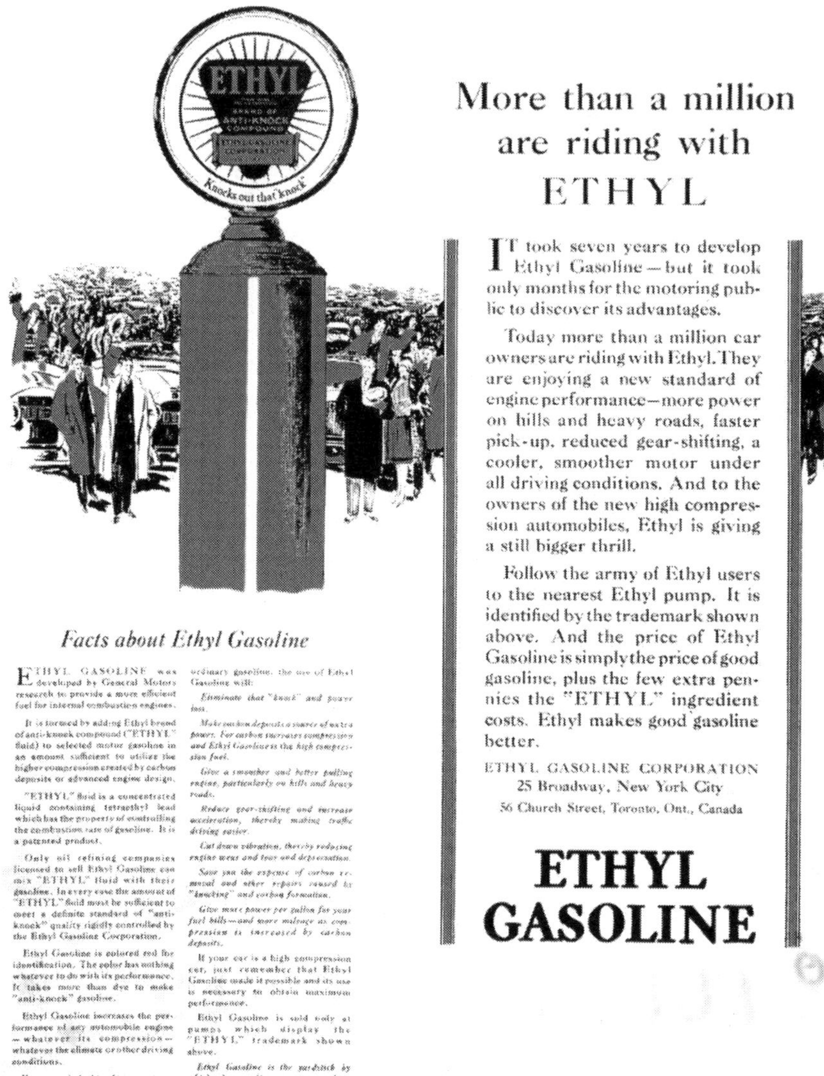

Figure 6.3 Facts About Ethyl Gasoline Advertisement[96]

Each one of these considerations should amplify our concerns about the conventional approach toward environmental risk regulation in the United States, which Chapters 2 and 4 have shown to treat uncertainty as a justification against regulating potential public health threats and which consequently incentivizes the sort of corporate irresponsibility that the case of TEL bears out.

6.4 Exercising Due Care

The standard of due care under conditions of uncertainty (see Chapter 5) would not permit emitters to skirt their responsibilities in the absence of evidence verifying actual dangers to public health. Indeed, as the discussion of possible mitigating or magnifying factors in Chapter 5 details, the standard of due care envisaged here would hold each of the considerations detailed earlier in the TEL example against the emitter, amplifying the obligation GM et al. would have had to exercise due care (precaution) to preventatively safeguard the public against what proved to be severe and irreparable harmful effects of occupational and environmental exposure.

The proposed standard of due care would have required, for instance, that companies involved in the manufacture and sale of TEL and leaded gasoline conduct thorough tests using available technologies to confirm the potential for adverse health effects, to forthrightly disclose this information to public health officials and environmental regulators, to comply with subsequent emission standards or to implement feasible substitutes (like ethanol) or alternatives (like smaller, more efficient engines), and to inform workers and the general public of any potential for harm (even if uncertain) that their manufacturing processes and products may entail. In short, had a comparable mandatory standard of due care existed at the time TEL was being prepared for mass production, had industry been required to take even some of these reasonable precautionary measures to mitigate the potential for harm, this public health crisis would have been avoided. While TEL is but one historical example, it speaks to the tens of thousands of uncertain environmental threats that the public currently faces, the continued irresponsible corporate practices that prioritize the bottom line over human health, and a narrow conception of risk that tolerates (and rewards) industry gambling with public welfare until the scientific community or regulatory agencies can corroborate actual health risks. Accordingly, as "justice delayed is justice denied, especially when it can kill people,"[97] the adoption of a precautionary standard of due care—whether the one proposed here or an alternative that can better withstand scrutiny—that is capable of preventing future public health crises does not just make for prudent public policy, it is rather morally required of us.

Now one might object that the companies in the TEL case could not have tested the health effects of lead in the ambient air, since blood lead level monitoring and epidemiological testing capabilities were not possible until the 1960s. One might insist that it is mistaken to indict industry for neglecting to try to prevent harm that it was not able to discern or foresee. As admitted earlier, the clinical (as opposed to "biochemical") tests that could have been conducted prior to the 1960s were highly limited and inaccurate.[98] Consequently, the data that public health experts or industry scientists could have collected may not have done much to protect the public from "subclinical" effects of lead exposure, that is, from the adverse health effects of long-term, low-level exposure. Indeed, standard clinical examinations—prior to the advent of more scientifically sophisticated dose-response testing capabilities—were predicated on observable characteristics of toxic exposure or "insensitive toxicity indicators," such as the ability to straighten or extend one's fingers ("extensor strength of the hand") and the blueish discoloration of one's gums ("lead line" or "Burton line").[99]

This objection, then, regards the relevance of our imperfect knowledge of harm, the distinction between reasons and duties, and the contextual sliding scale of the stringency of our obligations of due care that parallels the degree of uncertainty (see Chapter 3.4), such that if emitters lack compelling reasons to believe that the emission of and exposure to some substance may cause harm, they cannot rightly be held culpable for either the threats they create or the harm that may prove to materialize. However, this objection is ultimately misplaced. Enough was known about the dangers of high-level lead exposure as early as the late 19th century to give industry, policy-makers, regulators, and the public sufficient reason to infer the likely harmful effects that broadening the scope and degree of occupational and environmental exposure that the manufacture of TEL would entail. As but one example to augment the known effects of lead poisoning detailed in Section 6.1 earlier, consider that "[d]uring the 25-year period, 1875–1900, about 30,000 cases of lead poisoning were reported from the lead mines of Utah alone; more than 1,000 cases a year."[100] This is to say, in yet another context, that the argument from excusable ignorance is not persuasive.

The profit-driven incentives corporations have to engage in socially irresponsible practices at the expense of public health and safety not only undergird the intuition behind precautionary risk regulation under uncertainty, but they highlight the danger to an innocent and unsuspecting public that can follow from the absence of exercising due care. The disregard with which corporations gambled with the welfare of others and put innocent people in the way of possible injury in the case of TEL testifies to the need to hold emitters accountable—irrespective of prevailing uncertainty—by imposing on them reasonable measures to strive to prevent creating uncertain threats of environmental harm. "We must not let history repeat itself by neglecting effective prevention where it is most needed. It is a shame if action is not taken when all the ingredients for successful prevention exist."[101]

Notes

1. See Kristin Shrader-Frechette, *Taking Action, Saving Lives: Our Duties to Protect Environmental and Public Health* (Oxford: Oxford University Press, 2007): Chapters 1–3.
2. Samuel Epstein, *Cancer-Gate: How to Win the Losing Cancer War* (Amityville: Baywood Publishing, 2005): 107.
3. Alan Loeb, "Birth of the Kettering Doctrine: Fordism, Sloanism and the Discovery of Tetraethyl Lead," *Business and Economic History* 24 (1995): 77–8, 82–3; Sven Hernberg, "Lead Poisoning in a Historical Perspective," *American Journal of Industrial Medicine* 38 (2000): 251.
4. Bernardino Ramazzini, *Diseases of Workers: The Latin Text of 1713 Revisited*, Wilmer Wright, trans. (Chicago: Chicago University Press, 1940 [1713]).

5. George Baker, "An Inquiry Concerning the Cause of the Endemial Colic of Devonshire," *Medical Transactions: Published by the College of Physicians in London* 2 (1772): 419–70.
6. Carol Angle and Matilda McIntire, "Lead Poisoning during Pregnancy," *American Journal of Diseases of Children* 108 (1964): 436; also Asher Finkel, ed., *Hamilton and Hardy's Industrial Toxicology*, 4th ed. (Boston: J. Wright, 1983).
7. Thomas Oliver, "A Lecture on Lead Poisoning and the Race: Delivered to the Eugenics Education Society," *British Medical Journal* 1 (1911): 1096–8.
8. Hernberg, "Lead Poisoning in a Historical Perspective," 246. See also Finkel, *Hamilton and Hardy's Industrial Toxicology*.
9. Hernberg, "Lead Poisoning in a Historical Perspective," 246.
10. Alfred Garrod, "Second Communication on the Blood and Effused Fluids in Gout, Rheumatism and Bright's Disease," *Medical Chirurgical Transactions* 37 (1854): 49–61; Alfred Garrod, *Treatise on the Nature and Treatment of Gout and Rheumatic Gout* (London: Walton and Maberly, 1859).
11. J. Lockhart Gibson, "Plumbic Ocular Neuritis in Queensland Children," *British Medical Journal* 2 (1908): 1488–90; W. Dowling Prendergast, "The Classification of the Symptoms of Lead Poisoning," *British Medical Journal* 1 (1910): 1164–6.
12. Leslie Nye, "An Investigation of the Extraordinary Incidence of Chronic Nephritis in Young People in Queensland," *Medical Journal of Australia* 2 (1929): 145–59.
13. Hernberg, "Lead Poisoning in a Historical Perspective," 248.
14. Ibid.
15. Ibid., 245.
16. H.A. Waldron, "The Anaemia of Lead Poisoning: A Review," *British Journal of Industrial Medicine* 23 (1966): 83–100.
17. Centers for Disease Control and Prevention, *Preventing Lead Poisoning in Young Children* (Atlanta: U.S. Department of Health and Human Services, 1991): 9; Hernberg, "Lead Poisoning in a Historical Perspective," 247–8, 250; Robert Percival et al., *Environmental Regulation: Law, Science, and Policy*, 6th ed. (New York: Aspen Publishers, 2009): 554.
18. Herbert Needleman et al., "Lead Levels in Deciduous Teeth of Urban and Suburban American Children," *Nature* 235 (1972): 111–2; Herbert Needleman et al., "Subclinical Lead Exposure in Philadelphia School Children: Identification by Dentine Lead Analysis," *New England Journal of Medicine* 290 (1974) 245–8; Herbert Needleman et al., "The Long-Term Effects of Exposure to Low Doses of Lead in Childhood: An 11-Year Follow-up Report," *New England Journal of Medicine* 322 (1990): 83–8; David Bellinger et al., "Low-Level Lead Exposure, Intelligence and Academic Achievement: A Long-Term Follow-Up Study," *Pediatrics* 90 (1992): 855–61; Shilu Tong et al., "Declining Blood Lead Levels and Changes in Cognitive Function During Childhood: The Port Pirie Cohort Study," *Journal of the American Medical Association* 280 (1998): 1915–9; Shilu Tong et al., "Environmental Lead Exposure: A Public Health Problem of Global Dimensions," *Bulletin of the World Health Organization* 78 (2000): 1068–9; Gerald Markowitz and David Rosner, *Deceit and Denial: The Deadly Politics of Industrial Pollution* (Berkeley: University of California Press, 2002): 135–7.
19. Percival et al., *Environmental Regulation*, 305.
20. Sven Hernberg and Jorma Nikkanen, "Enzyme Inhibition by Lead under Normal Urban Conditions," *Lancet* 1 (1970): 63–4; Sven Hernberg et al., "δ-Aminolevulinic Acid Dehydrase as a Measure of Lead Exposure," *Archives of Environmental Health* 21 (1970): 140–5; Hernberg, "Lead Poisoning in a Historical Perspective," 250; Philip Landrigan, "Pediatric Lead Poisoning: Is There a Threshold?," *Public Health Reports* 115 (2000): 530–1; Bruce Lanphear et al., "Cognitive Deficits Associated with Blood Lead Concentrations <10 μg/dL in US

Children and Adolescents," *Public Health Reports* 115 (2000): 521–9; Percival et al., *Environmental Regulation: Law, Science, and Policy*, 305; Heda Dapul and Danielle Laraque, "Lead Poisoning in Children," *Advances in Pediatrics* 61 (2014): 313–33; World Health Organization, "Lead Poisoning and Health: Fact Sheet," http://who.int/mediacentre/factsheets/fs379/en/, last updated September 2016.

21. David Rosner and Gerald Markowitz, "A 'Gift of God'?: The Public Health Controversy over Leaded Gasoline during the 1920s," *American Journal of Public Health* 75 (1985): 344–5.
22. Jerome Nriagu, "The Rise and Fall of Leaded Gasoline," *Science of the Total Environment* 92 (1990): 15; Loeb, "Birth of the Kettering Doctrine," 81–2.
23. Free Alcohol Hearings, U.S. Senate Finance Committee, 1906, Statement of James S. Capen, Detroit Board of Commerce, 59; David White, "The Unmined Supply of Petroleum in the United States," *Paper presented at the Society of Automotive Engineers Annual Meeting*, February 4–6, 1919; George Smith, "Where the World Gets Oil and Where Will Our Children Get It When American Wells Cease to Flow?," *National Geographic*, February 1920: 202; "Declining Supply of Motor Fuel," *Scientific American*, March 8, 1919: 220.
24. Rosner and Markowitz, "A 'Gift of God'?," 348; Nriagu, "The Rise and Fall of Leaded Gasoline," 19; Alan Loeb, "Paradigms Lost: A Case Study Analysis of Models of Corporate Responsibility for the Environment," *Business and Economic History* 28 (1999): 100.
25. Loeb, "Paradigms Lost," 98, 103.
26. Loeb, "Birth of the Kettering Doctrine," 82; Loeb, "Paradigms Lost," 98.
27. Rosner and Markowitz, "A 'Gift of God'?," 347–8; Loeb, "Paradigms Lost," 99.
28. "DuPont Tells of the Gas: His Company Had Fatalities, But Has Lessened Dangers," *New York Times*, October 31, 1924: 15; Rosner and Markowitz, "A 'Gift of God'?," 347.
29. "Bar Ethyl Gasoline as 5th Victim Dies: City Health Authorities Forbid Its Use: Sold in 10,000 Filling Stations," *New York Times*, October 31, 1924: 1 (Rosner and Markowitz 1985 fn. 25).
30. Rosner and Markowitz, "A 'Gift of God'?," 348; Nriagu, "The Rise and Fall of Leaded Gasoline," 19.
31. Rosner and Markowitz, "A 'Gift of God'?," 348.
32. Hernberg, "Lead Poisoning in a Historical Perspective," 247; "Third Victim Dies from Poison Gas," *New York Times*, October 29, 1924: 1, 23.
33. Loeb, "Paradigms Lost," 99.
34. Jamie Lincoln Kitman, "The Secret History of Lead," *The Nation*, March 2, 2002: http://thenation.com/article/secret-history-lead.
35. Rosner and Markowitz, "A 'Gift of God'?," 346.
36. Ibid., 345; Nriagu, "The Rise and Fall of Leaded Gasoline," 19; Loeb, "Paradigms Lost," 100.
37. Rosner and Markowitz, "A 'Gift of God'?," 345; Agreement between the Department of Interior and General Motors Chemical Company, Dayton, Ohio, NA, RG 70, 101869, file 725.
38. Nriagu, "The Rise and Fall of Leaded Gasoline," 19.
39. Graham Edgar to Dr. Paul Nicholas Leech, July 18, 1924, NA, RG 70, 101869, File 725.
40. Loeb, "Paradigms Lost," 99–100; Hernberg, "Lead Poisoning in a Historical Perspective," 251.
41. Loeb, "Paradigms Lost," 100, 103.
42. Jerome Nriagu, "Clair Patterson and Robert Kehoe's Paradigm of 'Show Me the Data' on Environmental Lead Poisoning," *Environmental Research* 78 (1998): 74.

43. Ibid., 74–5.
44. Loeb, "Paradigms Lost," 100.
45. Rosner and Markowitz, "A 'Gift of God'?," 349. This qualified concession of responsibility and the principle that only environmental hazards that could be proven merited regulation became a defining feature of contemporary U.S. environmental risk management, and as some have noted, prevented "future controls on environmental lead hazards for nearly four decades" (Nriagu, "Clair Patterson and Robert Kehoe's Paradigm of 'Show Me the Data' on Environmental Lead Poisoning," 72). Apparently persuaded by this reasoning, the committee of seven scientists appointed by Cummings following the conference to independently ascertain the health effects of TEL and leaded gasoline concluded that "there are at present no good grounds for prohibiting the use of ethyl gasoline as a motor fuel, provided that its distribution and use are controlled by proper regulations" (Rosner and Markowitz, "A 'Gift of God'?," 350; Miscellany, "Committee Report of Ethyl Gasoline," *Journal of the American Medical Association* 86 (January 30, 1926): 370). Curiously, this eight-month study still concentrated on occupational exposure as opposed to exposure to TEL in the ambient air, its short duration precluded a proper examination of longer-term risks of exposure, its recommended regulations were largely limited to improving safeguards against workplace exposure, and no rationale was offered as to why the "opposite decision rule . . . that there were no good grounds for allowing leaded gasoline"—which would have been equally justified given prevailing uncertainties—was not adopted instead (Loeb, "Lost Paradigms," 102).
46. Nriagu, "Clair Patterson and Robert Kehoe's Paradigm of 'Show Me the Data' on Environmental Lead Poisoning," 74.
47. Loeb, "Paradigms Lost," 103.
48. See Chapter 2 for the distinctions between these different forms of uncertainty.
49. Nriagu, "Clair Patterson and Robert Kehoe's Paradigm of 'Show Me the Data' on Environmental Lead Poisoning," 75; Hernberg, "Lead Poisoning in a Historical Perspective," 252; Gerald Markoitz and David Rosner, "Corporate Responsibility for Toxins," *Annals of the Academy of Political and Social Science* 584 (2002): 165; Markowitz and Rosner, *Deceit and Denial*, 12–138. For specific examples of silencing see Felix Wormser, "Facts and Fallacies Concerning Exposure to Lead," *Occupational Medicine* 3 (1947): 135–44; William Graebner, "Private Power, Private Knowledge, and Public Health: Science, Engineering and Lead Poisoning, 1900–1970," in *The Health and Safety of Workers*, Ronald Bayer, ed. (Oxford: Oxford University Press, 1988): 15–71; Christopher Sellers, "The Public Health Services Office of Industrial Hygiene and the Transformation of Industrial Medicine," *Bulletin of Medical History* 65 (1991): 42–73; Jane Lin-Fu, "Vulnerability of Children to Lead Exposure and Toxicity," *New England Journal of Medicine* 289 (1973): 1289–93; Herbert Needleman, "Clair Patterson and Robert Kehoe: Two Views of Lead Toxicity," *Environmental Research* 78 (1998): 79–85.
50. Shrader-Frechette, *Taking Action, Saving Lives*, 109.
51. William Graebner, "Hegemony Through Science: Information Engineering and Lead Toxicology, 1925–1965," in *Dying for Work*, David Rosner and Gerald Markowitz, eds. (Bloomington: Indiana University Press, 1985): 140–59; Nriagu, "Clair Patterson and Robert Kehoe's Paradigm of 'Show Me the Data' on Environmental Lead Poisoning," 72, 74.
52. B. Ramirez-Cervantes et al., "Health Assessment of Employees with Different Body Burdens of Lead," *Journal of Occupational Medicine* 20 (1978): 610–7; Hernberg, "Lead Poisoning in a Historical Perspective," 248.
53. David Parkinson et al., "Occupational Lead Exposure and Blood Pressure," *British Journal of Industrial Medicine* 44 (1987): 744–8.

54. Shrader-Frechette, *Taking Action, Saving Lives*, 105; Robert Doll and Richard Peto, "The Causes of Cancer," *Journal of the National Cancer Institute* 66 (1981): 1191–308; Richard Clapp et al., *Environmental and Occupational Causes of Cancer* (Lowell: Lowell Center for Sustainable Production, 2005); Epstein, *Cancer-Gate: How to Win the Losing Cancer War*, 15; Philip Landrigan and Dean Baker, "Clinical Recognition of Occupational and Environmental Disease," *Mt. Sinai Journal of Medicine* 62 (1995): 406–11; Philip Landrigan et al., "Cancer Prevention in the Workplace," in *Cancer Prevention and Control*, Peter Greenwald et al., eds. (New York: Marcel Dekker, 1995): 393–410; Jack Siemiatycki et al., "Listing Occupational Carcinogens," *Environmental Health Perspectives* 112 (2004): 1447–59.
55. Rosner and Markowitz, "A 'Gift of God'?," 346–7.
56. Ralph Nader, *Unsafe at Any Speed: The Designed-In Dangers of the American Automobile* (New York: Grossman Publishers, 1965).
57. Loeb, "Paradigms Lost," 104.
58. Ibid.
59. Joseph Annest, "Trends in the Blood Lead Levels of the U.S. Population," in *Lead Versus Health: Sources and Effects of Low-Level Lead Exposure*, Philip Rutter and Robin Russell Jones, eds. (New York: John Wiley and Sons, 1983): 33–58; Joseph Annest et al., "Chronological Trend in Blood Lead Levels between 1976 and 1980," *New England Journal of Medicine*, 308 (1983): 1373–7; World Health Organization, *Inorganic Lead: Environmental Health Criteria 165* (Geneva: WHO, 1995); Ellen Silbergeld, "Preventing Lead Poisoning in Children," *Annual Review of Public Health* 18 (1997); Herbert Needleman, "Childhood Lead Poisoning: The Promise and Abandonment of Primary Prevention," *American Journal of Public Health* 88 (1998); Hernberg, "Lead Poisoning in a Historical Perspective," 252. See also Nriagu, "The Rise and Fall of Leaded Gasoline," 24, 26.
60. Loeb, "Paradigms Lost," 104–5.
61. Nriagu, "The Rise and Fall of Leaded Gasoline," 23–4; Percival et al., *Environmental Regulation*, 192–4.
62. Percival et al., *Environmental Regulation*, 191.
63. *Small Refiner Lead Phasedown Taskforce v. EPA*, 705 F.2d 506, 528 (D.C. Cir. 1983), in Percival et al., *Environmental Regulation*, 197.
64. *Ethyl Corp.* v. *EPA*, 163 U.S.App.D.C. 162, 501 F.2d 722 (1974, 1976).
65. Nriagu, "Clair Patterson and Robert Kehoe's Paradigm of 'Show Me the Data' on Environmental Lead Poisoning," 74.
66. National Health and Nutrition Examination Surveys (NHANES), in Percival et al., *Environmental Regulation*, 34.
67. Percival et al., *Environmental Regulation*, 192–3.
68. Ibid., 194.
69. Refer to Chapter 3.4 for a discussion on the distinction between reasons to exercise precaution and reasons that oblige us to exercise precaution.
70. Percival et al., *Environmental Regulation*, 213; Environmental Protection Agency, "Chemical Right to Know: High Production Volume Chemicals Frequently Asked Questions," EPA 745-F-09–002g (March 1999): HPV chemicals are those whose annual rate of domestic production and/or importation exceeds 1 million pounds.
71. Nriagu, "The Rise and Fall of Leaded Gasoline," 16: one tonne (metric ton) is equivalent to 1.1 tons.
72. Ibid., 16.
73. Federal Highway Administration, "State Motor Vehicle Registrations, By Years, 1900–1995," U.S. Department of Transportation (April 1997): https://fhwa.dot.gov/ohim/summary95/mv200.pdf.
74. Centers for Disease Control and Prevention, *Preventing Lead Poisoning in Young Children*, 1.

75. Clair Patterson, "Contaminated and Natural Lead Environments of Man," *Archives of Environmental Health,* 11 (1965): 344–60; Herbert Needleman, "The Removal of Lead from Gasoline: Historical and Personal Reflections," *Environmental Research* 84 (2000): 22–3.
76. Centers for Disease Control and Prevention, *Preventing Lead Poisoning in Young Children,* 1; Hernberg, "Lead Poisoning in a Historical Perspective," 250.
77. Centers for Disease Control and Prevention, *Preventing Lead Poisoning in Young Children,* 9.
78. Environmental Protection Agency, *Air Quality Criteria for Lead,* EPA Report No. EPA-600/8-83028aF-dF (Research Triangle Park: Office of Health and Environmental Assessment, 1986): Centers for Disease Control and Prevention, *Preventing Lead Poisoning in Young Children,* 20.
79. Lin-Fu, "Vulnerability of Children to Lead Exposure and Toxicity," 1289–93; Centers for Disease Control and Prevention, *Preventing Lead Poisoning in Young Children,* 11; National Research Council, *Measuring Lead Exposure in Infants and Children* (Washington, DC: National Academy Press, 1987): 187.
80. Agency for Toxic Substances and Disease Registry, *The Nature and Extent of Lead Poisoning in Children in the United States: A Report to Congress* (Atlanta: ATSDR, 1988); Centers for Disease Control and Prevention, *Preventing Lead Poisoning in Young Children,* 19–20, 23.
81. Centers for Disease Control and Prevention, *Preventing Lead Poisoning in Young Children,* 17.
82. Ibid., 9–12.
83. Jean Moore, "Community Aspects of Childhood Lead Poisoning," *American Journal of Public Health* 60 (1970): 1430–4; Hernberg, "Lead Poisoning in a Historical Perspective," 249.
84. As well as older homes with flaking lead paint.
85. Centers for Disease Control and Prevention, *Preventing Lead Poisoning in Young Children,* 12; Needleman, "Childhood Lead Poisoning"; Hernberg, "Lead Poisoning in a Historical Perspective," 249–50; Shrader-Frechette, *Taking Action, Saving Lives*, 129.
86. Shrader-Frechette, *Taking Action, Saving Lives*, 27. (Also note other scholars in p. 27, fn.122 on page 227.)
87. Farhad Nadim et al., "United States Experience with Gasoline Additives," *Energy Policy* 29 (2001): 1; Jamie Lincoln Kitman, "The Secret History of Lead: Special Report," *The Nation,* March 2, 2000; Valerie Thomas and Andrew Kwong, "Ethanol as a Lead Replacement: Phasing Out Leaded Gasoline in Africa," *Energy Policy* 29 (2001). As TEL was phased out of production in the late 1970s and early 1980s, butane proved to be an additional substitute (John Holusha, "The Troubles with Gasoline," *New York Times*, August 7, 1986).
88. Nadim et al., "United States Experience with Gasoline Additives," 1.
89. Nriagu, "The Rise and Fall of Leaded Gasoline," 15–6; Public Health Service, "Proceedings of a Conference to Determine Whether or Not There Is a Public Health Question in the Manufacture, Distribution, or Use of Tetraethyl Lead Gasoline," in *Public Health Bulletin No. 158* (Washington, DC: Government Publishing Office, 1925): 9.
90. Nriagu, "The Rise and Fall of Leaded Gasoline," 24; Nader, *Unsafe at Any Speed.*
91. Stan Luger, *Corporate Power, American Democracy, and the Automobile Industry* (Cambridge: Cambridge University Press, 2000).
92. Loeb, "Birth of the Kettering Doctrine," 82; Ethyl Gasoline Corporation, "More Than a Million Are Riding with Ethyl," *Popular Mechanics: Advertising Section* 49 (1928): 119.
93. Loeb, "Paradigms Lost," 98.
94. Ibid.

95. Centers for Disease Control and Prevention, *Preventing Lead Poisoning in Young Children*, 9–10; Rosner and Markowitz, "A 'Gift of God'?," 347–8.
96. Ethyl Gasoline Corporation, "More Than a Million Are Riding with Ethyl," 119.
97. Shrader-Frechette, *Taking Action, Saving Lives*, 97.
98. Hernberg, "Lead Poisoning in a Historical Perspective," 248.
99. Ibid.
100. Ibid., 246.
101. Ibid., 253.

References

Agency for Toxic Substances and Disease Registry. *The Nature and Extent of Lead Poisoning in Children in the United States: A Report to Congress*. Atlanta: ATSDR, 1988.

"Agreement between the Department of Interior and General Motors Chemical Company, Dayton, Ohio." NA, RG 70, 101869, File 725.

Angle, Carol and Matilda McIntire. "Lead Poisoning during Pregnancy." *American Journal of Diseases of Children* 108 (1964): 436–9.

Annest, Joseph. "Trends in the Blood Lead Levels of the U.S. Population." In *Lead versus Health: Sources and Effects of Low-Level Lead Exposure*, edited by Philip Rutter and Robin Russell Jones. New York: John Wiley and Sons, 1983.

Annest, Joseph, et al. "Chronological Trend in Blood Lead Levels between 1976 and 1980." *New England Journal of Medicine* 308 (1983): 1373–7.

"Bar Ethyl Gasoline as 5th Victim Dies: City Health Authorities Forbid Its Use: Sold in 10,000 Filling Stations." *New York Times*, October 31, 1924.

Baker, George. "An Inquiry Concerning the Cause of the Endemial Colic of Devonshire." *Medical Transactions: Published by the College of Physicians in London* 2 (1772).

Bellinger, David, et al. "Low-Level Lead Exposure, Intelligence and Academic Achievement: A Long-Term Follow-Up Study." *Pediatrics* 90 (1992): 855–61.

Centers for Disease Control and Prevention. *Preventing Lead Poisoning in Young Children*. Atlanta: Department of Health and Human Services, 1991.

Clapp, Richard, et al. *Environmental and Occupational Causes of Cancer*. Lowell: Lowell Center for Sustainable Production, 2005.

"Committee Report of Ethyl Gasoline." *Journal of the American Medical Association* 86 (January 30, 1926).

Dapul, Heda and Danielle Laraque. "Lead Poisoning in Children." *Advances in Pediatrics* 61 (2014): 313–33.

"Declining Supply of Motor Fuel." *Scientific American*, March 8, 1919: 220.

Doll, Robert and Richard Peto. "The Causes of Cancer." *Journal of the National Cancer Institute* 66 (1981): 1192–308.

"DuPont Tells of the Gas: His Company Had Fatalities, But Has Lessened Dangers." *New York Times*, October 31, 1924.

Environmental Protection Agency. *Air Quality Criteria for Lead*. EPA-600/8-83028aF-dF. Research Triangle Park: Office of Health and Environmental Assessment, 1986.

———. "Chemical Right to Know: High Production Volume Chemicals Frequently Asked Questions." EPA 745-F-09–002g, March 1999.

Epstein, Samuel. *Cancer-Gate: How to Win the Losing Cancer War*. Amityville: Baywood Publishing, 2005.

Ethyl Corp. v. EPA, 163 U.S.App.D.C. 162, 501 F.2d 722 (1974).

Ethyl Corp. v. EPA, 541 F. 2d 1 (D.C. Circuit 1976).

Ethyl Gasoline Corporation. "More Than a Million Are Riding with ETHYL." *Popular Mechanics*. Advertising Section 49 (1928).

Federal Highway Administration. "State Motor Vehicle Registrations, by Years, 1900–1995." Washington: Department of Transportation, April 1997. https://fhwa.dot.gov/ohim/summary95/mv200.pdf.

Finkel, Asher, ed. *Hamilton and Hardy's Industrial Toxicology*, 4th edition. Boston: J. Wright, 1983.

Garrod, Alfred. "Second Communication on the Blood and Effused Fluids in Gout, Rheumatism and Bright's Disease." *Medical Chirurgical Transactions* 37 (1854): 49–60.

———. *Treatise on the Nature and Treatment of Gout and Rheumatic Gout*. London: Walton and Maberly, 1859.

Gibson, J. Lockhart. "Plumbic Ocular Neuritis in Queensland Children." *British Medical Journal* 2 (1908): 1488–90.

Graebner, William. "Hegemony Through Science: Information Engineering and Lead Toxicology, 1925–1965." In *Dying for Work*, edited by David Rosner and Gerald Markowitz. Bloomington: Indiana University Press, 1985.

———. "Private Power, Private Knowledge, and Public Health: Science, Engineering and Lead Poisoning, 1900–1970." In *The Health and Safety of Workers*, edited by Ronald Bayer. Oxford: Oxford University Press, 1988.

Graham, Edgar. "Letter to Dr. Paul Nicholas Leech." NA, RG 70, 101869, File 725, July 18, 1924.

Hernberg, Sven. "Lead Poisoning in a Historical Perspective." *American Journal of Industrial Medicine* 38 (2000): 244–54.

Hernberg, Sven and Jorma Nikkanen. "Enzyme Inhibition by Lead under Normal Urban Conditions." *Lancet* 1 (1970): 63–4.

Hernberg, Sven, et al. "δ-Aminolevulinic Acid Dehydrase as a Measure of Lead Exposure." *Archives of Environmental Health* 21 (1970): 140–5.

Holusha, John. "The Troubles with Gasoline." *New York Times*, August 7, 1986.

Kitman, Jamie Lincoln. "The Secret History of Lead." *The Nation*, March 2, 2002. http://thenation.com/article/secret-history-lead.

Landrigan, Philip. "Pediatric Lead Poisoning: Is There a Threshold?" *Public Health Reports* 115 (2000): 530–1.

Landrigan, Philip and Dean Baker. "Clinical Recognition of Occupational and Environmental Disease." *Mt. Sinai Journal of Medicine* 62 (1995): 406–11.

Landrigan, Philip, et al. "Cancer Prevention in the Workplace." In *Cancer Prevention and Control*, edited by Peter Greenwald, et al. New York: Marcel Dekker, 1995.

Lanphear, Bruce, et al. "Cognitive Deficits Associated with Blood Lead Concentrations <10 μg/dL in US Children and Adolescents." *Public Health Reports* 115 (2000): 521–9.

Lin-Fu, Jane. "Vulnerability of Children to Lead Exposure and Toxicity." *New England Journal of Medicine* 289 (1973): 1289–93.

Loeb, Alan. "Birth of the Kettering Doctrine: Fordism, Sloanism and the Discovery of Tetraethyl Lead." *Business and Economic History* 24 (1995): 72–87.

———. "Paradigms Lost: A Case Study Analysis of Models of Corporate Responsibility for the Environment." *Business and Economic History* 28 (1999): 95–107.

Luger, Stan. *Corporate Power, American Democracy, and the Automobile Industry*. Cambridge: Cambridge University Press, 2000.

Markoitz, Gerald and David Rosner. "Corporate Responsibility for Toxins." *Annals of the Academy of Political and Social Science* 584 (2002): 159–74.

———. *Deceit and Denial: The Deadly Politics of Industrial Pollution.* Berkeley: University of California Press, 2002.

Moore, Jean. "Community Aspects of Childhood Lead Poisoning." *American Journal of Public Health* 60 (1970): 1430–4.

Nader, Ralph. *Unsafe at Any Speed: The Designed-In Dangers of the American Automobile.* New York: Grossman Publishers, 1965.

Nadim, Farhad, et al. "United States Experience with Gasoline Additives." *Energy Policy* 29 (2001): 1–5.

National Research Council. *Measuring Lead Exposure in Infants and Children.* Washington: National Academy Press, 1987.

Needleman, Herbert. "Childhood Lead Poisoning: The Promise and Abandonment of Primary Prevention." *American Journal of Public Health* 88 (1998): 1871–7.

———. "Clair Patterson and Robert Kehoe: Two Views of Lead Toxicity." *Environmental Research* 78 (1998): 79–85.

———. "The Removal of Lead from Gasoline: Historical and Personal Reflections." *Environmental Research* 84 (2000): 20–35.

Needleman, Herbert, et al. "Lead Levels in Deciduous Teeth of Urban and Suburban American Children." *Nature* 235 (1972): 111–2.

Needleman, Herbert, et al. "Subclinical Lead Exposure in Philadelphia School Children: Identification by Dentine Lead Analysis." *New England Journal of Medicine* 290 (1974): 245–8.

Needleman, Herbert, et al. "The Long-Term Effects of Exposure to Low Doses of Lead in Childhood: An 11-Year Follow-Up Report." *New England Journal of Medicine* 322 (1990): 83–8.

Nriagu, Jerome. "The Rise and Fall of Leaded Gasoline." *Science of the Total Environment* 92 (1990): 13–28.

———. "Clair Patterson and Robert Kehoe's Paradigm of 'Show Me the Data' on Environmental Lead Poisoning." *Environmental Research* 78 (1998): 71–8.

Nye, Leslie. "An Investigation of the Extraordinary Incidence of Chronic Nephritis in Young People in Queensland." *Medical Journal of Australia* 2 (1929): 145–59.

Oliver, Thomas. "A Lecture on Lead Poisoning and the Race: Delivered to the Eugenics Education Society." *British Medical Journal* 1 (1911): 1096–8.

Parkinson, David, et al. "Occupational Lead Exposure and Blood Pressure." *British Journal of Industrial Medicine* 44 (1987): 744–8.

Patterson, Clair. "Contaminated and Natural Lead Environments of Man." *Archives of Environmental Health* 11 (1965): 344–60.

Percival, Robert, et al. *Environmental Regulation: Law, Science, and Policy*, 6th edition. New York: Aspen Publishers, 2009.

Prendergast, W. Dowling. "The Classification of the Symptoms of Lead Poisoning." *British Medical Journal* 1 (1910): 1164–6.

Public Health Service. "Proceedings of a Conference to Determine Whether or Not There Is a Public Health Question in the Manufacture, Distribution, or Use of Tetraethyl Lead Gasoline." *Public Health Bulletin No. 158.* Washington: Government Publishing Office, 1925.

Ramazzini, Bernardino. *Diseases of Workers: The Latin Text of 1713 Revisited*, translated by Wilmer Wright. Chicago: Chicago University Press, 1940 [1713].

Ramirez-Cervantes, B. et al. "Health Assessment of Employees with Different Body Burdens of Lead." *Journal of Occupational Medicine* 20 (1978): 610–7.

Rosner, David and Gerald Markowitz. "A 'Gift of God'?: The Public Health Controversy over Leaded Gasoline during the 1920s." *American Journal of Public Health* 75 (1985): 344–52.

Sellers, Christopher. "The Public Health Services Office of Industrial Hygiene and the Transformation of Industrial Medicine." *Bulletin of Medical History* 65 (1991): 42–73.

Shrader-Frechette, Kristin. *Taking Action, Saving Lives: Our Duties to Protect Environmental and Public Health*. Oxford: Oxford University Press, 2007.

Siemiatycki, Jack, et al. "Listing Occupational Carcinogens." *Environmental Health Perspectives* 112 (2004): 1447–59.

Silbergeld, Ellen. "Preventing Lead Poisoning in Children." *Annual Review of Public Health* 18 (1997): 187–210.

Small Refiner Lead Phasedown Taskforce v. EPA, 705 F.2d 506, 528 (D.C. Circuit 1983).

Smith, George. "Where the World Gets Oil and Where Will Our Children Get It When American Wells Cease to Flow?" *National Geographic*, February 1920: 181–202.

"Third Victim Dies from Poison Gas." *New York Times*, October 29, 1924.

Thomas, Valerie and Andrew Kwong. "Ethanol as a Lead Replacement: Phasing Out Leaded Gasoline in Africa." *Energy Policy* 29 (2001): 1133–43.

Tong, Shilu, et al. "Declining Blood Lead Levels and Changes in Cognitive Function during Childhood: The Port Pirie Cohort Study." *Journal of the American Medical Association* 280 (1998): 1915–9.

Tong, Shilu, et al. "Environmental Lead Exposure: A Public Health Problem of Global Dimensions." *Bulletin of the World Health Organization* 78 (2000): 1068–77.

Waldron, H.A. "The Anaemia of Lead Poisoning: A Review." *British Journal of Industrial Medicine* 23 (1966): 83–100.

White, David. "The Unmined Supply of Petroleum in the United States." Presented to the Society of Automotive Engineers Annual Meeting. New York, NY, February 4–6, 1919.

World Health Organization. *Inorganic Lead: Environmental Health Criteria 165*. Geneva: WHO, 1995.

———. "Lead Poisoning and Health: Fact Sheet." Last updated September 2016. http://who.int/mediacentre/factsheets/fs379/en/.

Wormser, Felix. "Facts and Fallacies Concerning Exposure to Lead." *Occupational Medicine* 3 (1947): 135–44.

7 Demanding Higher Standards of Corporate Responsibility

We live in an era when exposure to environmental threats of harm has become so pervasive as to be accepted by most as commonplace and viewed as inevitable, where probabilistic risks and uncertain threats of harm are considered necessary by-products of life in organized society. This era is further defined by the failure of environmental laws and overtaxed regulatory agencies to safeguard the public from exposure to even *known* toxins and carcinogens; by our appraisal of industry's proactive efforts to avert environmental health crises as somehow supererogatory; and by the standard practice of legislators, regulators, analysts, and scholars to judge uncorroborated possibilities of environmental harm as tolerable or safe until a preponderance of evidence proves otherwise—even when we know that this burden of proof usually cannot be satisfied because crucial evidence is withheld or contested by industry. These features define a system of environmental risk management that is wholly untenable and testify to the need to revise our expectations of corporate responsibility and environmental health policies.

This notion is only bolstered by the Trump administration's efforts to substantially cut funding to environmental agencies and to institute industry-friendly rollbacks on diverse environmental protections—initiatives that are spearheaded by a president whose record as an entrepreneur and whose time in office exemplify the evasion of corporate responsibility and the disregard of public welfare. This destructive corporate culture and inherently flawed system of environmental risk management amplify the need to hold industry accountable for its obligations to prevent endangering public health, *irrespective* of the laxer standards to which existing environmental laws may hold emitters. This is to say that moral principles should be informing our environmental laws (and catalyzing stricter regulations), not vice versa: our moral appraisals should not be constrained by what laxer environmental laws are in place. In this vein, as this book has argued, environmental risk management is not foremost an issue of sound science (and empirically corroborating credible risks to human health), or of economic viability (and balancing the benefits of industrialized society with the costs to human and environmental health), or of political feasibility (and designing risk regulations that can achieve broad support and thus may be implemented). Rather, environmental risk management is chiefly an issue of morality, of what corporations owe to the public and those who they may expose to their emissions. Heeding the equal moral standing of others, and thus respecting them as ends in themselves, means refraining from gambling with their welfare and striving to mitigate the potential for harm by exercising due care.

7.1 Taking Responsibility for Uncertain Threats of Environmental Harm: An Overview

As Chapters 2 and 6 demonstrated, the regulation of uncertain environmental threats has conventionally been determined by appeals to the significance of our epistemic limitations. The significance, that is, of our inability to corroborate the severity of the adverse health effects of exposure (outcome uncertainty), or the likelihood that some foreseeable harm to human health will occur (probability uncertainty), or the complex causes of the adverse health effects that do materialize (causal uncertainty), which may result from scientific and technological limitations in our testing capabilities or from disagreement within the scientific community about how to interpret the best available evidence derived from available methods of analysis (scientific uncertainty). While ignoring the nuances of these different forms of uncertainty, and thus framing uncertainty in terms of risk (treating uncertainty narrowly as probability uncertainty), both proponents of and opponents to precautionary environmental risk regulation were shown to appeal to prevailing uncertainty to justify their antithetical policy positions, with proponents insisting that the uncertain probability of harm requires preventative safeguards to protect public health, and opponents insisting that until a preponderance of evidence can confirm a strong probability of harm to the public, any preventative measures are unjustified. Yet Chapter 2 argued that this puts any discussion about whether to regulate emissions that entail possible, albeit unverified, harm to public health at an untenable impasse—permitting but one of two alternatives.

One possibility was to accept that since conventional justificatory appeals to uncertainty are self-defeating, this stalled debate implies that no regulation of emissions under uncertainty can be justified. Rejecting the plausibility of this unqualified implication, the alternative was to ground an argument for precaution in something *other than* our epistemic limitations, that is, to develop a normative justification for preventatively regulating uncertain environmental threats to public health. After showing that existing defenses of a precautionary system of risk management have difficulty refuting common objections, Chapter 2 abandoned the traditional understanding of the precautionary principle—as a policy approach based on scientific knowledge about risk, whose broad aim is to manage uncertainty—and introduced a novel interpretation of the precautionary principle as a deontological principle based on moral equality, whose aim is to safeguard the public's right not to be exposed to potentially harmful and preventable threats of environmental harm.

This broadly Kantian principle, developed in detail in Chapter 3, suggests that if we take seriously the equal moral standing of others, we have an obligation to respect others as autonomous moral agents. Yet to expose others to uncertain, unconsented-to, and preventable environmental threats, which may ultimately cause them harm, is to gamble with their interests and welfare and thus to disregard their moral standing. And since it is untenable, for various reasons, to expect emitters to garner the consent of others (whether expressly, tacitly, or hypothetically) to uncorroborated threats of environmental harm, requiring emitters to exercise due care under uncertainty so as to mitigate the potential for harm is necessary to avoid wrongdoing. Yet it deserves repeating that when uncertainty prevails, there is no way to discern whether a threat poses a probable (imminent) risk of nontrivial (substantive) harm to others, which is traditionally how unreasonable and, thus wrongful, risk impositions are defined. Accordingly, it is not the uncertain threat itself that constitutes wrongdoing and the basis for assigning blame and culpability. Rather, those who are put in potential harm's way by emitters who fail to exercise due care under uncertainty are wronged because their interests and welfare are disregarded for the sake of the emitter's own interests, which is to say that such emitters assume they are not on equal moral footing with their fellows.

Vindicating this normative argument depends on demonstrating, however, that leading theories of moral responsibility and arguments from moral luck and the ethics of risk do not adequately account for the problem of uncertain threats, which was the focus of Chapter 4. Conventional theories of moral luck treat uncertainty narrowly as probability uncertainty and maintain that only those threats that entail strong probabilities of severe harm are unreasonable and thus warrant regulation. And since prevailing uncertainty precludes our ability to foresee whether the outcome of an uncertain threat will be harmful, as well as our ability to assess the probability that the outcome will cause harm, all uncertain threats are *ipso facto* morally permissible (that is, until evidence can prove otherwise). Arguments from moral luck, on the other hand, would have us believe that while the outcomes of uncertain threats may be morally wrong, actors should not be held culpable for the threats or harms they generate, given the unavoidable ignorance that prevailing uncertainty entails. Finally, arguments in the ethics of risk suggest that uncertain threats are trivial (highly improbable and/or would result in negligible harm) and thus that these unquantifiable threats should be presumed to be safe (treated as reasonable risks). This amounts to the same conclusion responsibility theorists draw, namely that exposing others to uncertain threats is permissible.

Each of these conventional accounts were subsequently shown to be inadequate. By couching culpability in causal responsibility and presupposing clear causal chains of events that permit us to identify the injury, the injured, and the injurer, theories of moral responsibility cannot account for most environmental harms, given their highly complex causal chains. Arguments from moral luck wrongly assume that one's ignorance under uncertainty is unqualified and unavoidable. Yet this overlooks the deducible reasons one may have to believe that a particular uncertain threat will produce some harm (recall the milk vs. motor oil example from Chapter 3.4 and how one may reasonably infer that exposure to a substance that resembles used motor oil is likely to cause harm), and it also ignores the salience of our knowledge that our environmental history is rife with examples of how the release of substances into the environment proved to be deleterious. Moreover, one's knowledge of her ignorance of circumstance may itself be a compelling reason to exercise due care and to deliberate about alternative courses of action that can still satisfy our ends, or to scrutinize the action to identify plausible outcomes, or to reevaluate the ends that motivate our performing the action in the first place if no feasible alternative action is possible. These considerations suggest that we have access to enough information about the potential for harm when uncertainty prevails that we cannot generally claim ignorance, which undermines the argument from moral luck that our epistemic limitations excuse us of culpability. Finally, by equating uncertain threats with trivial risks, arguments from the ethics of risk wrongly assume knowledge to which we do not have access under conditions of outcome and probability uncertainty.

Adequately defending the proposed *pro tanto* duty to exercise due care requires two important qualifications, however. The first qualification is that not all uncertain threats of environmental harm are the same. Outcome and probability uncertainty, in other words, vary across contexts and can be more or less pronounced, which should influence our judgments about when an obligation of due care actually exists and how strong the duty is. Consequently, Chapter 3 also differentiated between reasons and duties to exercise due care—noting that the more reasons one can infer to believe that an uncertain threat will materialize in some (undefined) harm to others, the stronger one's duty becomes to exercise precaution. This also means that as we approach genuine uncertainty, we may recognize fewer compelling reasons for taking due care, which may cast doubt on our corresponding duty to do so. However, it was stressed that the salience of our subjective judgments of the potential for harm are suspect, since the root of the moral problem that uncertainty creates is that we cannot reasonably draw inferences about that which remains unknown. The second qualification is that because any reasonable standard of due care must be sensitive to context, what the exercise of precaution under uncertainty requires and how one's obligation is discharged will also vary across contexts and actors.

Exploring this second qualification in detail, Chapter 5 developed a practical framework to define what reasonable precautionary measures industry's duty of due care may entail by exploring three broad scenarios in which uncertainty varies: (1) outcome and probability uncertainty are present, but the substance in question shares similarities to pollutants whose effects have been scientifically verified, and from which the effects of exposure to the uncertain environmental threat may be inferred; (2) toxicity testing could eliminate outcome and probability uncertainty (that is, the actual threat of exposure could feasibly be verified), but the substance in question has not yet been tested and thus its threat to public health remains uncertain; and (3) outcome and probability uncertainty are present and this uncertainty cannot currently be overcome, even with toxicity testing, using existing technologies and scientific standards. The degree of uncertainty that best characterizes a given circumstance—which is to say that the knowledge we can infer or empirically confirm about a particular uncertain threat, or the extent to which we can eliminate uncertainty about the health effects of exposure and the probability that exposure will entail adverse health effects—will shape what due care consists of and how the obligation can be discharged.

Beyond this central consideration, other morally relevant context-dependent factors include the availability of feasible substitutes, the involvement of vulnerable populations (like children, pregnant women, industrial workers, the poor, and racial or ethnic minority communities), the volume of production and emission of the substance that poses the uncertain threat, an emitter's history of delinquency with existing environmental regulations or of corporate social irresponsibility with regard to the uncertain threat, efforts to disclose to regulators and the public the potential harm that an emitter's emissions may entail, and efforts to implement best available control technologies (BACTs) to further mitigate the potential for harm. Should an emitter who exposes the public to an uncertain threat of environmental harm fail to take advantage of available substitutes that would not entail this threat to public health; should the emissions put vulnerable populations in the way of potential, albeit uncertain, harm; should the emitter have a history of violating existing environmental regulations and/or engaging in socially irresponsible practices like withholding data, manufacturing doubt, and misleading the public about the actual risks to human health that exposure would entail; and so forth, the requisite standard of due care to which we should hold the emitter would be higher than in the absence of these criteria. (This was illustrated in Chapter 6 with the historical example of tetraethyl lead and corporations like General Motors, Standard Oil of New Jersey, and Ethyl Gasoline Corporation.) Conversely, if one or more of these mitigating factors were present—if no vulnerable population were involved, if the emitter had a history of compliance with environmental laws and social responsibility, forthrightly disclosed the findings of industry-led studies that could confirm the actual risks of exposure, and strove to implement BACTS to avert public health crises—the emitter's duty to exercise precaution would be lessened.

This discussion prefaced a return to the policy-oriented and normative objections introduced in Chapter 2 that are commonly leveled against precautionary approaches to environmental risk regulation. And while demonstrating that this book's deontological defense of a precautionary standard of due care under uncertainty can convincingly refute these objections and that a precautionary approach can involve reasonable measures to safeguard the public, Chapter 5 also reiterated that precautionary risk regulations should only aim to augment, *not* replace, existing risk analysis. The exercise of precaution is justified when our knowledge of the potential for harm to public health is constrained enough that formal, quantitative risk assessments (QRAs) cannot be conducted—and thus when QRA inherently fails to prescribe reasonable thresholds of acceptable risk and adequate safety measures. Again, the regulation of arsenic in drinking water, particulate matter in the ambient air, and methylmercury in foods each lend credence to the usefulness of QRA as a policy tool in certain contexts. QRA, however, and its reliance on cost–benefit analysis (CBA), is no panacea; given the tens of thousands of chemicals grandfathered under the Toxic Substances Control Act (TSCA), manufactured and emitted into the environment, whose toxicity profiles are either absent or incomplete—and thus which pose uncertain threats of environmental harm to public health and welfare—the limitations of a QRA/CBA-based system of risk management and its ability to safeguard the public against environmental harm are stark.

Buttressing the plausibility of this flexible and context-dependent precautionary standard of due care, Chapter 6 explored a high-profile, contentious, and precedent-setting case of an uncertain threat of environmental harm: the protracted public health hazard that the manufacture of tetraethyl lead and leaded gasoline created. This case and the questionable actions over several decades by the oil and automotive industries to suppress knowledge about the health effects of low-level lead exposure from leaded gasoline exhaust and to prevent mandatory emission standards from being implemented underscored some of the adverse consequences of the absence of a requisite standard of due care.

7.2 Recent Developments

As is detailed in Chapter 5, one of the consistent (non–context-dependent) aspects of the obligation emitters have to exercise precaution under uncertainty—indeed, the central pillar of the proposed standard of due care—is their duty to take reasonable strides to discern the possible adverse health effects of their emissions to mitigate the potential for harm—since any finding that adverse health effects are likely would subject the substance and its emission to existing environmental regulations or would justify the implementation of a new emission standard. This means that corporations should be required to test for the toxicity of the substances they use in their production processes or discharge into the environment, to forthrightly disclose these data to regulators, and to provide details to the public on these findings in easily accessible and understandable ways for individuals to be able to better insulate themselves from potential harm.

These requirements and objectives were recently highlighted in The Lautenberg Chemical Safety for the 21st Century Act, which revised several problematic tenets of the TSCA. With the implementation of the Lautenberg Act in the fall of 2016, the burden of proof on regulators and public health scientists has been somewhat lightened, as it is no longer necessary for the Environmental Protection Agency (EPA) to empirically corroborate the presence of a credible risk or probable exposure before it can mandate companies to conduct toxicity tests. Moreover, the act expands the EPA's capacity to require testing of both new and existing substances,[1] it allows the EPA to designate substances as "high priority" whenever companies fail to provide adequate safety assessment data,[2] and it prohibits industry from manufacturing new substances unless corporations can demonstrate that the substance "is not likely to present an unreasonable risk of injury."[3] Beyond requiring companies to establish toxicity profiles for the substances they intend to manufacture and emit into the environment—which amounts to eliminating uncertainty and bringing more chemical substances under the umbrella of existing emission standards—the Lautenberg Act also explicitly requires that vulnerable populations (including infants, children, workers, and the elderly) be identified and protected from occupational and environmental exposure.[4] Finally, the act also promotes greater public disclosure of information pertaining to potential public health threats by substantively constraining the conditions under which companies can legitimately claim that the findings of industry-led toxicity tests are confidential.[5]

These promising developments to the regulation of substances whose health effects are uncorroborated or understudied closely overlap with the broad aims of this book project: to make toxicity testing mandatory to reduce the number of uncertain environmental threats we face, and to prevent corporate emitters from disregarding and gambling with the interests and welfare of the public. The Lautenberg revisions to the TSCA, which received overwhelming bipartisan support, lend credence to the precautionary measures defended earlier to better protect the public from the large subset of chemical substances that entail uncertain health effects—and that QRA and CBA cannot address. Moreover, the act alludes to the higher standards of corporate social responsibility that implementation of this proposed precautionary standard will require. Yet in the shadow of cases like tetraethyl lead, when the oil and automotive industries claimed ignorance of the health effects of exposure and manufactured uncertainty to undercut the justification for stricter environmental regulations—which parallels other controversial cases of corporate irresponsibility, such as the denial of the adverse health effects of exposure to ionizing radiation by the Department of Defense in the 1950s, of exposure to cigarette smoke by the American tobacco companies in the 1990s, and of the effects of greenhouse gas emissions by diverse companies in the oil, gas, coal, and automotive industries that continue today—it is unclear what lasting success the Lautenberg Act may have on improving public health and welfare.

Underscoring the need for practical national and global policy reform are three extensions of the ethical defense of precaution developed in this book: namely, the implications of uncertain environmental threats and duties of due care on food security and food justice, on environmental discrimination and global governance, and on climate ethics and historical emissions.

7.3 Implications and Prospects for Future Research

The burgeoning literature on food justice and protecting the human right to basic sustenance of food-insecure communities stresses the importance of eliminating food deserts and of empowering communities to become more self-reliant by establishing sustainable local food systems when structural reform is implausible. However, contemporary debates over the human right to food and the moral obligations we have to underprivileged and often marginalized groups and nations that are struggling with hunger assume that long-term solutions to food insecurity (as opposed to immediate food aid) primarily entail improving access to food. It is commonly overlooked, however, that a right to basic sustenance implies a right to food *that is safe to eat*. Yet in the food deserts of historically poor, urban, and racial and ethnic minority communities—as is also true of food-insecure communities in lesser-developed countries—healthier alternatives free of synthetic pesticides, preservatives, additives, and genetically modified organisms (GMOs)—many of which pose scientifically unverified human health effects—are generally unavailable. Bisphenol A (BPA) in the lining of canned foods and growth hormones (recombinant bovine growth hormone [rBGH]) in conventional dairy products are but two familiar examples of the more than 70,000 chemical substances manufactured in the United States and routinely (and lawfully) emitted into the environment for which toxicity data are either limited or absent. And as this foregoing discussion has established, such substances beget uncertain environmental threats, some of which may well prove to be harmful. In the context of food justice, the presence of these uncertain threats means that conventional efforts to mitigate food insecurity may well be counterproductive—exposing already vulnerable populations to myriad substances that may cause long-term adverse health effects. Extending this book's central argument would mean that even under conditions of uncertainty, corporations in relevant industries like agriculture, food production, and food packaging would do wrong by failing to exercise due care (and thus would be culpable to blame and punishment) and that regulators would be obliged to institute preventative measures to protect the public (and especially vulnerable groups) from the uncertain threats these industries beget, thus championing a meaningful human right to food would require that the implementation of precautionary environmental risk regulations that can safeguard vulnerable, food-insecure communities against exposure to uncertain threats of environmental harm (as well as the elimination of structural injustices that lead to inequitable exposure to environmental risk among vulnerable populations).

In a similar vein, scholars have shown that vulnerable populations like racial minorities and the poor face disproportionate levels of exposure to environmental threats of harm—an inequality that is especially prominent in developing countries, which lack the infrastructure, bureaucracies, technological expertise, and resources to adequately safeguard public health. The continued U.S. export of pesticides banned for domestic use and the global trade in hazardous and electronic waste testify to this persistent problem of global justice—a problem that is amplified by the pervasive outcome, probability, causal, and scientific uncertainty about the actual dangers to human health that many threats of environmental harm pose. Augmenting various arguments about our responsibilities to eliminate structural injustices, to reform policies and institutions that tolerate environmental injustice, and to assist those who are in need and unable to help themselves, an extension of the standard of due care under uncertainty would provide a novel argument for eliminating these global environmental inequalities. Applying the central argument developed in Chapters 3 and 4 that actions that create uncertain threats wrongfully gamble with the welfare of those who may be exposed and expanding the discussion in Chapter 5 on how emitters can discharge their duty of due care to strive to mitigate the potential for injury may reveal the responsibilities nonstate actors and international institutions—like multinational corporations, development organizations, human rights and humanitarian aid organizations, and so forth—have to prevent global inequalities in exposure to uncertain environmental threats.

Finally, it is conventionally argued that prior to 1990 and the report issued by the Intergovernmental Panel on Climate Change that confirmed the correlation between greenhouse gas emissions and climate change, emitters were excusably ignorant of the effects of their emissions—and thus are not culpable for their historical (pre-1990) emissions. Instead, conventional arguments in climate ethics develop other justifications of "common but differentiated responsibilities," such as the extent to which a country benefited from its emissions or its ability to shoulder a greater distribution of the costs of climate change. Having shown that the epistemic limitation excuse (or the claim of excusable ignorance) is highly problematic, this book project should have us reject the starting presumption of existing climate ethics scholarship. And applying the central normative argument that emitters have duties to prevent exposing others to potentially harmful emissions—even in the absence of a preponderance of evidence that corroborates the effects of exposure—may provide a novel justification for holding developed countries responsible for their historic emissions and, thus, for requiring that they absorb the costs of climate change. If it is possible to show that prior to 1990 developed countries had sufficient reason to believe that their greenhouse gas emissions would cause some harm in the future, and if it can be shown that developing countries failed to take reasonable measures to mitigate the potential for climate-related harm, then developed countries could be held to account. And in substantially shifting the distribution of the costs of these historical emissions back to wealthy countries, developing nations would be safeguarded against bearing an inequitable burden of the costs of mitigating and adapting to the effects of climate change.

Whatever the context, the notion that prevailing uncertainty should not give industry license to gamble with human health is, hopefully, an intuitive one. As has been suggested throughout, uncertain threats of environmental harm are pervasive, and they pose a unique and exigent moral problem in large measure because of the complex nature of environmental harms. The effects of long-term low-dose exposure are difficult to measure, in part because epidemiological and toxicity testing capabilities are limited and extrapolation from controlled animal studies are problematic. Diverse intervening causal factors, cumulative exposures, deferred effects, different pathways and timings and lengths of exposure, and varying physiological dispositions (vulnerabilities) to being harmed upon exposure all serve to alter the kind, magnitude, consistency, and observability of demonstrable harm. This is all to say that it is naïve to ground regulatory decisions about environmental health exclusively, or even chiefly, in the imperfect toxicological sciences when uncertainty prevails, and it is immoral for us to tolerate a system of environmental risk management that would have us delay regulation under uncertainty until the imperfect toxicological sciences can yield preponderances of evidence to verify actual risks to public health. "Justice delayed *is* justice denied,"[6] as any victim of preventable environmental harm can attest. And it is time that debates over the merits of precautionary environmental risk regulation table considerations of risk assessment, economic viability, and political feasibility and acknowledge that what is at stake is not the deterrence of statistical deaths, but rather the safeguard of human welfare and that what should shape decisions about whether or not to regulate uncertain threats (as well as environmental risks) is what we deserve and owe each other as moral equals—obligations of mutual respect that are not diminished by prevailing uncertainty.

Notes

1. Government Publishing Office, Frank R. Lautenberg Chemical Safety for the 21st Century Act, H.R.2576, 114th Congress Public Law 182 (June 22, 2016): §4(a).
2. Ibid., §§6(b)(1)(C)(iii), 6(b)(3).
3. Ibid., §§5(a)(1)(B), 5(a)(3), 5(g).
4. Ibid., §§3(12), 5(e)(1)(A), 5(f)(1), 6(a), 6(b)(4)(A), and 6(b)(4)(F).
5. Ibid., §§14(c)(2)(G), 14(c)(3).
6. Kristin Shrader-Frechette, *Taking Action, Saving Lives: Our Duties to Protect Environmental and Public Health* (Oxford: Oxford University Press, 2007): 97 (emphasis added).

References

Government Publishing Office. "Frank R. Lautenberg Chemical Safety for the 21st Century Act, H.R.2576." *114th Congress Public Law 182*, June 22, 2016. https://congress.gov/bill/114th-congress/house-bill/2576/text.

Shrader-Frechette, Kristin. *Taking Action, Saving Lives: Our Duties to Protect Environmental and Public Health.* Oxford: Oxford University Press, 2007.

Index

American Cancer Society 24

Best Available Control Technologies 141–2
bisphenol A 12–13, 23, 140, 193
blameworthiness *see* moral responsibility

California Proposition 65, 138–9
Chlorine Chemical Council v. EPA 34
climate ethics and historical emissions 194
conscientious and negligent drivers 104–5, 109–10
consent 40, 42, 46, 78–81; as hypothetical 80–1
consumer protection labeling schemes 138–41
Corrosion Proof Fittings v. EPA 6–7, 35
culpability *see* moral responsibility

DDT 1, **21**, 32–3, 144–5
Delaney Clause 5, 34–5, 135
diethylstilbestrol 23, 80, 98
due care: contextual mitigating or aggravating factors 10–11, 29–30, 76, 112, 153, 162–76, 189–90; duties of 49, 76, 83, 111–12, 127; and ignorance 83, 102–5, 107–11, 176; reasons *vs.* duties 71–2, 81–4, 85n9, 107, 189; and reciprocity or mutually-acceptable burden-sharing 96–7, 99, 111–12, 127–8, 133–4, 136–43, 147–51, 158n53; residual duty 138; standard of 112–13, 128–43, 149–50, 175–6, 191–2; and uncertainty 72, 76, 78, 107–8, 110–11, 113, 127–37, 191–2
DuPont 11–12, 164–6, 168–9, 173
Dworkin, Gerald 94, 103, 108–9, 111

endangering actions 27, 49, 72, 107–8, 111, 130, 133, 169
environmental discrimination 172, 193–4; *see also* vulnerable populations
environmental harm 21, 24–7
EPA 22, 34, 44–5, 112, 130–1, 136, 149, 168, 191–2
epidemiology *see* toxicology
epistemic limitation excuse *see* moral luck
ethics of risk 10, 72, 92, 97–102, 115, 188–9
Ethyl Corp. v. EPA 34, 169
Ethyl Gasoline Corporation 136–7, 165–9, 172–4
European Union Registration, Evaluation, Authorisation and Restriction of Chemicals 121–2n106, 131–2
ExxonMobil *see* Standard Oil of New Jersey

FDA 23–4, 135, 139–40
Federal Food, Drug, and Cosmetics Act *see* Delaney Clause
Feinberg, Joel 93, 97, 99
food justice 192–3
Food Quality Protection Act *see* Delaney Clause
formal risk assessment *see* quantitative risk assessment

Gardiner, Stephen 37–9
General Motors 11–12, 136–7, 152, 164–8, 172–3, 175
genetically modified organisms **21**, 32–3, 82, 145, 193
GM Chemical Company *see* General Motors

GM Research Corporation *see* General Motors
Goklany, Indur 33, 46–7

high production volume chemicals 44–5, 114, 142, 151, 171

Industrial Union Dept., AFL-CIO v. American Petroleum Institute 6, 35
intuitive toxicology *see* risk, lay perceptions of

Jackson v. Johns-Manville Sales Corp. 98

Kantian ethics 9, 47–8, 69; and autonomy 48–9, 72–5, 77–8; and consent 78–81; and moral enlightenment 73–5; and moral standing 48–9, 72–3, 75, 78, 135–6; and teleology 74, 87n30
Kehoe, Robert *see* Ethyl Gasoline Corporation

Lautenberg Chemical Safety for the 21st Century Act 112–13, 151, 191–2
lead *see* tetraethyl lead and corporate social *ir*responsibility
leaded gasoline *see* tetraethyl lead and corporate social *ir*responsibility

McMahan, Jeff 104–5, 109, 111
Midgley, Thomas *see* General Motors
moral equality 47, 49, 72–3, 78
moral luck 9–10, 72, 92, 102–11, 115, 188–9; and alternatives 109–10, 115; and excusable ignorance 102–5, 107–8, 110–11, 115; and foreseeability of environmental harms 106–8, 110–11, 175–6; McMahan on 104–5, 109; as option luck 109; Reid on 107–8; as resultant luck 103–4, 110; and uncertain threats of environmental harm 105–7, 110
moral permissibility 72, 83, 93–4, 102–5, 107–8, 110–11, 115
moral responsibility 10, 72, 84–5n3, 92, 115, 188–9; as answerability 77–8; and causal responsibility 92–6; and environmental threats 94–5, 130, 153; and excusability 93–4, 102, 119nn60–1; and ignorance 83, 87n39, 106–8, 110–11; and innocent and excused threats 104; and moral obligations 70–2, 92–6; and toxicity testing 130–1, 133–4, 149–51, 175–6, 191–2
Morgan-Knapp, Christopher 40–2

Nader, Ralph 168
Nagel, Thomas 70, 104, 110
Nozick, Robert 113, 133

Otsuka, Michael 109–10, 115

precautionary principle 3–7, 19–20; and conventional criticisms of 10–11, 30–6, 144–5; and conventional formulations of 28–30, 33, 36–8, 42–3, 46–50; normative defenses of 37–46; rights-based interpretation 22, 28, 46–50, 127, 146, 148–50; and rights-based rejoinders to conventional criticisms 143–55; as supplement to quantitative risk assessment 2–3, 27–8, 145–6, 161, 190–1
Public Citizen v. Young 5, 34–5, 135

quantitative risk assessment 6, 8, 27, 35, 46, 146, 154, 191; and precautionary principle 2–3, 7–8, 27–8, 145–6

rBGH **21**, 23–4, 139–40, 193
Reid, Thomas 103–4, 107–8
Reserve Mining Company v. EPA 34, 129–30
rights-based precautionary principle 46–50
Rio Declaration 22, 29
risk 22, 27, 128–34, 146; as *de minimis* or trivial 5, 34, 72, 99, 119n56, 132–3, 135; and environmental threats 100–2, 134–7; lay perceptions of 31, 41, 58n95, 81–4, 145–6; and moral obligations 97–9
risk assessment *see* quantitative risk assessment
risk impositions *see* risk

Scanlon, T.M. 72, 77–8, 115
Shrader-Frechette, Kristin 19–20, 25, 105, 147, 175
Sindell v. Abbott Labs 98
Standard Oil of New Jersey 11–12, 136–7, 152, 164–6, 172–3
Sunstein, Cass 31, 38, 146

tetraethyl lead and corporate social *ir*responsibility 3–6, 11–12, **21**, 137, 152, 162–76
Thomson, Judith Jarvis 98–9
toxicity studies *see* toxicology
toxicity testing and profiles *see* toxicology
toxicology 3, 24–7, 143, 149–51, 163–4, 175–6, 192, 194–5; and Screening Information Data Set 114, 130–1, 136
Toxic Release Inventory Program *see* Toxic Substances Control Act
Toxic Substances Control Act 44–5, 61n176, 103, 114, 130–1, 151, 191

uncertain threats of environmental harm 2, 27, 49, 69–70, 72, 88n46, 94–5, 101–2, 105–6, 108, 110; and moral equality 48–9, 72–3, 75, 78, 131–2, 135–6, 142, 146, 188; *vs.* traditional risk-impositions 22, 27, 97–102, 128–34, 153, 188
uncertainty: causal uncertainty **21**, 25–7, 39; and consent 42, 46; degrees of 10, 20, 51–2nn8–9, 52n16, 128–37; genuine uncertainty 9, 27, 52n16, 89n65, 113; and ignorance 27, 102–8, 110–11; and moral luck 105–8, 110–11, 176; outcome uncertainty **21**, 22–4, 25–6; and precaution 28, 34, 128–43; and "private-interest" science 83, 137, 162, 164–70; probability uncertainty 7, 21–2, 25–6, 50, 128; scientific uncertainty **21**, 24–6; and wrong-doing 49, 72, 75–8, 82–3, 114–15, 130–1, 164–70, 179n46
uncertainty public health warnings and the right to know 140–1
Universal Declaration of Human Rights 47

vulnerable populations 10, 12, 112–13, 138, 164, 171–2

Whiteside, Kerry 25, 37, 42–6